The *New* HOME *Medical* ENCYCLOPEDIA

The New HOME
Medical
ENCYCLOPEDIA

ILLUSTRATED

Samuel L. Andelman M.D., M.P.H., M.H.A.

DIRECTOR OF HEALTH, VILLAGE OF SKOKIE, ILLINOIS
FORMERLY COMMISSIONER OF HEALTH, CITY OF CHICAGO

FOREWORD BY
Walter C. Alvarez M.D.

EMERITUS PROFESSOR OF MEDICINE, MAYO GRADUATE SCHOOL OF
MEDICINE, UNIVERSITY OF MINNESOTA
FORMERLY SENIOR CONSULTANT IN INTERNAL MEDICINE, THE MAYO CLINIC
ROYAL SOCIETY OF MEDICINE

Volume 1 • A through C

NEW YORK / CHICAGO

Quadrangle Books, Inc.
A NEW YORK TIMES COMPANY

Lexicon Publications
DIVISION OF GROLIER INCORPORATED

EDITORIAL STAFF FOR DR. ANDELMAN

ADA P. KAHN

FREDERIC T. JUNG, M.D.

SHERIDAN L. HANSEN

PROCTOR R. ANDERSON, M.D. · FRANCES M. GATES
BEATA M. HAYTON · FRANCES HENKIN · LOU JOSEPH
ROBERT E. KOWALSKI · MARILYN VOSS LEYLAND
BARBARA MOCK · SANDEE L. PETERSON
DONALD F. PHILLIPS · ANNE M. SCHMID
KENNETH M. WYLIE, JR.

WAYNE G. BRANDSTADT, M.D.
LORRAINE L. KRUSE · LILA L. KRIST · SHELLEY ABELSON
JENNY TESAR · MARY VAN ARSDALE
MARY ELINORE SMITH

TYPOGRAPHY AND DESIGN

TRUDI JENNY

CYNTHIA PETERSON

MARK COWANS · RUSTY PORTER · VINCENT TORRE

PHOTOGRAPHS

SHERIDAN L. HANSEN

DRAWINGS

ELSIE LAURELL

Library of Congress Catalog Card Number: 71–116070
International Standard Book Number: 0–8129–0260–2

FOREWORD

by Dr. Walter C. Alvarez

This splendid encyclopedia reflects the expertise and concern of its editor. Dr. Samuel Andelman is an eminent public health official who has devoted most of his life to helping people stay healthy. His book will enable people to understand illnesses—their own and others'—and thus to cooperate intelligently with their doctors.

Often what a doctor tells his patients to do is almost unintelligible to them because they haven't the background to interpret his language. The physician himself may not always realize how unfamiliar laymen are with the words he uses. Even the wisest physician may say something like this to a patient: "Your trouble is that your NPN is too high"—forgetting that the average man has no idea what NPN means. Of course, the doctor might have been very explicit. He might have said that the amount of nonprotein nitrogen in the patient's blood was excessive, and as a result his kidneys were not performing as well as they should. Or he might have put it quite simply: "Your kidneys aren't working well."

I became particularly aware of this communication problem in 1951, when I began to write a syndicated newspaper column. During the first year, some 120,000 letters came to my desk. What interested me was that so many of the writers said something like this:

"My doctor took a brief history, made a brief examination, and quickly wrote a prescription. As he saw me to the door, he said, 'You have Addison's disease.' When I asked, 'But, Doctor, what is that? Is it serious? Do you doctors know the cause of it or have a cure?', the doctor said, 'Take the medicine I have prescribed. I can't talk to you now. My waiting room is full.' So please, Dr. Alvarez, tell me what the disease is and what I can do."

Dr. Andelman's excellent encyclopedia could have helped most of these puzzled letter-writers. This book is written in plain, easily understood language, while at the same time giving basic, up-to-date information. Its easy readability and simplified explanations will make the book attractive not just to laymen but to medical students and many physicians. The alphabetical arrangement of entries makes it possible for the reader to find quickly what he is looking for. Suppose it happens to be *adenitis*. In a medical textbook, adenitis might be described in several chapters discussing diseases that have inflammation or swelling of the glands. But here, in its proper place among the A's, the reader finds it defined in layman's terms.

This book will help the doctor-patient relationship in other ways, too. One problem every physician faces is how best to communicate with a patient who may be badly shocked by distressing news of his physical condition. Many doctors have found that giving the patient a booklet or a few pages of information about his disease can be more helpful than trying to explain it to him while he is upset.

A professor once expressed this idea vividly to a class of medical students: "A year ago my doctor told me that I had a fairly advanced case of pulmonary tuberculosis, and I would have to go into a sanatorium for several months. Then he went on for twenty minutes or more, giving me instructions, but I was so shocked that I did not remember a word. Think of that when you give a patient bad news. Don't expect him to remember anything you tell him. Give him some printed instructions that he can read after he has recovered from his shock."

Dr. Andelman's encyclopedia would be an ideal reference in such a situation. It can do much for people who need important information about their illness. It can do much, too, in the way of teaching laymen what the main danger signals of illness are. Too often a patient comes to his doctor's office with, say, advanced cancer of the lung, and learns it is incurable just because he ignored a bad cough for many months.

Too often, also, he is handicapped by lack of knowledge of his own body. A tragedy that need not have happened befell a man who described his persistent pain as a stomachache; when he found that he really had cancer of the rectum, he said, "Just think, I may lose my life simply because I never knew where my stomach was!" The first page of this encyclopedia tells where the stomach is, under the heading *Abdomen*. If the patient had had a chance to read it, he would have known how to describe his symptoms to a physician—and possibly save his life.

This book will also help its readers by showing, under various headings such as *Quackery,* the folly of wasting thousands of dollars on fad medicines, fad foods, and fad gadgets. We keep reading that our older citizens alone throw away millions of dollars a year on the products of quackery. Many have chronic arthritis and hopefully buy all sorts of advertised cures—a useless expense which they can ill afford. Years ago, one of San Francisco's ablest lawyers gave a notorious quack $5,000 to save his failing eyesight. When his vision did not improve, a puzzled friend said to him, "Surely you know that quack's unsavory reputation." The lawyer replied, "Yes, but if you are going blind, and no specialist will give you any hope, you are likely to gamble a lot of money on a 'guaranteed' cure."

Perhaps, too, a book like this can do good in another way—by combating the tendency of many men and women to distrust the doctor's opinion. They may undervalue the great diagnostic wisdom and skill of men like Dr. Andelman, while overprizing the results of various laboratory tests. Most people do not know that a number of nervous diseases, for example, simply cannot be diagnosed by means of ordinary laboratory tests. Nor do they know that there are some diseases that any wise, observant, and skilled diagnostician can recognize at a glance.

For instance, one day my old chief, a brilliant physician, was walking with me down a long ward in a huge city hospital. We stopped before a bed where a woman of thirty or so was propped up. "What's wrong with her?" my chief asked. I replied, "Because she is sitting up in bed and seems a little short of breath, I would guess that she has some form of heart disease."

"Good," he answered, "but what *form* of heart disease?"

"How can I tell from this distance?" I said.

"First," he said, "look carefully at the front of her neck. Under her necklace you will see the scar of a thyroid gland operation. Now look carefully at her eyes. You will see that they are slightly bulging. Next, look at the big artery there on the side of her neck. You will see that she has a fast, irregular pulse. Obviously, then, she has been operated on for an exophthalmic goiter, but she still has the 'fibrillating heart pulse' that sometimes goes with an exophthalmic goiter." All laymen should know that a diagnosis can sometimes be made at a glance, and that often the many laboratory tests which the patient says he wants are unnecessary.

Not only does Dr. Andelman's encyclopedia tell about diseases, but it gives the meaning of many words that a layman may hear often enough but does not really understand. We hear *biopsy* frequently, but we may not know that it means a microscopic study of tissue sections removed from a patient during life. *Necropsy* means a similar study of tissue removed after death. A *circadian rhythm* is a daily rhythmic change in a number of functions of a person's body (the word *circadian* has a very interesting derivation, which is explained in the article). And *atelectasis* means the collapse of a lung. Numerous medically used drugs that have long Greek names are likewise explained, with their origins. Any patient who uses these drugs may gain comfort from knowing where they come from and why they help people with certain diseases.

Of course, Dr. Andelman did not prepare this unique encyclopedia so that sick persons can prescribe for themselves; that could be dangerous. And that is why almost every one of the thousands of diseases and disorders discussed here includes a section on treatment which usually begins, "See your doctor." It then goes on to explain the various types of treatment the doctor may prescribe—step by step through the progress of the disease and its cure. Such in-depth coverage is only one of the features that make this the most complete home medical encyclopedia available to the layman. Its more than 2,500 articles cover not only well-defined physical diseases but also physiology, mental and emotional disorders, environmental influences (air and water pollution, altitude, and humidity, for example), and even sociological information closely related to health.

As in most other areas of science today, extraordinary advances continue to be made in all branches of medicine. Virtually every one that has any practical application for the layman is recognized in Dr. Andelman's book. Some of these advances have been sudden and dramatic, such as those made possible by the electron microscope. Others have been less spectacular but no less significant, impelled by years of painstaking research, such as the discovery of means to control more and more communicable diseases. Through physicians and other members of the health team, new medicines, new treatments, and new techniques for diagnosis are bringing hope and health to victims of disease. It is now possible, for example, by a process called mass screening, to identify a greater number of diseases in their early stages than has ever been done before—including heart disease, diabetes, cancer, sickle-cell anemia, lead poisoning, and even diseases of newborn infants, such as PKU (phenylketonuria).

These and other medical services will continue to expand tremendously. But how, the reader may ask, will the public pay for them? How will medical care be financed? Undoubtedly prepaid health insurance will be available in many forms, in programs financed by government and by private companies. In fact, health insurance may well be required by law, like automobile insurance, rather than remaining a voluntary choice. The group practice of doctors and the number of Health Maintenance Organizations (HMO's) will increase, with support from prepaid insurance plans.

The distribution of good health care, and its high cost, are problems that will not be easily or quickly solved. A similar problem is how to get up-to-date health information to the public at large, and how to *use* advanced medical knowledge as widely as possible in the medical profession. Computerized medicine may help to solve both these problems. In fact, the use of computers for diagnosis and treatment may revolutionize medical services, both in doctors' offices and in hospitals. Not only can computers assimilate facts about a patient's past history, symptoms, laboratory test results, and other data, but they can provide answers —accurate, dependable answers—for the patient's medical problem, its nature and treatment. Furthermore, this computerized information can be rapidly duplicated and disseminated to everyone concerned—doctors, nurses, technicians, therapists, and public health officials. To be sure, a computer will never replace the creative, intuitive physician who arrives at a diagnosis by a combination of sixth sense, close observation, and long experience. But no physician is infallible, and the computer can be a reliable aid by substantiating the doctor's conclusions.

Because medicine is so closely interrelated with other sciences, new techniques in such fields as physics and chemistry will broaden our understanding of the physiological functions of the human body in the years ahead. With improvements in electronic and nucleonic equipment, and with information obtained in the space program, new knowledge may be applied to the diagnosis and treatment of various ailments. Hyper- and hypothyroidism are good examples. These disorders are now detected by means of a "radium cocktail," which so effectively improves upon older methods that it often replaces surgery. Because certain radioactive materials have an affinity for certain organs of the body, they can be used to detect organic disease with a simple device similar to a Geiger counter.

Surgery has made enormous strides in recent years; space medicine, an infant branch of medical science, is growing at an astonishing rate. In the future we may expect biochemical research to produce further revelations about the structure and physiology of individual cells. Our concepts of immunology may be altogether changed by research in immunologic phenomena. Physical medicine, rehabilitation, and occupational and industrial health will benefit greatly from research in their own and other fields.

In the almost fantastic area of organ transplants, the trend will be toward supplanting diseased internal organs with mechanical ones, much as we have done in the past with dentures, hearing aids, and artificial arms and legs. Ingenious research will be needed, but we are almost certain to see a marked increase in the successful use of artificial substitute organs.

The articles in Dr. Andelman's book have been composed with an awareness that, in medicine, today's spectacular achievements are tomorrow's commonplaces. Wherever possible, only the most current information is provided. (Future editions of the book will, I am told, take note of new discoveries in medicine which have meaning for the layman.) I cannot think of a better medical encyclopedia for the American home than the one Dr. Andelman has so expertly given us here. I wish it the widest possible usage.

The New HOME Medical ENCYCLOPEDIA

Abasia. When a person is unable to walk due to a defect in coordination, the condition is known as abasia. (*See* LEG, PARALYSIS.)

Abdomen. Externally, the part of the body between the ribs and the pelvis is called the abdomen, though some people inaccurately call it the stomach. (An honest old word for it is belly.) Internally, the abdominal cavity, which is lined with a protective membrane called the peritoneum, contains the stomach, the intestines, the liver, the spleen, the pancreas, the kidneys, the bladder, and, in women, the reproductive organs.

The abdominal organs constitute the body's food-processing plant, distribution center, and garbage-disposal unit. Unlike the heart, lungs, and brain, they have—with the exception of the liver and the spleen—no bony shielding.

The abdomen is often accidentally injured, and is subject to many diseases. Moreover, diseases and injuries in other parts of the body, from the head to the feet, are quite likely to cause abdominal distress.

No one is likely to get through life without experiencing some sort of abdominal pain. If it is at all severe, it generally frightens people into getting immediate medical attention. The fear is justified. A hundred years ago, before the development of modern surgery, severe abdominal pain often meant that the patient's condition was hopeless.

The interpretation of abdominal pain may be extremely difficult, even for the experienced physician. Differential diagnosis—the process of selecting the right cause among many possible causes—requires all the doctor's training, experience, and powers of observation, plus all the scientific aids that modern laboratories can provide.

As a rule, the so-called stomachache, a generalized feeling of discomfort that goes away after a few hours, is more likely to be due to nervous tension or unwise eating than to serious disease. (*See* STOMACHACHE.) However, if the pain continues, or if it keeps coming back, the time for self-diagnosis and self-treatment with household remedies is past. In the early stages of some serious diseases, including cancer, the pain is not particularly severe. Thorough investigation by a physician is required, whether or not there are other signs of ill health, such as loss of weight, abdominal enlargement, and blood in urine or stools.

The problem of severe, localized abdominal pain, especially when it concerns what to tell the doctor on the telephone, may be simplified by a system that divides the abdomen into six areas: the pit of the stomach (epigastrium), the area around the navel, and four corners or quadrants—upper right, upper left, lower right, and lower left.

Burning pain in the pit of the stomach, relieved by food or antacids, is one of the symptoms of an ulcer in the stomach or duodenum. (*See* ULCERS.) Sudden, overwhelming pain is a sign of perforation, a critical surgical emergency. The pain of pneumonia or heart attack is sometimes felt in the abdomen.

Pain in the right upper quadrant may be due to disease of the liver or gallbladder. Agonizing colicky pain, with nausea and vomiting, is a sign that a gallstone is stuck in the narrow passage leading from the gallbladder to the intestine. The pain of gallbladder disease may also be felt in the right shoulder or shoulder blade. A gallbladder attack is not usually a real emergency; it only feels like one. However, there is only one preventive: removal of the gallbladder. (*See* GALLBLADDER.)

Pain in the left upper quadrant may be due to intestinal disease, particularly of the colon, or to injury or enlargement of the spleen.

Sharp cramping pain around the navel is a common symptom of gastroenteritis due to virus infection or food poisoning. (*See* ENTERITIS.) Pain around the navel can also be an early sign of appendicitis. (*See* APPENDICITIS.) Pain localized in the right lower quadrant means that inflammation is well advanced. Temporary relief, followed by increasingly severe pain and abdominal swelling, is a sign that the appendix has ruptured and peritonitis has set in.

In a woman of childbearing age, sudden severe pain in either of the lower quadrants may be a sign of a ruptured tubal pregnancy, a critical emergency. Various diseases of the ovaries or fallopian tubes can cause pain in either or both sides of the abdomen.

Violent, colicky pain on either side is an indication that a kidney stone is stuck in the ureter, the tube leading from the kidney to the bladder. Pain low down in the abdomen may be due to intestinal or bladder disease. In women this kind of pain may be associated with essentially normal menstruation or with a disease of the uterus. In men, there may be enlargement of the prostate, or inguinal hernia.

Other causes of severe, colicky pain are intestinal obstruction or obstruction of the stomach outlet. Obstruction is a critical emergency and may be due to a serious underlying disease, such as ulcers, cancer, or long-standing inflammation.

Another cause of intense abdominal pain is lead poisoning. The common name for this condition is painter's colic, because lead compounds are a common ingredient in paint. In recent years attention has been directed toward lead poisoning in children, who become ill after eating bits of paint from walls or woodwork. (*See* LEAD POI-

SONING.) Lead is not easily eliminated by the body. A single small dose will do no harm, but after repeated doses enough lead can accumulate to cause severe symptoms and even death. The lead glaze formerly much used on pottery is also a source of danger, to both the worker and the user.

Enlargement of the abdomen may be due simply to the accumulation of fat or, in women, to pregnancy. In a thin child, however, a "potbelly" is a sign of advanced malnutrition. In affluent societies this is likely to be due to faulty absorption; in poor ones starvation is still all too common.

Temporary enlargement may be due to the gassiness of a minor upset or to a nervous condition, usually in women, in which a sudden swelling goes down as quickly as it appears. This has been called "accordion abdomen," and it does not seem to have any great significance.

The swelling that accompanies intestinal obstruction or peritonitis is, of course, one of the indications of a really critical situation.

Less immediately critical, but indicative of serious organic disease, is the accumulation of fluid in the abdomen, called *ascites,* or dropsy. Among the conditions that produce it are some forms of heart disease, cirrhosis of the liver, kidney disease, and advanced cancer. (*See* CANCER; CIRRHOSIS OF THE LIVER; HEART.) Additional information may be found in the various entries dealing with abdominal organs and their diseases.

Aberration. Deviations from what is considered normal behavior are sometimes called aberrations. (*See* MENTAL HEALTH; PHOBIA; SEXUAL ABNORMALITIES.)

Abortion. The termination of a pregnancy at any stage before the fetus could survive outside the womb is known as abortion. Generally a fetal weight of less than 500 grams (somewhat more than one pound) is considered the limit in defining this condition. (*See* PREMATURE BIRTHS.) Thus abortion usually takes place before the twentieth week of gestation.

Abortions may develop spontaneously or they may be induced. (*See* ABORTION, INDUCED; ABORTION, SPONTANEOUS.)

The problem of induced abortion elicits a great deal of emotional response. Recent liberalization of abortion laws in America and elsewhere remains controversial. Where abortion is illegal, both the woman and the abortionist are liable to prosecution.

Abortion laws were not always as strict as they are now. Until 1803, abortion was either lawful or widely tolerated in both the United States and Great Britain. In that year, as part of a general overhaul of British criminal law, abortion was made a crime. In 1821 Connecticut became the first state to enact an abortion law. Similar laws subsequently were enacted throughout the country. Canon law, establishing as dogma that no circumstance justified abortion, was not promulgated for Catholics until 1869 by Pope Pius IX.

In 1943 the New York Academy of Medicine became one of the first medical organizations to recognize the need for abortion law reform. In 1959 the American Law Institute developed a Model Penal Code regarding abortion. Great Britain enacted in 1967 a permissive abortion statute which, if liberally construed, allows virtually unrestricted abortion.

The chief abortion arguments today concern the stage at which an embryo or fetus has an inherent right to life, versus the woman's right to control her own body.

Abortion advocates in the United States continue to argue for abortion "on demand," while those who oppose abortion, for religious or other reasons, view it as an immoral act. (*See* ABORTION, INDUCED.)

Abortion Complications. Serious complications of abortion are usually, though not always, associated with criminal abortion. Uterine perforation and subsequent bleeding, hemorrhage, bacterial infection, kidney failure, and shock can all be associated with abortion. Chemical poisoning, blood poisoning, and anemia can also result, depending on the method used. (*See* ABORTION.)

Death from abortion most frequently results from postabortion bacterial endotoxic shock—a combination of bacterial infection and blood loss. If the kidneys also become affected, the mortality rate may range up to 70 percent or higher.

The combined effects of infection can sometimes cause persistent renal failure sufficient to require some form of dialysis.

Accidental perforation of the uterus may happen during dilatation and curettage. Severe bleeding and infection of the peritoneal cavity can result. Abdominal surgery might be required.

All infected abortions can be classified as septic. This designation also implies the presence of a fever of 100.4° F. or higher.

In places and at times where abortions are illegal, both the patient and the abortionist are held legally responsible.

Abortion, Induced. Abortions are either spontaneous or induced; the latter is the deliberate termination of a pregnancy by delivery of the fetus before maturity. A therapeutic abortion is an abortion induced to safeguard the life of a pregnant woman. Many abortions are induced for other reasons, such as the desire to prevent the birth of a severely malformed infant or of an infant conceived as a result of rape or incest. Whether an induced abortion is legal or illegal, licit or criminal, depends on how it is defined by the law in force in a given state at a given time; the distinction is juridical, not medical.

As social attitudes and laws regarding abortion undergo change, the incidence of induced abortions has been mounting rapidly. Though for obvious reasons only guesses are possible, the rate of illegal abortions in the past was placed at between 15 and 25 percent of all live births. It is because of the high risks involved in such abortions—too often performed by unqualified persons under unsanitary, disease-producing conditions—that abortion laws in many states are being liberalized. A notable example is the New York State abortion-reform law, which went into effect on July 1, 1970.

Traditionally, laws prohibited abortion except when the woman's life or health was in jeopardy, although pregnancies resulting from rape by force or from incest could also sometimes be legally aborted. Today, most therapeutic abortions are performed when the pregnant woman has a serious physical or mental disorder or when the fetus has potential abnormalities. If a pregnant woman has advanced hypertensive vascular disease, severe heart disease, or cancer of the cervix, a therapeutic abortion is clearly indicated. Or if her physician has been able to diagnose genetic or enzymatic disease or other abnormalities early in the development of the fetus, or if she has had rubella (German measles) in the first two or three months of pregnancy, these conditions can be grounds for therapeutic abortion. (*See* AMNIOCENTESIS; RUBELLA SYNDROME.)

A rather large number of women request, and are given, abortions for psychiatric reasons. By the very nature of their mental condition, some of them suffer further psychiatric disturbances as a result of guilt and remorse following the abortion—unless they have received competent counseling to prepare them for the experience.

The techniques used in abortions depend on the age of the fetus. During the first twelve weeks of pregnancy, vaginal abortion may be performed by the traditional method of dilatation and curettage or by a suction system. (*See* D & C.) After that period, the fetus has grown too large for these techniques. When a more advanced pregnancy is to be terminated, the injection of a strong salt solution into the amnion will usually stimulate labor. At times, a hysterectomy or abdominal hysterotomy will be performed, using a type of anesthesia comparable to that used in normal deliveries. (*See* CHILDBIRTH.)

Criminal abortions sometimes involve the use of coat hangers, knitting needles, and other strange objects, or soap or chemicals. Not only are these frequently ineffective, but they can lead to infections, bleeding, pain, and even death. (*See* ABORTION COMPLICATIONS.)

At the present time, when sexual mores and morals are in a state of flux, and out-of-wedlock pregnancies are no longer rare, the legalizing of abortion has become a serious issue. Throughout the United States, it is being discussed by laymen, religious leaders, and professionals in fields of human and social welfare.

The layman's point of view, and particularly the woman's, often centers on the principle that women should have the right to control their own bodies. This of course implies that they have a right to use contraceptives, but since no contraceptive is 100 percent effective, they may still become pregnant. At that point, many women believe, the pregnant woman should be free to decide whether or not to bear a child, and to make that decision rationally and realistically, with full consideration for the child's future as well as her own and her family's.

Certain religious leaders and certain laymen hold that abortion at any stage of fetal existence means destroying a life, which no human being has a right to do.

Some professional persons interested in improving the quality of family living, and alarmed at the worldwide trend toward overpopulation, favor legalized abortion, as do many others who are worried about the ever-increasing number of criminal abortions.

Thus, the issue has many sides. How it

is resolved will affect the welfare and well-being of both present and future generations.

Abortion, Spontaneous. The termination of pregnancy through natural causes, without mechanical or medicinal intervention, before the fetus is viable (able to live on its own) is known as spontaneous abortion. This occurrence is sometimes referred to as a miscarriage, since that word carries less stigma. But the medically correct term is spontaneous abortion.

Recent studies have indicated that from 10 to 15 percent of all pregnancies may terminate in spontaneous abortion between the fourth and twentieth weeks of fetal development—most frequently in the first trimester.

In the early months, the death of the fetus usually precedes spontaneous abortion. Such death may be the result of abnormalities in the ovum or the generative tract or of maternal (or, more rarely, fetal) disease. The most common cause of fetal death is a developmental abnormality incompatible with life.

As a rule, studies have shown, the embryo has been dead for about six weeks before abortion is completed. Thus the frequently held notion that a fall or some other physical injury leads to miscarriage is largely unfounded.

Generally, physicians are unable to prevent spontaneous abortions occurring in the early months. Because of the relation of various fetal abnormalities to this condition, physicians usually prefer to let nature take its course. Spontaneous abortion seems to be nature's way of ridding itself of a defective embryo.

Spontaneous abortions are sometimes grouped as *threatened, inevitable, incomplete,* and *missed.* Any bloody vaginal discharge or definite vaginal bleeding that appears during the first half of pregnancy can indicate a threatened abortion. The condition may or may not be accompanied by mild cramps similar to those of a backache or menstrual period. Twenty percent of all pregnancies show evidence of threatened abortion. At least half of these actually terminate in abortion, while the remainder continue to full term. Heavy vaginal bleeding, cervical dilation, abdominal pain, and passage of blood clots indicate that abortion is imminent.

Inevitable abortion takes place when there is a rupture of the membranes, in the presence of cervical dilation, making it impossible for the fetus to survive.

If any part of a fetus or placenta remains in the uterus after abortion, the condition is termed an incomplete abortion. Since profuse bleeding and possibly infection may result, prompt attention is urgently demanded.

If a dead fetus is retained in the uterus for more than two months, the condition is termed a missed abortion. In most cases the fetus will ultimately be expelled spontaneously.

If spontaneous abortion occurs in three or more pregnancies, the woman is said to be a habitual aborter. Faulty maternal conditions are said to contribute in large part to habitual abortion. Among the possible causes are incompatible blood groups (*see* RH FACTOR), incompetent cervix (early dilation followed by rupture of the membranes), anatomic uterine defects, hormonal abnormalities, hypertensive vascular disease, syphilis, or poor nutritional status. In most instances the precise cause cannot be determined, though psychological factors may play a part.

Recently, spontaneous abortion has been linked to occupational conditions that expose a woman to harmful gases or infections.

Abrasions. The most superficial kind of wound is an abrasion, caused when the topmost layers of skin or the mucous membranes are scraped or rubbed off. Skinned knees, scraped elbows, and floor burns are all abrasions.

Abrasions are common accidental injuries. Although they are not as serious as deeper wounds, they can bleed and become infected. Whenever the skin is broken, infection is a possibility. To prevent infection, the abrasion should be washed with plain soap and water. Generally no bandage is required for an abrasion, because bleeding is minimal. (*See* FIRST AID; WOUNDS.)

Abscesses. A pocket of pus is called an abscess. Pus is a white, yellowish, or pink material composed of leukocytes (white blood cells) and other material from the blood.

In an infection, the leukocytes are involved in the fight against bacteria. Thus when there is a severe local infection, there will be many leukocytes, and much pus. (*See* BLOOD CELLS.)

There are a hundred or more types of abscesses, named for the part of the body infected or for the disease causing them: for example, pulmonary (lung) abscesses, syphilitic abscesses (from venereal disease), and alveolar abscesses (in the alveolus or body socket, of a tooth).

Destruction of tissue can be found by an X-ray picture, which can discover disease that otherwise could not be detected, as in this abscessed tooth.

American Dental Association

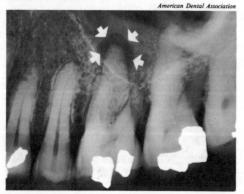

Abscesses are treated by draining the pus and eliminating the basic infection or disease.

Acanthosis. A thickening of the prickle cell layer of the skin is called acanthosis. (*See* KERATOSES; SKIN.)

Acapnia. When the carbon dioxide content of the blood is diminished, a condition called acapnia occurs. (*See* BLOOD; BLOOD CIRCULATION.)

Accidents. Every ten minutes, two persons are killed and more than 200 are injured in accidents in the United States. For persons aged one to thirty-eight, accidents are the leading cause of death. For persons of all ages, accidents are the fourth leading cause of death, following heart disease, cancer, and stroke.

Every year thousands of people are injured or killed in accidents that occur at home, on the job, at school, on the road, and in leisure-time activities. Most of these accidents could have been prevented.

According to National Safety Council statistics, almost half of the accidental deaths in 1970 involved cars and other motor vehicles. However, an accident can be serious without being fatal. Many accidents leave their victims disabled, sometimes permanently.

Although traffic accidents annually claim the most lives, accidents in the home cause the highest number of disabling injuries. In 1970, 54,800 persons were killed in traffic accidents, and 2,000,000 were disabled. In the same year, 26,500 persons were killed in home accidents—but 4,000,000 were disabled.

The most common causes of accidental deaths, based on statistics assembled by the National Safety Council, and in order of the number of lives claimed in 1970, are motor vehicle accidents, 54,800; falls, 17,500; drowning, 7,300; fires, burns, and deaths associated with fires, 6,700; suffocation by

Where Accidents Happen to Children in the United States:
Percentage Distribution July 1965–June 1967

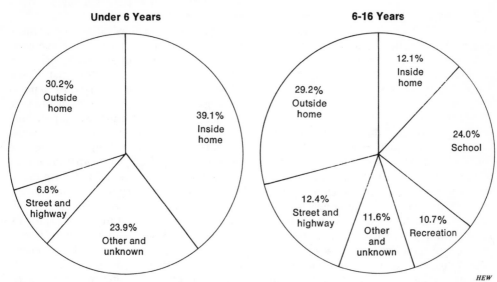

Under 6 Years

30.2% Outside home

39.1% Inside home

6.8% Street and highway

23.9% Other and unknown

6-16 Years

12.1% Inside home

29.2% Outside home

24.0% School

12.4% Street and highway

11.6% Other and unknown

10.7% Recreation

HEW

ingested objects, 3,400; poisoning by solids and liquids, 3,000; firearms, 2,300; and poisoning by gases and vapors, 1,600. In addition, 17,400 persons died in other types of accidents in 1970, including electric shock, being hit by a falling object, mechanical suffocation, and train and plane accidents.

Motor vehicle accidents most often involve young people, particularly those in the fifteen- to twenty-four-year age group. In 1970, deaths caused by auto accidents to that age group represented 30 percent of the total motor vehicle fatalities among persons of all ages.

Among infants under a year old, suffocation is the major cause of deaths in the home. Bedclothes, plastic bags, and abandoned refrigerators can be fatal to young children.

Accidents in the home take a high toll. In 1970, one person in fifty in the United States was disabled one or more days by injuries from home accidents. About 100,-000 of these injuries produced some permanent impairment.

Falls are the leading cause of accidental

deaths in the home, and more than four out of five of the victims are sixty-five years of age or older. Most of the fatal falls occur at floor level, caused by something slippery spilled on the floor, a small rug that skids, or objects, especially toys, left on the floor. The two most dangerous rooms in the house are the kitchen and the bathroom. Stairways are another danger area, especially if they are not well lighted or the treads are loose. Using chairs or tables as stepladders is also dangerous.

Many home accidents can be avoided if homes are properly maintained, well lighted, and cleared of obstacles. (*See* FIRST AID.)

Accommodation. Usually the term accommodation refers to adjustments the eye makes to provide both near and far vision. (*See* EYE; FARSIGHTEDNESS; NEARSIGHTEDNESS.)

Acetylsalicylic Acid. Introduced into medicine in 1893 and widely used for reducing fever and relieving pain, acetylsalicylic acid (aspirin) is today a common household pain reliever. (*See* ASPIRIN.)

Achalasia. When the smooth muscle fibers of the gastrointestinal tract fail to relax at a point where they join with another part of the tract, the condition is known as achalasia. (*See* COLON; DIGESTION; GASTROINTESTINAL SYSTEM.)

Aching. A dull, throbbing pain with varying degrees of discomfort, located in deep tissues of the body rather than at the surface of the skin, is usually referred to as aching. The pain may be in a distinct area or may be widespread, often to a point where it may be hard to put one's finger on the place that hurts. This is characteristic of certain types of tissues such as bones, joints, and muscles. (*See* PAIN.)

Aching, then, differs from other types of pain in the quality of the pain. This difference is thought to be caused by varying kinds of stimulation of pain nerve endings. (*See* NERVOUS SYSTEM.) Other reasons may be how various locations of the body react to similar stimuli, or variations in the actual pain receptors.

Like all pain, aching is useful to the well-being of the individual. Simply stated, it occurs when something is wrong and thus is primarily a warning signal. Aching may result from a decayed tooth, a broken bone, or a badly bruised bone or muscle. Without the pain, a person would not know that he should seek dental or medical care. There are, in fact, individuals who, because of injury to the spinal cord, are unable to feel any kind of pain. Although this may at first seem a blessing, it is not. Such persons must constantly examine themselves to make certain they have not had an injury.

The degree to which one feels aching (as is true for other pains) depends on one's "pain threshold"—that is, the amount of stimulus one needs in order to sense a pain. Some people have a very high threshold, while others have low thresholds. Actually, when monitored electronically, the nervous

impulses registering pain are alike in practically all persons. However, some may be able to "take" it better, denying to themselves or others that "it hurts."

A phenomenon may occur in which an injury is sustained in one area of the body while another area, often distant, seems to ache. This is known as "referred" pain. Most often the original injury is to an internal organ but the pain is felt at or near the surface. A physician must have a thorough knowledge of referred pain so that when patients complain of aching in one part of the body, he can consider other causes.

Headaches are a specialized form of referred pain from deeper structures to the surface of the head. Most of them result from pain inside the cranium or skull cap, but some may be from elsewhere in the body. The brain itself is incapable of feeling pain, but the covering or attachments of the brain can bring on intense aching. Thus even brain tumors do not cause aching of the brain but rather of the capsule and vessels around it. Headaches may also be brought on by meningitis, low spinal fluid, an alcoholic binge, constipation, eye disorders, nasal problems, and muscular spasms. (*See* HEADACHE; MIGRAINE.)

Aching may also develop after a buildup of toxic products in the body. We have all experienced the aching that follows too much exercise. When sugars are used for energy in muscle contraction, lactic acid and other wastes are produced. Normally these are regularly cleared through the blood and voided or rebuilt chemically to be used again. But excessive waste production brings with it a general feeling of achiness. Only with time can the body get rid of the wastes and the aches, hopefully reminding the victim not to overexercise again.

Wastes from toxic products may similarly build up during disease. The person with a bad cold and fever "aches all over" while the body is fighting off bacteria and leaving wastes as a result. And those whose kidneys do not function properly develop uremia, in which wastes cannot be disposed of and of which general aching is often a symptom. (*See* KIDNEY; UREMIA.)

When aching becomes intense pain, physicians may prescribe drugs to relieve it. Aspirin may work but how it works is still not understood. Narcotic drugs or their synthetic counterparts deaden pain by reducing the brain's recognition of nerve impulses. The pain is still there, but one does not feel it. Muscle relaxants may be the drug of choice for aching due to muscle injury. Drugs primarily designed for treatment of the aching type of pain are known as analgesics. (*See* ANALGESIC; ARTHRITIS; ASPIRIN; NARCOTICS.)

Achlorhydria. When chemical testing of a patient's gastric (stomach) juice shows that it contains little or no hydrochloric acid, he is said to have achlorhydria.

Hydrochloric acid aids digestion by activating the enzyme called pepsin in the stomach. In people with achlorhydria the stomach seems to empty more rapidly than in normal people. The acid, however, is not absolutely necessary for digestion, and the lack of it may produce few symptoms, or none at all. Some people who are born without the ability to secrete hydrochloric acid can manage very well.

The important thing about achlorhydria is that it may be a sign of serious disease. In some cases, failure of acid secretion may be part of the aging process. In others, however, achlorhydria is due to cancer or to destruction of the stomach lining by inflammation. Pernicious anemia, in which the stomach fails to manufacture a substance necessary for absorption of vitamin B_{12}, is associated with achlorhydria. The test for gastric acidity is important in distinguishing pernicious anemia from other forms of anemia. (*See* ANEMIA; DIGESTION; STOMACH.)

Achondroplasia. Achondroplasia or osteochondrodysplasia is a form of inherited dwarfism caused by retardation of bone

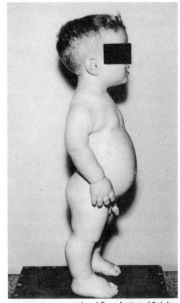

Armed Forces Institute of Pathology

Achondroplasia is a disorder in which the bones do not develop properly in the fetal, or unborn, state. If the problem continues after the child is born, he may become a dwarf.

formation. Most often affected are the long bones of the arms and legs, the bones of the fingers, the nose, the base of the skull, and, to a lesser extent, the vertebrae—all bones which arise from cartilage. The skull develops normally; only the length of the bones is affected. The dwarf's final height is usually under four and one-half feet.

The disease is apparent in X-ray films even before an infant is born, and many affected infants are stillborn. In spite of their unusual appearance, achondroplastic dwarfs have normal intelligence and are able to live normal, useful lives. (*See* DWARFS.)

Achylia. When the stomach produces little or no digestive juice (chyle), the condition is called achylia. It is associated with atrophy (wasting away) of the stomach lining. The same word is sometimes used to describe a lack of digestive juice from the pancreas. (*See* DIGESTION; HYDROCHLORIC ACID; PANCREAS; STOMACH.)

Acidosis.   A clinical term referring to a number of conditions in which the acid/base balance of the blood is toppled to the acid side is acidosis. (*See* ALKALOSIS.)

The acid/base balance, or pH, in the body hovers around the neutral point, neutral being 7. Actually, the pH of the plasma and extracellular fluid ranges between 7.35 and 7.45. The pH is normalized despite wide variations in the dietary load of acid or alkali. Many body functions are influenced by the pH, and disturbances may have disastrous effects on metabolic activity, circulation, and the central nervous system. To keep the balance constant, the body employs a number of elaborate buffering systems so that when the scales tip either to the acid or to the base, buffers return the fluids to normal. However, the body is not always capable of maintaining the balance. If the fluids become acidic, the result is acidosis.

Metabolic acidosis comes about when acid is added to the body, when alkali is lost, or when the kidney is malfunctioning and keeps down the normal excretion of acid through the urine. The fluids lose the bicarbonate or alkali content and the acid content increases, thus lowering pH below the normal point of 7.4.

A large number of diseases or disturbances can lead to acidosis in the body. These include diabetes, salicylate (aspirin) poisoning, ethylene glycol (antifreeze) poisoning, methyl alcohol (rubbing alcohol) poisoning, lactic acid buildup in muscles, renal failure, diarrhea, drainage of pancreatic juice, and several chemical difficulties involving loss of alkali.

LOSS OF ALKALI. Severe diarrhea often brings on acidosis because the liquid stools contain inordinate amounts of alkali. Loss of pancreatic juice, which is also very alkaline, has a similar effect. This loss may result from diseases of the pancreas or of the upper portion of the small intestine, into which the pancreas secretes its fluids.

KIDNEY MALFUNCTIONING. Diseased kidneys cannot deal with a normal chemical balance in the diet or dispose of the acids which accumulate in body fluids. In acute or short-lived difficulties the problem is mild, but in chronic or long-lasting diseases the acid overbalance builds continually. In chronic kidney failure the organ cannot excrete normal quantities of ammonium. The bicarbonate ion content falls precipitously and an acid condition results.

DIAGNOSIS OF ACIDOSIS. Acidosis is very difficult to diagnose without a complete chemical study. External symptoms are vague in most cases, and are extremely variable. Hyperventilation (rapid, deep breathing) is the only typical clinical finding, but even this is difficult to detect. If the condition has persisted for some time, patients may show nearly normal breathing. Diabetic individuals may have acidosis symptoms, including sluggishness and coma. (*See* COMA.) (But coma can have a great many other causes.) Blood studies will show reduced bicarbonate levels giving a tentative diagnosis of acidosis. Subsequent monitoring of pH will tell whether the treatment is alleviating the condition.

Once acidosis has been established, the exact cause must be determined. Obviously, if the imbalance is due to poisoning, the condition will have to be treated differently from ketoacidosis in diabetes. (*See* DIABETES MELLITUS; INSULIN; KETOACIDOSIS.) In some patients the syndrome may have multiple causes, and each must be treated.

TREATMENT OF ACIDOSIS. In less severe cases, treatment aimed at correcting the chemical imbalance can be administered unless, of course, the acidosis has been brought on by ketosis or shock. In such cases the physician will attempt to find and treat the underlying cause rather than directly altering body chemistry with drugs. But if the acidosis is so severe as to threaten life or if treating underlying causes is not possible, chemical alterations must be initiated immediately. The main problem in this treatment is the amount of alkali to be given so as to balance off the acid. This is determined by the amount of bicarbonate loss plus the amount of acid in the body fluids. In most cases it is best to proceed gradually, monitoring the pH, until normalcy is established. Rapid administration of large amounts of alkali may produce alkalosis. Electrolyte balance of positive and negative ions must also be watched carefully. The two chemicals used to restore balance are sodium bicarbonate and sodium lactate, given intravenously. Sodium bicarbonate and sodium citrate can also be given orally, but may lead to nausea and vomiting.

Acids.   A great number of widely diverse chemicals, some vital for health and life and others causing poisoning and burns, are collectively called acids. Although acids may be organic or inorganic, both kinds release hydrogen ions when in solution. This is the acidic factor.

Chemically, acids are the opposite of alkalis, which yield hydroxyl ions (oxygen and hydrogen bound together). When acids and alkalis are placed together, they react to form a salt and water. Acids turn litmus paper red and alkalis turn it blue.

Amino acids are the basic units of proteins. Other acids are also important in the food we eat. One of these, ascorbic acid or vitamin C, is found in citrus fruits, tomatoes, and other fresh fruits. Deficiency of this vitamin leads to scurvy. Nicotinic acid is also called niacin and is part of the vitamin B complex. It is necessary to prevent pellagra. (*See* NIACIN; VITAMINS.)

Many other forms of inorganic and organic acids are normal components of the body. A proper balance of hydrogen ions is necessary to maintain the proper pH or acid/base level. Although the pH differs in different parts of the body, that of the plasma, which is easily measurable, is about 7.4. This is achieved by the buffer systems that keep acidity lowered in much the same way that aspirin may be buffered. (*See* ELECTROLYTES.)

Many end-products of metabolism are acidic in nature. Breakdown of fats produces acids which are detected in the blood and the urine. In diabetic individuals the body uses fats for energy since it cannot metabolize carbohydrates properly, thus creating excessive levels of acids and producing a condition called acidosis. (*See* DIABETES MELLITUS.) Other metabolic difficulties can similarly produce excessive acids; in gout there is a high level of uric acid. Acid levels may also rise due to kidney failure.

In addition to acids in the body, a large number of acid chemicals are used by individuals and in industry. Properly utilized, these are greatly beneficial, but careless use can lead to burns or poisoning.

The caustic action of acid is determined largely by the release of hydrogen ions and the oxygenating power of the substance. Thus we can swallow vinegar, which is dilute acetic acid, but a drop of sulfuric acid will burn the skin badly.

Immediate first aid for acid burns is to quickly neutralize the chemical's action. Since alkalis are the chemical opposite of acids, these are used to neutralize the burning effects of the latter. If nothing else is available, soap will help minor acid burns when accompanied by copious amounts of water for dilution. If available, a paste of magnesium sulfate (Epsom salts) and water should be spread over the burn. Severe acid burns require medical care. (*See* BURNS.)

When acid is accidentally swallowed, its burning action continues from the mouth through the digestive tract to the stomach. Large amounts of water should be administered promptly to dilute the acid and thus cut down its burning properties. Vomiting should not be induced as is done with other poisons since this will bring the acid back up through the tract, burning as it comes. Call a physician immediately after administering the water. (*See* POISONING.)

Like other chemicals we use, acids should be handled carefully. The label should always be read thoroughly, and the substances should be kept far from the reach of children.

Acne. The skin problem known as acne begins with the thickening and drying of sebum, the otherwise oily and liquid secretion of the sebaceous glands. A plug of this thick material, called a blackhead (*comedo;* plural, *comedones*), forms in the gland opening, or follicle. This stops the normal flow of sebum and results in swelling and unsightly pimples.

Unless the comedones are removed, other complications can develop. Elevated lumps *(papules)* may appear, and bacterial infections may set in. Cysts of infection may form in the skin. Some acne cases are accompanied by greasiness of the skin and hair, a general sluggishness in the behavior of the individual, and menstrual irregularities in girls.

Acne is very common. Surveys have shown that about one in every five young people visit a dermatologist because of it. The disease is primarily one of adolescence, but there are cases among older persons, and even among the newborn. It has been estimated that 80 to 90 percent of teenagers suffer from acne at one time or another. This fact, however, offers little consolation to the high school youngster who feels that the acne blemishes keep him from getting dates or otherwise being accepted socially.

Just what causes acne? Medical science is not quite sure, but there is evidence that it is related to the effect of sex hormones on the sebaceous glands and the pilosebaceous units (combinations of hair follicles and sebaceous glands). A castrated person normally will not develop acne, but it can be induced by injections of androgen, the male hormone.

Acne in women frequently becomes more severe in the premenstrual period, for reasons not completely understood.

Not all persons with acne have the same reactions to various foods. Some authorities surmise that hormonal factors in cow's milk may aggravate acne. In general, it is theorized that foods are not a direct cause, but rather can make the acne flare up from a relatively dormant state.

Bromides and iodides taken internally can produce the lesions of acne and should be avoided by persons with the disease. Acne has also been reported among babies who are fed too much butterfat or cod-liver oil.

Psychic and emotional factors play a part in acne, perhaps not in the cause, but frequently in the severity. Students find that their acne flares up at times of stress, such as before examinations. And physicians report that the patient's attitude can speed or retard a cure. Some cases of acne have markedly improved or cleared up with treatment by placebos (that is, harmless pills containing no medicine), an understanding doctor, and a cooperative patient. The individual with a hopeless attitude toward his acne is particularly hard to cure.

Acne vulgaris is the complete name for the condition when it seemingly results from internal body chemicals or hormones. It often appears first on the forehead, along with abnormal greasiness here and elsewhere on the scalp; then blackheads or pimples appear. Acne also is found on the face, upper arms, and chest—areas where the sebaceous glands are particularly well developed and active. What looks like acne on the upper thighs and the buttocks may actually be another skin ailment.

When acne appears under the arms, around the anus, or in the genital regions, the problem may lie in the apocrine glands. These are similar to sweat glands, but yield a more milky fluid. Another disease of the sebaceous glands is seborrhea, an excess of sebum without the typical plugged pores of acne. Disorders of sebaceous and other skin glands may be related to other disease conditions of the body. (*See* APOCRINE GLANDS; SEBACEOUS GLANDS; SEBUM; SWEAT.)

Climate and the seasons have an effect on acne. In the temperate zones, the disease usually is more severe during the winter months. In tropical regions, where humidity and temperature are high, acne is complicated by the effects of much sweating and secondary infections. Soldiers have suffered from the problem during the Vietnam conflict and in the humid areas of the Pacific during World War II.

While common acne apparently results from problems inside the patient's body, a variety of the disease can be induced by chemical agents on the skin surface. Paraffin, bug-killers like DDT, lubricating and cutting oils, crude petroleum, creosote and other coal-tar derivatives, chlorinated compounds used in electrical insulation, and asbestos are industrial products known to produce or aggravate acne in some individuals.

Petrolatum, greasy ingredients in some hair dressings, and some cheap cosmetics may provoke acne symptoms. Small acne cysts and comedones have sometimes developed behind the ears of persons who have failed to rinse well after using shaving soap containing paraffin.

Medical preparations applied to the skin or taken internally have sometimes been found responsible for acne-like lesions. Again, only some individuals seem susceptible. Others use the same medications without a skin reaction. Steroids and adrenocorticotrophic hormones (ACTH), taken internally, are among medications that sometimes produce acne symptoms. (*See* HORMONES; CORTICOSTEROIDS.)

TREATMENT OF ACNE. If the acne patient and his doctor are lucky enough to find the reason for flareups of the disease, then obviously the best treatment is to eliminate it. If the irritant is from an outside source, such as an industrial chemical, exposure can be cut down or eliminated. But most acne seems to be caused by factors in the body's internal chemistry. In these cases, cure may be difficult until the disease has run its course. This usually occurs when the adolescent passes into full adulthood.

Trial-and-error elimination of suspected foods in the diet is sometimes successful. Consumption of chocolate, peanuts, milk, and ice cream can be stopped, one by one, for periods of perhaps a few weeks or a month. If the acne improves and if the relation of the food to the problem is still uncertain, the patient might resume eating one of the foods. If it is an aggravating cause, the acne could flare up within one or two days.

Some diets for acne patients restrict the consumption of nuts, caffeine beverages (coffee, tea, cola drinks), and animal fats, but seldom restrict meat, fish, vegetables, cereal products, fruits, and nonchocolate candy. Drastic diets, unless followed under a physician's supervision, can cause nutritional problems far more severe than the discomfort of acne.

Skin cleanliness, while important in preventing and treating acne, has been overemphasized by popular misconceptions of the disease. Many uninformed persons still cling to the idea that an unclean skin causes acne. They point to the dark spots of the pimple and blackhead as evidence that "dirt" has clogged the pores. The darkening of the blackhead, however, is simply caused by the chemical reaction of the comedo to light and air.

Washing with mild soap, rather than hard scrubbing, is recommended. Special "acne soaps" may be of little additional value unless they help exfoliation, or the shedding of skin. Exfoliation is one object of acne "remedies" sold over the drugstore counter, and of prescriptions by the doctor. Some contain sulfur, resorcinol, zinc oxide, or salicylic acid, which may prepare the skin for easy removal of the comedones.

But it is doubtful that any ointment alone can cure the disease.

Cosmetics are useful for the acne patient, as they mask the lesions and thus help reduce the embarrassment and emotional stress that often accompany acne. The cosmetics must be chosen with care, lest they irritate the already inflamed skin.

Ultraviolet rays, by lamp or by direct sunlight, may seem to help acne, though the tanning and reddening of the skin may simply make the acne less noticeable. Remember that tanning by sun or lamp always carries with it the hazard of overexposure. Too much basking in the sun, in fact, could result in "summer acne," which apparently starts with the thickening of the skin produced by tanning. Summer acne improves or disappears in the fall.

Part of the treatment for acne is the removal of comedones. Doing this at home, particularly when there are more than just one or two blackheads, is hazardous. The procedure is best done by a doctor or some other trained medical person. The skin is first covered with a poultice, or towel soaked in hot water. Alcohol or another antiseptic is applied to the lesion. With pressure inward and downward with the fingernails, the comedo may be popped out. Some physicians use an instrument called a comedo-expressor for this task.

Too frequent popping of comedones, as well as fussing with, squeezing, and scratching pimples and blackheads, can make matters worse. So can attempting to hide acne on the forehead or cheeks by combing hair over it. Acne under overhanging hair often becomes more difficult to clear up.

Some physicians advocate tetracycline and dimethylchlortetracycline, or other antibiotics, for acne. These fight bacteria, a complication of simple acne, and are taken in capsules. Vitamin A, applied in a topical ointment, reportedly affects the cells lining the follicle. Horny cell production increases, helping to expel comedones and preventing the formation of new ones.

Some contraceptive pills have proven of value for acne in adult women. These contain the female hormones estrogen and progesterone, which counteract the effect of male hormones, stimulators of sebaceous glands.

X rays are sometimes advocated to reduce the size and activity of the sebaceous glands. In the amount used for acne treatment, the radiation is rated as harmless to the patient. With the development of other methods of treatment, however, X-ray therapy has been used less frequently for acne, is usually reserved for stubborn cases, and is safe only in the hands of experts.

Acne almost always leaves scars, minor or severe, but they do become less apparent with the passage of time. After the active symptoms of acne have disappeared, the more extensive scars may be removed by dermabrasion (also called planing), a surgical procedure in which a thin layer of skin is taken off with an abrasive electrical device similar to a sander.

Hair and sebaceous follicles are also subject to folliculitis, an inflammatory disease. Acne keloids is another name for keloid folliculitis keloiditis, in which there is formation of new tissue and scarring. (*See* FOLLICULITIS; HAIR; SKIN.)

Acrocyanosis. The term acrocyanosis means bluing (cyanosis) of the extremities (acro). The medical problem also involves coldness of the hands and feet, occasionally sweating, but very rarely pain.

The cause of acrocyanosis is not clear. It usually affects women and is sometimes associated with emotional reactions such as hysteria. (*See* HYSTERIA.) The small blood vessels (arterioles) of the hands and feet apparently contract, for reasons unknown, in response to some unidentified stimulus.

The disorder may last for many years, even a lifetime, and does not develop into anything more serious than discoloration and coldness of the extremities, especially in cold weather. There is no known cure. (*See* RAYNAUD'S DISEASE.)

Acrodynia. Chemical compounds containing the element mercury can cause a reaction in young children characterized by irritability, inability to sleep, loss of teeth, high blood pressure, and redness of the fingers, toes, nose, cheeks, and buttocks. This disorder is called acrodynia, or pink disease. Fever, increased numbers of white blood cells, and protein in the urine also occur with acrodynia. If there is doubt about the diagnosis, the amount of mercury excreted each day in the urine can be measured. High mercury levels point toward mercury intoxication.

The child with acrodynia must be removed from contact with mercury compounds, found around the house in calomel and mercury ointments, and in some paints. (Mercury-containing agents have been added to paint to prevent mold from growing on the painted surface.) Children eating paint chips will thus ingest the mercury.

A drug called penicillamine will increase the excretion of mercury from the body, but recovery from acrodynia is somewhat slow. Advanced cases do very poorly, and damage to the brain may leave permanent impairment. In one reported series, only 15 percent of seriously ill patients eventually recovered fully.

Acromegaly. If production of the pituitary growth hormone continues after adolescence, or begins again, the bones cannot grow longer; instead they can get thicker and the body tissues can continue to grow in a condition called acromegaly.

The bones that enlarge abnormally are particularly those of the hands, feet, cranium, nose, and forehead. Some vertebrae also enlarge. As a result the jaw protrudes, the forehead slants forward, the nose grows to as much as twice normal size, the foot may grow to size fourteen, and the person begins to look hunched. Soft tissues, such as the tongue, also thicken.

Irradiation of the pituitary gland will stop the production of growth hormone, but although this treatment is effective in arresting the disease, it cannot change the growth that has already taken place.

Acrophobia. People with a morbid dread of going up in airplanes because they fear great heights or open, high places are suffering from acrophobia. This condition should not be confused with airsickness, which is a bodily disturbance. (*See* PHOBIAS.)

Acrosclerosis. One form of a disease known as scleroderma (progressive systemic hardening of tissues) that affects the skin of the hands and the blood vessels leading to them is called acrosclerosis. Scleroderma is one of several diseases that involve the connective tissues of the body and are known as collagen diseases. The cause of scleroderma is unknown, and most forms of therapy are unsatisfactory.

In acrosclerosis the skin becomes waxy, smooth, leathery, and tight—most prominently on the fingers, hands, and ankles. The face becomes fixed in a masklike expression. Weakness and loss of weight frequently occur. The other important aspect of acrosclerosis is the sudden onset of decreased blood supply to the fingers, toes, nose, and ears. This is called Raynaud's phenomenon; the cause for this is unknown but attacks are often precipitated by exposure to cold. During an attack the affected parts become blue and painful.

Fortunately people with acrosclerosis seldom develop severe scleroderma. (*See* ACROCYANOSIS; RAYNAUD'S DISEASE; SCLERODERMA.)

ACTH. Secretion of the corticosteroids is stimulated by one of the hormones of the anterior pituitary gland, corticotropin, or ACTH. This hormone acts upon the cortex region of the adrenal glands, bringing on secretion of both the mineralocorticoids and glucocorticoids. (*See* ADRENAL GLANDS; CORTICOSTEROIDS; HYPOPHYSECTOMY; PITUITARY GLAND.) The secretion of ACTH is probably controlled by an area located in the lowest and posterior portions of the hypothalamus, a part of the brain located above the pituitary gland.

Actinomycin. This is an antibiotic substance that is available in two different forms. Actinomycin A is soluble in ether and alcohol, is red in color, and inhibits the growth of bacteria. Actinomycin B is soluble in ether but not in alcohol, is colorless, and kills bacteria. (*See* ANTIBIOTICS; DRUGS.)

Actinomycosis. A chronic, generalized disease affecting primarily the face, neck, chest, and abdomen and caused by the fungus Actinomyces israeli is termed actinomycosis. This organism normally inhabits the mouth and intestinal tract without causing disease, but injury to the mouth area or the intestine, or inhalation of the organism, can bring on actinomycosis.

This disorder is found in all parts of the world. During the first part of this century actinomycosis was the most common systemic disease caused by a fungus. Men are afflicted about twice as often as women. People in rural areas, especially farmers, have a high incidence of this illness.

The fungus does its damage by directly invading the involved tissue and then spreading into and damaging surrounding tissue. Pockets of the infection develop in combination with certain bacteria and pus, forming abscesses.

The face-and-neck variety of the disease (cervicofacial actinomycosis) accounts for about one half of all cases. The organism enters the facial tissue after injury to the mouth, or after removal of teeth or tonsils. The tissues around the jaw area are usually damaged and have a characteristic "woody" or lumpy feeling. (*See* LUMPY JAW.) The abscesses that form often drain pus to the level of the skin, but there is little if any pain.

Fifteen percent of the cases involve the chest region (thoracic actinomycosis). The

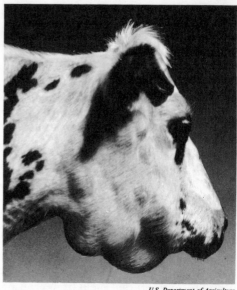

U.S. Department of Agriculture

Actinomycosis is an infectious disease which may be passed between man, cattle, and swine. When it affects the lymph nodes, as in the cow shown here, it is also called lumpy jaw. Pockets of pus (abscesses) form in the neck, face, lungs, or abdomen. The disorder is caused by *Actinomyces,* a fungus.

lungs and air passages become involved after some of the fungi are inhaled. Early in the illness the patient may have a slight cough or low fever. As more lung tissue becomes damaged he loses weight, sweats at night, and has a high fever.

Abdominal actinomycosis occurs after such disorders as appendicitis, intestinal infection, or a rupture of the stomach or bowel. Usually a mass or large abscess can be felt in the abdomen; the abscess may drain pus to the outside.

Rarely, cases of actinomycosis may affect the brain, the valves of the heart, or the region of the anus. Cases have been reported in which the skin of a person's hand had become infected after he had struck another person in the mouth.

Before the advent of penicillin, most people with actinomycosis died of it. Today penicillin in high doses usually stops the disorder. Other antibiotics, such as tetracycline, chloramphenicol, and streptomycin, may be used in addition. Often large abscesses are removed by surgery.

Acupuncture. An ancient oriental medical treatment in which long, fine needles are inserted into various parts of the body is known as acupuncture. This procedure, devised in China around 2700 B.C., has continued to be used in both China and Japan.

The procedure itself consists of the insertion of silver, gold, or steel needles, one to ten inches long, into various places on the body. The specific places, about 365 of them, are reportedly mapped on the body. The needles can be either hot or cold.

According to Chinese doctrine, the body must receive two special "humors," or vital principles, called yin and yang. Many diseases, it is felt, result from obstruction of the supply of yin and yang. Needling, or acupuncture, supposedly relieves the obstruction and thereby cures the disease. This treatment has been used for treating arthritis, headache, convulsions, and a variety of other disorders. Heart attacks are reportedly prevented by this procedure. Surgery has been accomplished with no other apparent anesthesia than an acupuncture.

Acute. When an illness is diagnosed as acute, this means that it is sudden and severe. An acute disease, or stage of a disease, should be treated quickly. An acute attack of appendicitis, for example, can be fatal if not treated in time. (*See* CHRONIC.)

Adam's Apple. Two wings of cartilage (the right and left thyroid cartilages), meeting at a right angle in the front of the larynx, or voice box, make the lump on the neck in men that is called the Adam's apple. The lump appears in adolescence as the larynx grows larger and the voice deepens. Through confusion over two similar Hebrew words, the lump got its picturesque name—a reminder of the biblical first man and the forbidden fruit he tasted. (*See* LARYNX.)

Adaptation. The ability of animals (including human beings) and plants to adjust to their environment is called adaptation. Certain forms of life can more easily adapt to a wider variety of environments than others. Human beings are capable of living in all kinds of climates. On the other hand, polar bears need very specialized conditions —cold climates—for their existence. Living things that cannot adjust to their environment usually die—a fate the dinosaurs met when the swamps they lived in dried up, and the climate and food changed.

A population of animals or plants may adapt to a changing environment through evolution, or gradual development over many generations, or they may adapt within their own lifetime by changing their behavior or body chemistry in some advantageous way. Evolutionary adaptation requires mutations in the genetic structure, while adaptation made during a lifetime requires sensitivity on the part of the organism. (*See* BIOCLIMATOLOGY; ECOLOGY; POPULATION GROWTH.)

Addiction. When a person surrenders himself to the habit of taking a drug without medical supervision, to such an extent that sudden withdrawal of the drug causes mental and/or physical trauma, he is said to be addicted. Drug addiction is defined as a compulsive use of a drug accompanied by mental or physical dependence upon it. (Addiction to a drug does not always involve a physical dependence.)

If an addict is withdrawn from a drug that causes physical dependence, he will exhibit characteristic withdrawal symptoms specific to the particular drug taken. If the addiction is mental (psychic), the user may suffer trauma as great as that of addicts experiencing physical withdrawal symptoms.

Glossary of Popular Drug Terms

Acapulco gold marijuana smuggled in from Mexico to the U.S.
acid LSD
barbs barbiturates
bennies Benzedrine tablets (prescription)
Bernice cocaine
blue birds or **blues** Sodium Amytal capsules
blue devils Amytal capsules
blue heavens Sodium Amytal tablets
blue velvet paregoric and antihistamine mixed and injected
boy heroin
caballo heroin
candy barbiturates
cartwheels amphetamine sulfate (double-scored tablets)
charge marijuana
coast-to-coast amphetamine sulfate capsules
copilots amphetamine tablets
corrine cocaine
crystals Methamphetamine
dexies Dexedrine tablets
dollies Dolophine tablets
doojee heroin
double trouble Tuinal capsules
downers sedatives, alcohol, narcotics, and tranquilizers
drivers amphetamines
dust cocaine
eye-openers amphetamines
flake cocaine
gage marijuana

gold dust cocaine
goofballs barbiturates
grass marijuana
gasshopper marijuana
greenies green, heart-shaped tablets of dextroamphetamine sulfate and amobarbital
H heroin
happy dust cocaine
hard narcotics opiates (heroin and morphine)
Harry heroin
hash hashish and marijuana
hay marijuana
hearts Benzedrine or Dexedrine heart-shaped tablets
hemp marijuana
horse heroin
jive marijuana
jolly beans pep pills, amphetamines
joy-powder heroin
L. A. turnabouts amphetamine sulfate capsules
lid proppers amphetamines
locoweed marijuana
M morphine
Mary Jane marijuana
mesc mescaline
meth Methedrine (also known as Desoxyn)
mezz marijuana
Mickey Finn chloral hydrate
Miss Emma morphine
muggles marijuana
muta marijuana
nimby Nembutal capsules
oranges Dexedrine tablets
pack heroin

peaches Benzedrine tablets
peanuts barbiturates
P.G. or **P.O.** paregoric
pinks Seconal capsules
pot marijuana
purple hearts Dexamyl capsules (Dexedrine and Amytal)
rainbows Tuinal capsules
red devils Seconal capsules
rope marijuana
roses Benzedrine tablets
scat heroin
schmeck heroin
seccies barbiturates
seggy Seconal capsules
snow cocaine
stardust cocaine
STP a highly potent hallucinogen
T marijuana
tea marijuana
Texas tea marijuana
tooies Tuinal capsules
truck drivers amphetamines
turps Elixir of Terpin Hydrate with codeine (cough syrup)
uppers stimulants, cocaine, and psychedelics
wake-ups amphetamines
weed marijuana
whites amphetamine sulfate tablets
white stuff morphine
yellow jackets Nembutal capsules (brand of pentobarbital)
yen shee opium ash

Physical dependency can occur pharmacologically with only specific drugs: barbiturates, alcohol, and narcotics, all of which are depressants. These three drug groups produce tolerance and a withdrawal sickness in the addict. The term *tolerance* means that the drug user undergoes a physiological change wherein the body cells change daily and adapt to the drug so that a greater dosage is required for the addict to obtain the same "high" as he obtained the first few days with a moderate dosage.

This buildup of physical tolerance continues until the addict volunteers or is forced to withdraw from his habit. The body then reacts violently with symptoms specific to the user's particular drug habit. (*See* DRUG WITHDRAWAL).

Drugs, such as tobacco, cause psychological dependence often referred to as habituation. This type of addiction occurs when the drug user becomes so mentally accustomed to his habit that he will exhibit symptoms similar to physical dependency. Restlessness, irritability, and anxiety are symptomatic.

Whether obtained by prescription or from an illegal supplier, drugs can become addictive if abused. Among these are certain stimulants that physicians may prescribe for persons who have so little energy that they cannot function without help: Dexedrine, Drinamyl, Benzedrine, Methedrine, and Preludin, to name a few. These "pep pills" can also be illegally obtained. (*See* AMPHETAMINE.)

Also prescribed as well as illegally available are the barbiturates and other drugs which sedate and relieve tension. Some of these are Librium, phenobarbital, pentobarbital, sodium amytal, and Soneryl. Then there are the narcotics, which are analgesics used to relieve pain and induce sleep. These include opium and its derivatives, such as morphine, codeine, and paregoric. Heroin, formerly used by physicians but now outlawed in medical practice, is obtainable illegally. Another misused narcotic is cocaine, once widely used in dentistry as an anesthetic but now replaced by safer medications. (*See* BARBITURATES.)

The hallucinogens are LSD (lysergic acid diethylamide), DMT, STP, mescaline, peyote, psilocybin, and psilocin. Some of these are used by psychiatrists in treating patients. (*See* DRUG ABUSE.)

Addison's Disease. When the adrenal cortex fails to produce adrenocortical hormones, the result is Addison's disease. Its symptoms include loss of appetite, low blood pressure, weak muscles, gastrointestinal disturbances, skin discoloration, and, eventually, death. The disease was named after Thomas Addison, who first described it in 1855.

Patients afflicted with Addison's disease can live for years if given small amounts of the missing hormones. Small pellets of solid deoxycorticosterone can be implanted in fatty areas of the back, and such treatment can last from six months to a year. Full treatment must also include glucocorticoids such as cortisone, cortisol, or prednisolone, as well as the mineral corticoids. (*See* ADRENAL GLANDS; ADRENAL HORMONES.)

Patients with this disease can be detected by the almost complete lack of 17-ketosteroids, one group of the steroid compounds normally secreted in the urine.

In normal persons, physical or mental stress conditions are met by an increased secretion of glucocorticoids to increase blood glucose. However, the person with Addison's disease cannot produce the excessive amounts of the hormones his body requires at such times. Therefore the patient must be given many times the normal quantities of glucocorticoids. "Addisonian crisis" is the term used to describe this critical need and the resulting severe debility during such periods.

Adenitis. Although the word adenitis can mean inflammation or infection of any glandular tissue, it most often refers to an inflammation of the lymph glands or nodes. (*See* LYMPH.) This irritated condition, which can be found in the lymph glands throughout the body, is caused by a general infection. Usually, however, the inflammation is more localized. The glands or nodes with the adenitis condition are those that drain the specific part of the body most seriously affected by the infection.

Scarlet fever, for example, causes cervical adenitis, in which the lymph nodes of the neck are inflamed, swollen, and tender to the touch. A form of adenitis affecting the genital region is venereal lymphogranuloma, or adenitis tropicalis. Another form, acute salivary adenitis, makes the salivary and other glands around the mouth inflamed.

Infectious mononucleosis, the ailment popularly called "glandular fever" and "kissing disease," is known in medicine as acute epidemic infectious adenitis.

Adenocarcinoma. A malignant tumor mass which originates from the glands or ducts of the epithelial lining of body cavities or surfaces is termed an adenocarcinoma. (*See* MALIGNANT.) These neoplasms (new growths) are the malignant counterpart of the adenoma. (*See* ADENOMA; CANCER; NEOPLASM.)

Adenoids. In the nasopharynx or upper part of the pharynx is a mass of lymphoid tissue called the pharyngeal tonsil. It is similar in function to the palatine tonsils, located in the fauces area at the rear of the mouth. Both help trap and destroy bacteria that enter the body through the mouth and nose. (*See* PHARYNX; TONSILS.)

The pharyngeal tonsil normally is largest when a child is five years old, diminishing in size until it almost disappears at about the age of twenty.

When it becomes infected and inflamed, the pharyngeal tonsil is referred to as adenoids. This condition can cause a blocking of the nasal passages so that the child has trouble breathing normally and speaks with a whine or twang. He may have a discharge from the nose, either similar to the discharge that accompanies a cold, or bloody.

If a child in your family develops these symptoms, take him to the doctor promptly for examination. Infections may spread from the adenoids to the middle ear through the eustachian tubes. (*See* OTITIS MEDIA.)

Removal of the adenoids by surgery—adenoidectomy—is the most common treatment. After this surgery, the child, through habit, may continue to breathe through his mouth and speak in a nasal fashion. Speech therapy can correct this.

Often the palatine tonsils and adenoids are removed at the same time. This is called "adenotonsillectomy." (*See* TONSILLECTOMY.)

After adenoidectomy, the tonsil or lymphoid tissue sometimes grows again. If it interferes with breathing or becomes infected, the tissue may be removed by surgery or controlled by irradiation.

Adenoma. A benign, or nonmalignant, tumor mass which arises from epithelial tissue (that covering external and internal body surfaces) and which either appears glandular microscopically or has grown from a true gland, is designated as an adenoma. Although these tumors are benign, they may grow to enormous size, crowding vital body organs and requiring surgical removal. They can occur in the bronchus, breast, colon (large bowel), gallbladder, kidney, liver, or thyroid.

Some adenomas are believed to be direct forerunners of malignancy and hence must be removed. Among these premalignant types are those of the bronchus, colon, and breast. Adenomas are quite common. As a rule they are easily removed before they encroach on other organs or change to a malignant form. (*See* CANCER.)

Adenosis. Diseases of the glands and development of glandular tissue are both referred to as adenosis. When one of the glands becomes overactive, this can be due to pathogenic production of glandular tissue, often in the form of a tumor. Such growth, which can occur almost anywhere in the body, is called adenoma. (*See* CANCER.)

Adhesions. Abnormal attachments between surfaces of the membranes which line the abdominal wall and enclose the abdominal organs, either after inflammations or following surgery, are termed adhesions. This sticking together of the membranes or peritoneum may also be the result of inherited traits, presence of foreign bodies, or trauma (mechanical injury). But for the most part adhesions are seen after inflammations or following surgery. (*See* SURGERY.)

The attachment is composed mainly of fibrous tissue. Surgical procedures often promote such fibrous growth by improper handling of the organs, sponges, and instruments, and by secondary infection. To some extent the formation of adhesions is a normal process by which the body localizes irritants—the same mechanism by which a particle of glass or a splinter will become coated with a whitish, fibrous membrane if left embedded in the flesh.

Problems begin with adhesions, however, when their growth obstructs the intestines. Typically the small intestine is the most affected. The symptoms are similar to those of other intestinal obstructions, with pain in the area and, in severe cases, difficulties in digestion.

Although the severity and frequency of adhesions after surgery have been greatly reduced, it is impossible to completely eliminate this side effect since, as mentioned earlier, fibrous formation is a normal process. But today's surgeons keep adhesions to a minimum by removing blood from the cavity, using moist, warm sponges, and handling tissues gently.

The term adhesion is also sometimes used in dentistry to describe the ability of the jaw to hold an artificial denture in place by the vacuum formed between the tissue and the denture. (*See* DENTISTRY; DENTURES.)

Adiposis. When fatty tissue anywhere in the body accumulates excessively, this condition is called adiposis. It may be simply due to overeating, or it may be pathologic. A number of diseases are accompanied by fatty deposits; when the fat is

deposited in the brain, death may follow. In other parts of the body it may cause intense pain. (*See* OBESITY; TUMORS.)

Adolescence. Adolescence is defined as the period from puberty (the age when reproductive organs become functional) to full sexual maturity (which is different in each person).

The striking difference between adolescents on the one hand and little children and adults on the other is the rapidity, variety, and extent of their growth and maturation. At no other time of life, except during the first year, is growth as fast. The changes come about because of a gradual but considerable increase in various hormone levels that previously were both low and stable.

As a result of these changes, the adolescent grows rapidly in height, weight, muscle mass, and sexual maturity. The changes also create new and greater nutritional requirements. For instance, in some girls who have only a minor degree of anemia, menstruation may further increase the body's nutritional demands that had already been imposed by their growth in height and weight. Such a girl may now require supplemental iron, especially if she follows inadequate fad diets because she wants to avoid even a normal gain in weight. (*See* ANEMIA; MENSTRUATION.)

The adolescent growth spurt in girls begins, on the average, between ten and eleven years of age and reaches its peak during the thirteenth year. It is very closely related to the onset of menstruation. In boys, these maturational events occur about two years later.

The great variation in the age at which different boys and girls reach physical and sexual maturity brings problems for the early- or late-maturing youngster. As girls start the adolescent spurt, nearly all their measurements are temporarily larger. About two years later, when the boys' spurt begins, that of the girls recedes. Boys tend to grow with greater speed, and at maturity are about 10 percent taller and 15 to 20 percent heavier than girls.

A number of adolescents, especially girls, become "overweight" and appear fat during early adolescence, but later, when they grow taller, become more slender again. Early-maturing girls tend to grow more rapidly in both height and weight than late-maturing girls, but their growth in weight is greater than their growth in height. Those girls who start their adolescent growth late are already taller and near to adult size. Their growth spurt is briefer and less intense.

Adolescence also brings an increase in strength and muscle size, though this occurs later than the greatest height or weight gain. Motor coordination, too, tends to increase, especially in boys, and follows closely after their growth in body size and weight.

Adolescence brings the child face to face not only with physiological processes leading to maturity, but also with psychological ones. Sex is new and disturbing to many boys and girls, and adjusting their thinking and behavior to it may be difficult. Some girls who find growing up a frightening prospect may make themselves unattractive by overeating or persisting in tomboyish habits. Some boys, doubting their own masculinity, may seek to prove it by behaving in an uncharacteristic manner. Still others may be confused when they discover that the values they have been taught are not always in accord with many practices of adults whom they respect.

All of us must remember, however, that adolescence is characterized by a great capacity for change in boys and girls, and their behavior vacillates widely in response to their physiological state. (*See* PUBERTY; TEENAGER.)

Adoption. A generation ago most children who were born out of wedlock (and these are still the majority of adoptable children) were reared in institutions or orphanages. Today, adoption is encouraged in our society. Its goal is to protect children by placing them in a family setting where they can develop more fully. Adoption also gives childless couples a socially sanctioned opportunity to have children.

Usually, adoption of children by people not related to them is accomplished through social agencies, though many unwed mothers make their own arrangements. The goal of all good adoption agencies is to place a healthy baby or child in a stable, secure home where he will have a warm family life and a decent upbringing. Half of all adopted infants are under three months of age when placed; 82 percent of them are under one year of age. Recent statistics show that three-fourths of all adoptions are by nonrelatives, and more than four of every five adopted children were born out of wedlock.

Generally, parents adopt a child because they have a great desire for children but are unable to have one (about one-sixth of all couples are said to be sterile). Whatever the reasons for their sterility, these couples have been found to make good parents. However, they are usually older than natural parents, since they probably have tried for some time to have a child of their own. Like most older parents they tend to be overaffectionate, overanxious, overprotective and overindulgent. Sometimes, however, the child is unaccustomed to the attention of affectionate parents and does not know how to respond. Especially if he has been in an institution for a long period before adoption, he may be suffering from emotional deprivation.

Realistically, the most important influences on the outcome of any adoption are the adoptive parents' biological or psychogenic reasons for infertility and their motives for adopting a child. Assuming that the child is normal and healthy, their own attitudes are crucial to the success or failure of the adoption. Most adopted children grow up with quite normal feelings toward their adoptive parents. Even if the adoptive parents have children of their own, the

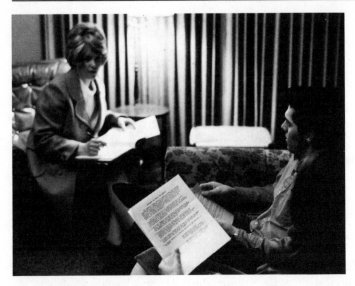

A case worker from an adoption agency conducts a preliminary interview with prospective parents.

adopted child is usually fully accepted.

When a child is adopted during infancy, his adoptive home is the only one he has ever known, and the adoptive parents are the first people to whom he becomes emotionally attached. A child of three or four is acutely aware of the change in his life but can forget the past rather quickly. An older child, however, may resent the change, even if his previous home was inferior in many ways.

Parents should know that at times the child will ask questions about his being adopted. If they anticipate the questions, they will be ready to reassure him lovingly and warmly—telling him only what he wants to know and in words he can understand. The child may become worried or anxious, for example, when he starts school. His parents have already told him, perhaps many times, about how they chose him as their child because they loved him "at first sight," but he needs to hear it all again, with renewed expressions of their love and support. Again, in early adolescence, when the child's desire to be like everyone else is very strong and when being adopted means being "different," he may ask questions, once more pleading for reassurance. In later adolescence or after mar-

riage, he may be concerned about his "real" family's background.

While a two-parent family is still considered to be the best of all choices for an adoptable child, it is recognized that such families cannot always be found for all the children who need the security of a permanent home. Therefore, not too many years ago, some states made it possible for a single man or woman to adopt a child. Usually these adults had experience with children, either through their own families or through their employment. Thus, many children who might otherwise never have had a happy home life now have a family of their own.

In the past, adoption agencies avoided placing children in one-parent homes because of the notion that it was necessary for children, especially boys, to have a father figure to serve as a model. But the child in a single-parent home can identify with other adults, friends or relatives of his parent. A boy, aware that he possesses the observable physical properties and attributes of a male, learns that society will expect him to behave as a boy. His mother (or father) will also respond to him as a boy and encourage appropriate behavior.

Recently, social agencies have also

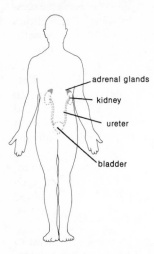

adrenal glands

kidney

ureter

bladder

placed children for adoption with older mothers, some over fifty years of age. At first, this was permitted only with members of racial minorities, but it is now being done with all groups. Children have also been placed for adoption with women who are working full time. Today, the working mother is a commonplace at all levels of society, so an emotionally stable woman, with the means to support a child, can still become a parent and offer a child a permanent home. There is also a small but growing number of young people, concerned with population problems, who are having one or two children of their own and then adopting others, giving—in a new way—opportunities for stability and nurture to children who would not otherwise have these benefits.

Adrenal Gland Disorders. Secretions of the adrenal glands are extremely important to the body, and either excessive or insufficient amounts of the hormones result in adrenal gland disorders. (*See* ADRENAL GLAND TUMORS; ADRENAL GLANDS; ADRENOCORTICAL INSUFFICIENCY; ADRENOGENITAL SYNDROME; ALDOSTERONISM; CORTICOSTEROIDS; HYDROCORTISONE STEROIDS; HYPERADRENALINISM; HYPOADRENALINISM.)

Adrenal Glands. Lying above each kidney is a gland which secretes a number of hormones vital to life; these endocrine glands are the adrenals. Each is composed of two distinct parts with distinctly different hormones. The inner part (medulla) produces adrenalin and noradrenalin and the outer part (cortex) secretes the corticosteroids, including both the mineralocorticoids and glucocorticoids. (*See* ADRENALIN; CORTICOSTEROIDS.)

Adrenalin is called the "fight or flight" hormone since it is secreted in times of stress. Both of the hormones produced by the medulla affect muscle contraction, gastric secretions, heart rate, and especially blood pressure.

Unlike any of the other endocrine glands, the medulla of the adrenal glands can be removed without apparent injury to the body, since other systems can take over the roles played by its two hormones.

The cortex portion of the adrenals secretes a rather large number of steroid hormones. These are vitally important in metabolism of minerals and carbohydrates, hence their names (the mineralocorticoids and the glucocorticoids). Removal of the cortex results in death within ten to fifteen days, if the complete structures are lost from both adrenal glands. Loss of cortex function produces problems, the degree depending on the amount of function lost. (*See* ADDISON'S DISEASE; ADRENOCORTICAL INSUFFICIENCY; ADRENOGENITAL SYNDROME; ALDOSTERONISM.)

Adrenal Gland Tumors. When cells within the adrenal glands proliferate abnormally, the result is excessive secretion of hormones from the tumors thus formed. The patient suffers from hyperadrenalism. Treatment for the condition is surgical removal of the offending tumor. (*See* ADRENAL GLANDS; ADRENAL HORMONES; ADRENALIN; ADRENOGENITAL SYNDROME; ALDOSTERONISM; CUSHING'S DISEASE AND SYNDROME; HYPERADRENALISM.)

Adrenal Hormones. These hormones are secretions from both the inner and outer parts of the adrenal glands, located on top of the kidneys. The cortex (outer part) secretes hormones which control metabolism and the medulla (inner part) produces the hormones adrenalin and noradrenalin. Adrenalin and noradrenalin are also known as epinephrine and norepinephrine. *(See* ADDISON'S DISEASE; ADRENAL GLANDS; ADRENALIN; ADRENOCORTICAL INSUFFICIENCY; ADRENOGENITAL SYNDROME; ALDOSTERONISM; CORTICOSTEROIDS; NOREPINEPHRINE.)

Adrenalin. Most commonly referred to as the "fight or flight" hormone, adrenalin is produced by the inner region of the adrenal glands. Scientists call it epinephrine. Adrenalin, along with norepinephrine, causes an increase of metabolic rate and cardiac output. Their action is similar to the effect brought on by stimulating the sympathetic nervous system, but the effect is more intense and longer lasting. *(See* ADRENAL GLANDS; ADRENAL HORMONES.)

Adrenalin has tremendous metabolic effects and is stronger in this respect than norepinephrine. *(See* NOREPINEPHRINE.) It brings on increased oxygen consumption, elevation of body temperature, hyperglycemia, and increased lactic acid in the blood. The hyperglycemia results from release of glycogen from the liver to produce glucose in the blood, and the rise in lactic acid is caused by breakdown of muscle glycogen to lactic acid.

The effects of adrenalin are practically instantaneous. A fright brings on pounding heart, sweating palms, gastric constriction, and muscular strength in less time than it takes to read this sentence. There are documented cases showing almost fantastic reactions. These include the woman who, seeing a child pinned beneath the wheels of a car, was able to lift the car and free the child. Afterward she was totally exhausted and experienced extreme muscular aches.

This case and others like it reflect an excessive secretion of adrenalin, which allows people to perform superhuman feats without really pausing to think about them.

Adrenocortical Insufficiency. Persons whose adrenal glands are unable to produce enough mineralocorticoids and glucocorticoids are said to suffer from adrenocortical insufficiency. Mineralocorticoids are important because they affect the balance of electrolytes such as sodium, potassium, and chlorides; glucocorticoids are important because they affect the blood glucose levels. (*See* ADRENAL GLANDS; ADRENAL HORMONES.)

Loss of adrenocortical secretion causes death within three days to a week, unless the patient is given extensive salt therapy or mineralocorticoid therapy. Without such treatment, a patient's cardiac output diminishes, shock ensues, and death follows. Although mineralocorticoid treatment will save a patient's life, glucocorticoids must also be administered to normalize the metabolism of carbohydrates, proteins, and fats.

Adrenogenital Syndrome. Tumors of the cortex of the adrenal glands cause the secretion of excessive amounts of adrenal sex hormones, which in turn bring on intense masculinizing effects throughout the body. This is called "adrenogenital syndrome." Normally, only minute amounts of sex hormones are produced by the adrenal cortex. (*See* ADRENAL HORMONES.)

A female with an adrenogenital syndrome develops manly characteristics such as beard growth, deepened voice, masculinized muscular growth, body hair, possibly baldness, and growth of the clitoris to resemble a penis. Young males with the same affliction will develop both primary and secondary sexual characteristics precociously, and may have the sexual organs and drives of an adult. The problem is more difficult to diagnose in the adult male because of normal development of virility.

However, adrenal tumors can sometimes create feminizing effects in the male, such as excessive breast growth. The syndrome can also be brought on by enormous growth of the adrenal cortex.

Treatment may be administration of cortisol to inhibit production of adrenal androgen, or by surgical removal of the pathogenic tumor.

Aerophagia. Swallowing air is known as aerophagia. People who eat rapidly, chew a lot of gum, talk a good deal, or are under nervous strain often gulp a considerable amount of air. Air bubbles trapped in the digestive tract cause abdominal discomfort, which is relieved by belching (eructation) or by passing gas (flatus) from the anus. (*See* BELCHING.)

Aerophobia. The fear of air in motion (drafts), which is rare among psychiatric patients but does not seem to be uncommon in people generally regarded as normal, is called aerophobia.

Aerophobia is thought to be related to the fears of primitive people regarding airborne demons. In our society persons suffering from this phobia seem to feel that there are harmful influences in the air. Or they may fear the odors carried by one's own body, such as odors from perspiration or from flatus.

An aerophobic person suffering from a true mental illness, such as paranoia, may suspect that others are trying to harm or kill him by creating "bad air" around him. (*See* PHOBIAS.)

Aerosol Addiction. Fluorocarbon 12 is a volatile liquid widely used as a refrigerant.

Several deaths have been reported from misuse of this substance. (One person died after inhaling fluorocarbon 12 vapor from a balloon.) If inhaled in the absence of oxygen or taken as a liquid in sufficient quantity, fluorocarbon 12 damages the larynx and respiratory system, often causing death.

Aerosols. Hundreds of products used in the home come in spray cans—from shaving cream to oven cleaners to insect killers. Most consumers like to use products that can be sprayed because they are quick, efficient, and usually less messy than the same products in nonspray form. However, they can be more dangerous, too.

Spray cans are full of pressure. The product is suspended in gas, so that when a button is pushed the gas is released and the contents come out in a spray. All sprays are aerosols, which means they are solutions containing particles suspended in a gas.

There is always the danger that the spray can may explode, because of a flaw in the can or because its contents may be under too much pressure. Perhaps the valve is defective or the contents got too hot. Whatever the reason, the chances for explosion will be less if the directions on the container are followed exactly.

Federal and state laws require manufacturers to print warnings on the can telling how the product should be used and stored. These warnings are futile, however, unless the user reads and follows them.

Know the products you bring into your home and garage; read the labels carefully. Most of the cautions on spray cans state: "Contents under pressure. Exposure to heat could cause bursting. Do not puncture or incinerate can."

Never set a spray can on the stove or a radiator, or store it in direct sunlight or any place where the temperature may go above 120°. When a spray can bursts, it becomes a hurtling missile capable of seriously injuring anybody or anything in its path.

When you are ready to discard the spray container, keep it separate from garbage that will be incinerated. Even though the contents of the can have been used up, gas remains and an explosion will result.

All the spray products in your home

should be stored in a cool, dry place, out of children's reach. Children should stay at a distance when adults are using sprays and other materials which send a vapor of liquid into the air. Because sprays may be dangerous when they get into the eyes or are breathed into the lungs they should be used only in a well-ventilated room.

Some sprays are doubly dangerous because both the gas, or propellant, and the product itself are harmful chemicals. Here again, reading the instructions on the label is your best guide to what to do if the spray gets into your eyes, on your skin, or in your lungs, causing discomfort.

If a child inhales or swallows the contents of a spray can and signs of poisoning are present, call the local hospital or poison control center immediately for emergency advice. If you take the victim to the hospital, bring the can whose contents you suspect caused the poisoning, so the doctor can treat the victim properly. Until medical attention is available, keep the victim quiet and in fresh air. (*See* POISONING.)

Afterbirth. Following the birth of the child, the mother is also delivered of the placenta or afterbirth, which has served as the connection between the developing child and the mother's uterus. The same conditions that stimulate delivery also displace the afterbirth. Its function completed, it follows the child out of the uterus, attached to the child by the umbilical cord. (*See* PLACENTA.)

Agalactia. On rare occasions a new mother finds that she is totally unable to produce milk for her infant. This complete lack of breast fluid is known as agalactia. In general, however, a mother will secrete at least a small amount of milk within several days after delivery. (*See* BREAST FEEDING.)

Agar. A by-product of seaweeds, agar (also known as agar agar) has a variety of

uses. For example, it is a biological culture medium used to grow penicillin, it is used for paper and silk production, it is added to food to thicken it, and is also used as an emulsifier.

Agglutination. When cells within a fluid clump together, the phenomenon is known as agglutination. (*See* BACTERIA; BLOOD; BLOOD CELLS; BLOOD TYPES; RED BLOOD CELLS; RH FACTOR; VASCULAR PROBLEMS; WHITE BLOOD CELLS.)

Aging. A gradual loss of energy, initiative, creative imagination, a narrowing of interests, an increase in egocentricity, and personality changes are often part of the normal process of aging.

Some people are fortunate enough to escape the mental and physical deterioration that this process involves. They remain active, alert, and zestful until the end. But those to be discussed here are less fortunate, presenting medical and psychiatric problems to both their families and their doctors.

With advancing age, there is a progressive loss of physical and mental resources that makes the older person feel helpless. Learning becomes more difficult and other noticeable physical changes, such as loss of teeth and impairment of hearing and sight, add to the person's feelings of anxiety.

Along with these stresses are feelings of loneliness—often because of the loss of his spouse or friends—and perhaps rejection by his children. As he tries to protect himself against his sense of isolation and insecurity, the older person may become ill-natured and quarrelsome, suspicious, or domineering.

From the mild changes of old age, a person may gradually slip into what is known as senile dementia, but this condition should not be confused with the behavior changes resulting from cerebral arteriosclerosis. The psychoses resulting from cerebral arteriosclerosis are due to insufficient blood supply to the brain, because of the narrowing of cerebral blood vessels. Only a physician can differentiate between arteriosclerosis and senile dementia, since both have many similar symptoms.

Although organic changes take place in the brain tissue of patients with senile dementia, there is no certain correlation between the amount of tissue damage and atrophy and the degree of senile dementia. The senile psychoses are frequently produced by an interaction of organic and psychological factors.

Meal Plan for an Elderly Person

Breakfast
Fruit or juice
Cereal with milk and/or an egg
Bread with butter or margarine
Beverage

Lunch
Meat, egg, or cheese dish
Vegetable—raw or cooked
Bread with butter or margarine
Fruit
Milk

Dinner
Meat, poultry, or fish
Potato or substitute
Vegetable or salad
Bread with butter or margarine
Fruit or dessert
Milk

Often the person with senile psychosis is one who has never felt secure and has followed a rigid pattern of living throughout his life. Psychiatrists feel that a person with a cheerful disposition who has always adjusted well to the stresses of life has the best outlook for escaping the psychological deterioration of old age. For the person who has always been unhappy and maladjusted, the stresses of retirement, the death of friends and relatives, and the other in-

securities of old age will be more likely to produce mental symptoms.

It is difficult to say just when the common changes of old age can actually become those of senile dementia, since the changes are so gradual.

Often the earliest clinical sign of senile dementia is the loss of memory for recent events. The person may pay less and less attention to the courtesies of social life, and will begin complaining that he is neglected. Some people may show greater dependence on others, coupled with hostility and fear. Their normal affection for members of the family may gradually turn to hatred.

With this gradual deterioration, the aged person may become more isolated, selfish, and irritable, as well as prying or suspicious, with further loss of memory. He may grow careless about dress and cleanliness. Hoarding and delusions of theft, of poisoning, of poverty, or of not being wanted are common.

Often the personality traits of earlier years become exaggerated in senile psychosis. Feelings of anxiety, irritability, timidity, and other personality changes are not caused only by changes in the brain cells. Rather they are the result of a realistic sense of uselessness and dependency, perhaps because of social or financial pressures. The fact that the person is not needed, important, or productive leads to these regressive changes.

As degeneration continues, the aged person begins to live more and more in the past. He may speak of parents and grandparents as still living, and misidentify living persons. Past events he recalls in great detail, while his memory of recent events is lost.

He becomes confused and may wander away. Since his judgment is impaired, he may become the victim of unscrupulous persons. He forgets where he has put an article and then accuses other persons of having stolen it.

Although there are no cures for senile

psychosis, there are preventive measures. Psychiatrists advise older people to maintain a feeling of emotional security and a sense of dignity. The aged person's family should fill his need for affection, for a sense of belonging, achievement, and recognition.

On the brighter side, adequate nutrition and early care of physical illnesses can retard mental deterioration in the aged.

Aglycemia.   An absence of sugar in the blood is called aglycemia, from the Greek *a* (meaning no or not), *glykys* (sweet), and *haima* (blood). This may be a disorder of the metabolism of sugar. (*See* SUGAR.) The normal sugar content of the human blood supply at any given time is about a fourth of an ounce, enough for only about thirty minutes at ordinary levels of activity.

Agnosia.   A loss of perception is known as agnosia. The loss may be failure to recognize familiar objects by touch, hearing, taste, sight, or smell. In many cases of mental illness, especially schizophrenia, patients will disclaim any recognition of members of their family, stubbornly maintaining that they have never seen them before —even when standing in front of them. This type of agnosia is also seen in victims of stroke, in depressed patients, and in epileptics.

Agoraphobia.   When a person has an abnormal fear of being in open spaces, he has agoraphobia. Sometimes just the thought of open spaces will cause him to panic, but usually the feeling arises when he faces an actual visit to an open space. To protect himself, he may choose to remain indoors and be near a comforting person. (*See* PHOBIAS.)

Agranulocytosis.   One of the most serious diseases affecting the white cells of the blood is agranulocytosis. In this disease the white blood cells are destroyed faster than they are produced—just the opposite of

leukemia, in which white cells are produced so fast that they crowd out other elements essential to life. (*See* LEUKEMIA.)

Agranulocytosis is an acute disease that in the days before antibiotics was fatal to about 90 percent of those who developed it. The cause is extreme sensitivity and reaction to chemical substances such as certain drugs. It is still serious, but death from agranulocytosis today is uncommon.

Sometimes agranulocytosis is referred to as an extreme form of leukopenia, a general class of blood diseases in which white cells are attacked and reduced in number; sometimes it is classed as a separate condition. However it is classified, it is the most serious of the ailments that destroy leukocytes. This is because it destroys specifically the types of white cells that attack infectious agents and protect the body against illness.

The white cells are grouped under two broad headings, granulocytes, making up about 75 percent of the total white cell count, and lymphocytes, the remaining 25 percent. The granulocytes are further classified into three types: neutrophils, eosinophils, and basophils. Of these the neutrophils are by far the most important in fighting disease. They make up about 60 to 75 percent of all the white cells and are the cells that move amoeba-like to the site of any wound and fight the invading elements.

In agranulocytosis the neutrophils are destroyed. The normal white cell count of the blood ranges from 5,000 to 10,000 per cubic millimeter. Counts of less than 5,000 are considered to indicate leukopenia. Agranulocytosis reduces the number to less than 1,000 per cubic millimeter. White cell development in the bone marrow is greatly decreased, and granulocyte cells disappear from the circulating blood. The patient is left completely vulnerable to the development of infection. And this is exactly what happens.

Fever begins. There is a state of sepsis or general infection throughout the body, causing open sores of the skin, the mouth, throat, gastrointestinal tract, and other tissues.

A number of drugs, including the sulfonamides, can be agents that trigger the extreme sensitivity reaction that results in agranulocytosis. Avoiding such "toxic" substances—if the person's sensitivity can be anticipated—is the best preventive. Once the condition has developed, the best treatment is the use of an antibiotic such as penicillin to combat the infection.

Other names for agranulocytosis include agranulocytic angina, essential granulopenia, sepsis agranulocytica, malignant leukopenia, malignant neutropenia, granulopenia, granulophthisis, mucositis necroticans agranulocytica, and Schultz's angina.

Ague. The shaking chills associated with malaria, whether due to malaria itself or to some other disease, are referred to as ague. Symptoms are recurrent, involving violent shaking spasms. Time intervals between chills vary widely. (*See* MALARIA; NEURALGIA.)

Ainhum. Natives of Africa are sometimes afflicted with a syndrome in which the fifth toe becomes encircled with tough, horny tissue causing a stricture that leads to spontaneous amputation of the toe in a phenomenon known as ainhum. The problem occurs mainly in dark-skinned persons, usually between the ages of thirty and forty. Tissue begins to harden at the base of the toe and gradually encloses the area, cutting off circulation. Within months to years the toe drops off bloodlessly.

Although the cause is unknown, the practice of going without shoes may have something to do with it. The only cure is the eventual natural amputation or else surgical removal. Complications involving infection sometimes occur.

Air. Surrounding the earth is a transparent mixture of gases called air, or the atmosphere. Without it, neither plants nor animals could live on the earth. Pure air has no color, taste, or smell, but it has weight and exerts pressure. Air resistance to motion is the basis for flight by birds and airplanes. (*See* ATMOSPHERIC PRESSURE.) Just as there is an ocean of water on the earth, there is an "ocean" of air that covers the earth, and it is larger in area than all the oceans of water put together.

The most abundant gases in air are nitrogen, which makes up more than 78 percent of the air's volume, and oxygen, which accounts for nearly 21 percent. The remaining 1 percent of air is almost entirely the inert gas argon. Small amounts of other gases are also found in air: neon, helium, xenon, krypton, hydrogen, ozone, carbon dioxide, nitrous oxide, methane, carbon monoxide, and hydrogen sulfide.

The composition of the air, especially its oxygen content, is vital to health. A decrease in oxygen content, as at high altitudes, can place a burden on the human circulatory system. This is why some people are subject to heart attacks in the mountains or in nonpressurized airplane cabins. Physicians usually advise patients with weak hearts to avoid exertion and stress when in high-altitude regions.

Pollens, dust, and other pollutants in the air can seriously affect persons with allergies and lung troubles. And the amount of moisture in the air is important to the well-being of many, including those with lung and upper respiratory diseases. (*See* AIR CONDITIONING; AIR POLLUTION; ALLERGY; ALTITUDE; HUMIDITY; OXYGEN.)

Air Conditioning. Control of the temperature, moisture, cleanliness, and movement of indoor air is called air conditioning. *Summer air conditioning* cleans, cools, and removes moisture from the air. *Winter air conditioning* cleans and heats the air and adds moisture to it. *Year-round air conditioning* cleans and controls the temperature and moisture of air throughout the year.

By permitting people to live and work in clean, healthfully moist air at comfortable temperatures, well-regulated air conditioning is beneficial both physiologically and psychologically. When our surroundings are too hot or too cold for comfort, our bodies are subject to certain strains. These, of course, vary in intensity according to each person's ability to adapt and according to the degree of heat or coldness. But it is often difficult for us to concentrate on our work or to enjoy our indoor activities if we are overheated or chilled. The same is true if the air around us is too moist or too dry (although we are often unaware of the influence humidity can have upon us), or if it contains dust, pollen, or other irritating particles. Moreover, uncomfortable variations in the temperature, humidity, and cleanliness of the air can have unfavorable effects on the sick, the elderly, and the very young.

Air conditioners clean the air in a variety of ways. Some of them force air through filters made of closely packed fiberglass, wool, or metal fibers that have been coated with a sticky substance to trap dirt. Air can also be cleaned by blowing it through water sprays or air washers. Another means is the electrostatic precipitator, which puts an electric charge on particles of dirt in the air so that they will be attracted by oppositely charged collector plates.

Air is cooled by blowing it through sprays of cold water, often the same sprays that clean it. In some air conditioners the air is passed over coils filled with cold water or a chemical refrigerant. In the same manner, air is heated by blowing it over coils filled with hot water or steam. Some air conditioners warm the air as it passes over wire screens that are heated by electricity.

Air conditioners remove moisture from (dehumidify) air in different ways. When they cool the air by passing it over cooling coils, the water or refrigerant in the coils can be made cool enough to cause the moisture in the air to condense. This happens because cold air cannot hold as much moisture as warm air can. Other air conditioners use desiccants or chemicals that remove moisture from the air. In cold weather, the air contains little moisture, and when heated it becomes dry and irritating to breathe. To prevent this, air conditioners add moisture to the air by passing it through sprays of water or over pans of heated water which evaporates into the air. (*See* HUMIDITY.)

Air Pollution. The contamination of air by dust, fumes, smoke, soot, gases, and other substances has been increasing rapidly over the years. Air pollution is a major problem in cities and industrial areas because of the tremendous amounts of pollutants that are generated by the burning of fuels for heat or energy. Geographical factors also affect air pollution conditions. (*See* TEMPERATURE INVERSION.)

Air pollution is much more than a mere nuisance that soils our clothes or irritates our eyes. High concentrations of pollution in the air can be harmful to our health—so harmful that it may be a contributing cause of death, especially in elderly persons with respiratory or heart disease. (*See* LUNGS; PAN.) Air pollution also costs millions of dollars each year in damage to fruit and vegetable crops, corrosion of metals, and erosion of stone buildings.

The sources of air pollution include the automobile and other forms of powered transportation, industrial plants that disperse wastes through smokestacks, heat-generating plants, the burning of garbage and trash, and building or road construction activities that create dust. (*See* CARBON MONOXIDE; NITROGEN OXIDE; OZONE; SMOG; SULFUR OXIDE.) When crops are sprayed, the air can become contaminated with dust and liquid droplets of the insecticides that are released into the atmosphere. (*See* PESTICIDES.) Particles of radioactive material created by nuclear energy processes also add to the air pollution problem. (*See* ATOMIC BOMB; FALLOUT; RADIATION.)

In the past decade, great efforts have been made to clear the air. Automobiles are now being equipped with devices that

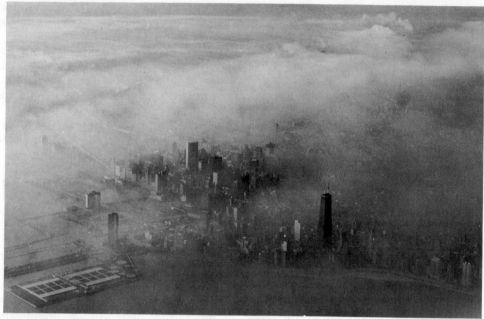

Argonne National Laboratory

A smoggy morning in downtown Chicago. The smoke, on this otherwise clear day, is generated by industry upwind of the city; it is held close to the surface of the earth by a temperature inversion. Some air, though apparently clear, may be dangerously polluted.

reduce the amount of exhaust gases. Filters, settling and washing chambers, and other electrical and mechanical methods of removing industrial wastes have been designed and used.

Despite the progress made by scientists and engineers, many antipollution methods are costly or else remove only the largest polluting particles. In some states and cities, the air pollution problem has become so serious that strict laws have been passed to regulate incineration or waste-disposal techniques, as well as the choice of fuels. National laws have also been passed to promote interstate cooperation in air pollution control.

Airsickness. Like seasickness, airsickness is caused largely by unaccustomed motion that overstimulates the semicircular canals, the center for the sense of balance in the inner ear. Sickness is more likely in turbulent air when the plane rises and drops abruptly. Anxiety and a sensitive stomach may also contribute to the problem.

Big jet planes have reduced the likelihood of airsickness because they fly more smoothly and more quietly. Choosing a seat between the wings may provide a little more stability. Reclining in the seat, with the head still and the eyes closed or fixed on the ceiling, may also help. (*See* MOTION SICKNESS.)

Akinesthesia. A loss or impairment of the sense of position and movement of the body is called akinesthesia.

Our awareness of our body's position and movement depends partly on a mechanism in the inner ear that controls our sense of balance and partly on nerve endings, called proprioceptors, that report the positions and movements of muscles, joints, and tendons. This sense can be impaired in certain disorders such as locomotor ataxia, multiple sclerosis, and pernicious anemia, when the disease attacks the proprioceptive pathways in the spinal cord. (*See* NERVOUS SYSTEM.)

Albinism. When the pigment-forming cells (melanocytes) of the skin fail to produce pigment (melanin), albinism results. People who suffer from albinism are called albinos.

Melanin is the dark pigment which gives color to skin, hair, and eyes and helps to protect the skin from the harmful rays of sunlight.

The chief characteristic of albinism is the distinctive appearance of the skin, hair, and eyes. The skin is white or pinkish and may have a yellowish tinge. The hair is platinum blond or white. The eyes are pink. The pink color of the skin and eyes is due to blood circulating in small blood vessels close to the surface. The yellowish tinge results from carotenes—yellowish pigments deposited in the skin when certain foods, such as carrots, are eaten.

Sometimes albinism does not affect all of a person's body; when it is partial and spotty it is called piebaldism. The so-called white forelock results when the condition is limited to a patch of hair.

Albinism is not a disease. It is an inherited trait in which the melanocytes are present in the skin but, for some unknown reason, do not function. Fortunately it is quite rare, occurring in only one in 10,000 people. Furthermore, it is a recessive trait; that is, both parents must carry the recessive gene responsible for albinism in order for a baby to be born with the defect.

The most serious problem associated with albinism is severe hypersensitivity to the sun. Since melanin is not present to help protect the skin from the harmful effects of sunlight, direct exposure to the sun can cause severe sunburn and destructive changes in the skin. These changes include excessively aged skin, keratoses, skin cancer, and destruction of the skin's connective tissue. An albino may look like a very old person by the time he is twenty.

Other defects that may occur in conjunction with albinism include mental retardation, deafness, short stature, and infertility (inability to conceive offspring). Albinos usually die at an early age.

There is no treatment for albinism except avoiding exposure to the sun to minimize its destructive effects.

Albinos. People with little or no pigment in their skin are called albinos. Their skin color is white or pink, their hair is white, and their eyes pink. (*See* ALBINISM.)

Albumin. Biochemically, the albumins are a specific class of proteins which are water soluble and composed of nitrogen, carbon, hydrogen, oxygen, and sulfur. They occur in animal and vegetable juices and tissues. When spelled "albumen," the word means the white of an egg or the part of an organism which surrounds a seed and nourishes it.

The most widely known albumins are ovalbumin (egg white), blood serum albumin, and lactalbumin (present in milk). Blood serum albumin maintains the body's osmotic blood pressure; therefore human serum albumin is used for the treatment of shock. (*See* SHOCK.)

Because animal and human albumins are similar, scientific efforts have been made to use albumin from cattle blood to treat human shock victims. Unfortunately, unfavorable reactions in test cases have shown it to be unsafe. However, the purified bovine albumin has been used to expand man's knowledge of protein, thus aiding in protein research. (*See* ANIMAL RESEARCH.)

Albuminuria. When the doctor finds that excessive amounts of the protein albumin have appeared in a patient's urine sample, he is said to have albuminuria. Extreme loss of protein from the body causes serious damage, and loss of even small amounts can affect the metabolism. The condition of albuminuria usually, but not always, indicates malfunction of the kidney. (*See* ALBUMIN.)

Alcohol. The substances known as alcohols are chemicals that have the same single characteristic in their makeup—a hydrogen atom attached to an oxygen atom, which in turn is attached to a carbon atom. This property gives them the unusual power to dissolve many organic compounds, and alcohol is used in industry for that very purpose.

Ethanol, or ethyl alcohol, the basis for wines and hard cider, is made by the fermentation of fruit juices. Industrial ethyl alcohol is made from potatoes or grains, chiefly corn, the starch in corn is treated with malt to convert it into fermentable sugar. Since the freezing point of ethanol is $-170°$ F. (-117 C.) it is used as the liquid in thermometers and as an antifreeze in cars (because mixtures of ethanol and water remain liquid at very low temperatures). Ethanol is an excellent fuel which burns with a high heat release, but without soot.

Since ethanol dissolves many organic compounds, it is the base for many toilet and drug preparations; it is also an ingredient in lacquers. Rubbing alcohol is usually ethanol, useful for sterilizing surgical instruments because it kills many bacteria. A number of important chemicals are made from ethanol, including the anesthetic ether and other solvents.

When alcohol is added to beverages, they may have pronounced effects on the drinker's central nervous system, as explained in the article ALCOHOLISM. If methyl (wood) alcohol is used in a beverage, the results may be tragic. Methyl-alcohol poisoning can lead to total blindness.

Alcoholics Anonymous. The fellowship of Alcoholics Anonymous was founded in 1935 to give men and women an opportunity to help one another solve their common problem of alcoholism. The organization now has more than 400,000 members in over 14,000 local groups in the United States and abroad. Although not affiliated with any particular religious body, the fellowship is based on shared spiritual experience and dependence on God, as each member understands him. Medical treatment is not used. (*See* ALCOHOLISM.)

Alcoholism. In the United States, about 4,500,000 people are afflicted with a chronic disorder marked by an uncontrollable urge to drink alcoholic beverages. The disease of alcholism is found in all walks of life and is considered a major public health problem.

No one really knows what causes alcoholism. Only 6 percent of an estimated 70 million adults who drink alcohol in America become chronic alcoholics. Some experts maintain that the disease has a physiological basis. Others believe just as strongly that it stems from psychological disturbances; that the alcoholic drinks to escape from the demands and anxieties of reality with which he apparently cannot cope.

Alcohol is rapidly absorbed throughout the entire body, but its effects are most noticeable in the central nervous system. Contrary to popular belief, alcohol is a depressant, not a stimulant. As sensitivity is reduced in the nervous system, the higher functions of the brain are dulled, leading to impulsive actions, loud speech, and lack of physical control. The drinker's face may turn quite red or, conversely, quite pale. He may feel nauseous and have fits of vomiting.

While drinking, the alcoholic gains more and more self-confidence, loses any sense of embarrassment or guilt, and throws off his inhibitions as the alcohol deadens the restraining influences of his brain. Large quantities impair his physical reflexes, coor-

Are You an Alcoholic?

1. Do you drink alone?
2. Does your work suffer because of drinking?
3. Does your family feel the effect of your drinking?
4. Has drinking affected your social reputation?
5. Do you feel remorse after drinking?
6. Has your work drive decreased because of drinking?
7. Do you feel less shy with people when you drink?
8. Do you drink because you are ill at ease with others?
9. Have you lost a job because of drinking?
10. Have you incurred financial difficulties?
11. Do you seek drinking companions of a lower social standing?
12. Do you crave a drink at a definite time daily?
13. Do you have a drink the first thing in the morning?
14. Does drinking cause an inability to sleep?
15. Has your efficiency decreased since you began drinking?
16. Do you drink to escape from reality?
17. Has drinking ever resulted in a loss of memory?
18. Does drinking build up your self-confidence?
19. Has a physician ever treated you for drinking?

If you have answered yes to more than four of the questions, this is a warning that you could become an alcoholic.

These test questions are adapted from those used by Johns Hopkins University, Baltimore, Maryland, in deciding whether or not a patient is alcoholic.

dination, and mental acuteness. The toxic effects of the alcohol may produce the delusions of delirium tremens. (*See* DELIRIUM TREMENS.) If the concentration of alcohol in his blood reaches 0.45 percent, he will lapse into a coma; if it reaches 0.5 percent, he may die.

The excessive and prolonged use of alcohol can lead to other diseases as the alcoholic starts to substitute alcohol, which is rich in calories, for other foods. Vitamin and mineral deficiencies and liver ailments are common among alcoholics. (*See* CIRRHOSIS OF THE LIVER.)

The treatment of alcoholism is lengthy, complex, and often involves psychological assistance. Relapses are so frequent that many people believe alcoholism is incurable. (*See* ALCOHOLICS ANONYMOUS.)

Alcoholomania. A person with a constant morbid craving for alcoholic beverages, to the exclusion of everything else, has alcoholomania. However, not all alcoholics are alcoholomaniacs. (*See* ALCOHOLISM.)

Aldosteronism. When the body secretes excessive amounts of the mineralocorticoid aldosterone the result is a syndrome called aldosteronism. Among the symptoms are an increased volume of extracellular fluid, high blood pressure, and low potassium levels, which may cause occasional periods of muscular paralysis.

Usually a patient urinates so often that he keeps losing sodium chloride through his kidneys, despite a low concentration of the compound in his urine. In mild cases this will prevent the development of edema—that is, the buildup of fluid in the body tissues—but in severe cases edema is pronounced.

Treatment generally consists in removing part of the adrenal cortex on both sides, the amount removed depending on the severity of the affliction.

Algae. An alga is a simple plant without true leaves. Algae grow in ponds, rivers, oceans, and soils in almost every region of the world.

For many fish and other water animals, algae are almost the only source of food. Man may also have to learn to use algae as a source of his food—to avert the food shortages that may develop as the world's population increases.

Some forms of algae may be harmful to health. They may contaminate the water in public bathing areas or in reservoirs. Here, through proper drainage, shading from the sun's rays, and the use of dilute solutions of certain chemicals, they may be eliminated. Then, too, algae, in their life and decomposition processes, can threaten a lake by using up available oxygen in the water. The lake then begins to fill up with decaying matter and weeds. (*See* EUTROPHICATION; WATER POLLUTION.)

Alimentary Canal. This complicated tube, about thirty feet long, extends all the way from the mouth to the anus. The alimentary canal includes the pharynx, the esophagus, the stomach, and the intestines. Its function is the processing of food—intake, swallowing, digestion, absorption —and excretion of waste. (*See* DIGESTION.)

Alkali. In chemistry, an alkali is a compound of oxygen and hydrogen with any one of certain metallic elements, especially sodium and potassium. The hydroxides of sodium (NaOH) and potassium (KOH) are very soluble in water, and the solutions will turn red litmus blue. They will neutralize strong acids like sulfuric and nitric. In contact with the skin and other tissues, they are extremely corrosive. The hydroxides of several other metals and of the ammonium radical have similar properties.

The alkalies are of fundamental importance in the chemical industries. They are used on a large scale in the manufacture of soap, glass, and many other products, and must be handled with due care. Household lye is mainly sodium hydroxide. Because of its effectiveness in "cutting" grease, opening clogged drains, and rinsing glassware, its use is widespread in spite of the accidents that have resulted, especially to children.

Alkaloids. Many nitrogenous compounds in plants have no food value but are medically useful for treating a variety of disorders and diseases. These compounds are called alkaloids, and among them are morphine, quinine, strychnine, reserpine, and nicotine. Although more than 900 alkaloids are known to man, only about twenty are used for medicinal purposes.

Alkalosis. A clinical term for a number of conditions in which the acid/base balance of the blood and other body fluids leans to the base or alkaline side is alkalosis. (*See* ACIDOSIS.)

The pH of blood plasma and extracellular fluids is normally close to 7.4, with a range of 7.35 to 7.45. The pH is kept normal despite wide variations in the dietary load of acid or alkali. Many body functions are influenced by the pH, and when it is disturbed the effects on metabolic activity, circulation, and the central nervous system may be disastrous.

Alkalosis can be brought on either by an abnormal loss of acid or by an excessive retention of alkali. Its causes are many and varied, including vomiting or gastric drainage, diuretic therapy, Cushing's syndrome, aldosteronism, adrenal steroid therapy, and the ingestion of excess alkali. (*See* ALDOSTERONISM; CUSHING'S DISEASE AND SYNDROME.)

The kidney has the major responsibility of maintaining or restoring a proper acid/base balance. When the bicarbonate concentration in body fluids increases or decreases, the kidney has the ability to reabsorb more- or less-than-normal amounts of bicarbonate. But the kidney may not be able to cope with particularly high overloads of alkali. In vomiting, primarily the hydrogen ion is lost, leaving too much alkali. Diuretics stimulate excessive loss of acid. Adrenal steroid therapy has the side effect of causing the kidney to excrete too much of the balancing hydrogen ions. Also, if there is a deficiency of potassium (hypokalemia) the kidney will excrete large amounts of hydrogen ions and keep the bicarbonate.

DIAGNOSIS OF ALKALOSIS. As with acidosis, there are no signs or symptoms which specifically point to alkalosis. Rather, the physician may suspect the problem because of certain aspects of the patient's history. When a patient has been vomiting chronically, or has been treated with adrenal steroids, or has been taking antacids, or has shown a potassium deficiency for any reason, the doctor may feel that chemical studies are in order to determine if any of these other conditions have led to alkalosis.

TREATMENT OF ALKALOSIS. When the administration of adrenal steroids has caused a patient to have alkalosis, the treatment is of course withdrawal of the steroids. Other causes are treated by restoring the electrolyte balance and correcting the dehydration brought on by vomiting or drainage. Potassium chloride is given to supply the deficiency.

If the patient must take diuretics for the treatment of other conditions, his physician may prescribe acidifying chemicals to be taken simultaneously with them and thus to prevent alkalosis.

When alkalosis is due to adrenal disease resulting in excessive secretion of natural adrenal steroids, treatment is removal of the proper amount of adrenal tissue. But if steroid treatment is absolutely necessary, the physician may again prescribe potassium chloride along with the steroids.

Hyperventilation, a symptom of acidosis, may also be the cause of alkalosis. (*See* HYPERVENTILATION.) Excessive, rapid breathing reduces the amount of carbon dioxide in the blood, bringing on an alkalizing effect. If anxiety is the cause of the hyperventilation, leading to alkalosis, obviously the anxiety must be treated.

Alkaptonuria. Presence of alkapton, a nitrogen waste product, also called homogentisic acid, in the urine is termed alkaptonuria. The chemical nature of alkapton gives the urine a particularly vile odor, and causes it to darken considerably when left standing. (*See* KIDNEY; URINE.)

Allergen. When a person has an allergy, this means that repeated contact with a certain substance irritates his skin or other parts of the body. The irritating substance is called an allergen.

There are innumerable varieties of allergens, such as pollen, foods, industrial and household chemicals, feathers, animal hair, drugs, fungi, and so forth.

Allergens must be distinguished from primary irritants, like mustard, that exert their effect at first encounter with them. Before a person reacts to an allergen, he must first be sensitized. This means he must have been exposed to it one or more times before his body develops a marked reaction to it.

Allergy. A person is said to have an allergy if he has acquired a special sensitivity to a substance that is harmless to the average person. The substance that produces the allergic reaction is called an allergen. (*See* ALLERGEN.)

The body normally has an efficient system to fight off foreign substances such as viruses or bacteria. It manufactures antibodies to destroy or neutralize the effects of the invaders. This is one means by which we ward off disease. But the body of the allergic individual seemingly overreacts to certain substances for reasons not yet clear to medical researchers. Antibodies are produced in great quantities, along with a product from the tissues called histamine.

The role of histamine in body chemistry

Cosmetic Allergens and Irritants

The following irritating and allergenic ingredients are commonly used in cosmetic preparations.

Compound	Often Found in	Allergic Reactions
Acetone	Nail polish remover	Nails peel and split Dermatitis of the fingers
Almond oil	Creams, lotions, soaps, perfumes, shampoos	Rhinitis Dermatitis venenata
Alum	Anhidrotics * Astringents	Dermatitis venenata
Aluminum acetate Aluminum chloride Aluminum sulfate	Astringents Anhidrotics Deodorants	Dermatitis venenata
Ammonium carbonate	Permanent wave preparations	Dermatitis of the hands, hairline area, and scalp
Antimony compounds	Hair dye	Dermatitis venenata
Arrowroot	After-bath powder Dry shampoos	Rhinitis Conjunctivitis
Arsenic	Hair tonics, dyes	Dermatitis venenata
Balsam of Peru	Perfume	Dermatitis venenata Rhinitis Hay fever
Barium sulfide	Hair removers (depilatories)	Dermatitis venenata
Benzaldehyde	Creams and lotions	Dermatitis venenata
Betanaphthol	Hair dyes, skin-peeling preparations	Dermatitis venenata
Bismuth	Bleach, freckle creams	Dermatitis venenata
Calcium sulfide	Hair removers	Dermatitis venenata

Compound	Often Found in	Allergic Reactions
Cornstarch	Dusting powders Face powders	Conjunctivitis Hay fever Rhinitis
Dibromflorescein	Indelible lipsticks	Cheilitis and/or respiratory symptoms, dermatitis Gastrointestinal distress, as in colitis
Gum arabic	Wave-sets Rouge and powder compacts	Atopic coryza Atopic dermatitis Gastrointestinal distress Asthma
Gum karaya	Wave-sets Toothpaste Denture adhesive powder Hand lotion Rouge and powder compacts	Hay fever Atopic coryza Atopic dermatitis Gastrointestinal distress Asthma
Gum tragacanth	Wave-sets Hand lotions Rouge and powder compacts	Atopic coryza Atopic dermatitis Gastrointestinal distress Asthma
Lanolin	Creams or pure lotions Shampoos Hand lotions Ointment bases	Dermatitis venenata
Lead	Hair dyes	Dermatitis venenata
Lycopodium	After-bath powders	Rhinitis Hay fever
Mercury	Bleach and freckle creams Hair tonics Medicated soaps	Dermatitis venenata

* Anhidrotics close pores to stop perspiration; are stronger than deodorants.

Compound	Often Found in	Allergic Reactions	Compound	Often Found in	Allergic Reactions
Methy heptine carbonate	Perfumed cosmetics Perfumes Toilet water	Asthma Rhinitis Hay fever Dermatitis (from skin contact)	Potassium carbonate Potassium sulfite	Permanent wave solutions	Dermatitis of hairline, scalp, and hands
			Pyrogallol	Hair dye	Dermatitis venenata
Oil of bergamot, cananga, coriander, geraniol, heliotropine, lemon, lavender, hydroxycitronella, lemon grass, neroli, linalool, orange peel, orris root, origanum, ylang ylang	Perfumes Perfumed cosmetics Toilet water	Rhinitis Hay fever Photosensitivity Contact dermatitis Asthma	Quinine sulfate	Hair tonics	Dermatitis venenata
			Resorcinol	Hair tonics	Dermatitis venenata
			Rice starch	Face powder Dusting powder	Conjunctivitis Hay fever Rhinitis
			Rosin	Hair sprays	Dermatitis venenata
Oil of cassia Mint oils	Perfume Toilet water Toothpaste Tooth powder Perfumed cosmetics	Rhinitis Asthma Hay fever Contact dermatitis	Salicylic acid	Deodorants Hair tonics	Dermatitis venenata
			Sodium carbonate	Permanent wave solutions	Dermatitis of hairline, scalp, and hands
			Strontium sulfide	Hair removers	Dermatitis venenata
Oil of citronella	Perfume and toilet water Perfumed cosmetics Mosquito repellent Creams and lotions	Rhinitis Hay fever Asthma Contact dermatitis	Sulfonamide resins	Nail polish	Eyelid dermatitis Pruritis Dermatitis venenata
			Tetrabromfluorescein	Indelible lipsticks	Cheilitis, respiratory distress, gastrointestinal discomfort
Orris root powder	Toothpaste Dry shampoos Sachets Some face powders	Hay fever Infantile eczema Rhinitis Conjunctivitis Asthma	Thioglycollic acid salts	Cold permanent wave preparations	Dermatitis venenata
			Wheat starch	Dusting and face powders	Conjunctivitis Rhinitis Hay fever
Paraphenylenediamine	Hair, eyebrow, and eyelash dye	Dermatitis venenata	Zinc chloride Zinc sulfate	Astringents	Dermatitis venenata
Phenol	Hand lotion	Dermatitis venenata			

AR-EX Products Company.

is unclear but important. It causes dilatation (expansion) of blood vessels, a drop in blood pressure, an increase in the heart rate, and a rise in the temperature of the skin.

During an allergic reaction, histamine escapes from body cells, producing inflammation and irritation. It can cause a flow of mucus in the lungs and nasal passages, resembling one of the symptoms of a cold. It also can provoke headaches, dizziness, and other discomforts. Thus drugs to counteract histamine (antihistamines) are helpful in some allergies.

Just as there are many allergens, there are many possible responses to them. Some persons, for example, may become nauseated or break out with hives if they even enter a home that harbors a furry animal. Another person may have breathing difficulties, chills, or tightness in the throat, on contact with a normally harmless chemical or plant pollen. Some alcoholics are allergic to the liquor they drink.

An individual with an allergy to one substance tends to be allergic to others as well. The pattern will differ from person to person. A tendency toward allergies seems to run in families, but members of the same family often are allergic to quite different things. No one really knows why this is.

COMMON ALLERGIES. Asthma is an allergic disease that affects the lungs. It may be caused by a wide variety of allergens. (*See* ASTHMA.) House dust, certain foods, feathers, and many other things may start the asthmatic patient wheezing.

Foods can set off reactions. Eggs, even in tiny quantities, make many persons ill. If you have an allergy and suspect that food is responsible, you can leave one item at a time out of your diet for periods of several weeks, then reintroduce it until you discover the allergen or allergens.

Milk allergy is common. It can produce violent reactions among some babies: diarrhea, vomiting, hives, and breathing difficulties. Switching to a milk substitute may

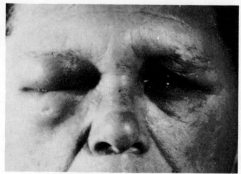

J. B. Kahn

A hair dye caused this allergic reaction. There are both swelling and conjunctivitis, an inflammation of the membrane covering the eyeball and lining the eyelid.

be necessary. Other common food allergens are nuts, chocolate, grains, meats, seafood, and certain vegetables and fruits.

While most of the common allergies are the result of exposure to organic (plant and animal) material, inorganic chemicals may cause allergies, too. Cosmetics, soaps, drug products, industrial solvents, paint, and so on, may produce allergic reactions. Many persons become extremely allergic to penicillin.

Allergic contact dermatitis is a skin condition produced by substances that touch the skin directly, in contrast to eruptions that occur on the skin from an internal or systemic reaction. Fabrics and dyes may do this. Poison ivy is another example of allergic contact dermatitis. (*See* POISON IVY.)

Some persons develop a sensitivity to stings from bees, wasps, hornets, or yellowjackets. In rare cases the reactions are so strong and rapid that the patient dies within a half hour after being stung. Emergency kits for stings are available. (*See* BEE STINGS.)

Emotional stress appears to be related to allergy. Though apparently not a direct cause, it can trigger allergic attacks. If you are prone to allergies, chances are you will have much less trouble with them if you avoid tension and worry.

PREVENTION AND TREATMENT. Allergists (doctors who specialize in the problem) have determined that most allergies begin during childhood, some 80 percent before the age of fifteen years. A survey concluded that one child in five has a major allergy. However, only slightly over one-third of these children receive any treatment.

It is very important that a person have professional help when he first develops an allergy. Children who are untreated often grow up with complications of their simple allergies, and may face a lifelong problem with asthma, emphysema, or some other respiratory disease.

The first thing to be done is to identify the allergen. The next is to remove the allergen from the patient's environment if possible, or take the patient away from the allergen. A change of climate sometimes works, but too often this proves a costly waste of time. Some hay fever sufferers, for example, have moved their families to the opposite end of the country, only to find a new allergen waiting there to harass them.

Air conditioners and filters are a great help to persons allergic to pollen. A change in occupation or the use of face masks on the job can help others. Hypoallergenic cosmetics are available—preparations that are compounded without the most common allergens.

If you and your doctor cannot determine by simple trial and error the irritant that gives you trouble, then skin tests may be made. A minute amount of various materials is exposed to the skin to see which one causes a reaction.

Some people can be desensitized to allergic substances by exposing them to minute amounts of an allergen over a period of time. Usually the person will then develop some type of resistance to this allergy, and not be so ill later when he is faced with the allergen in larger quantities.

Take medicine for allergies only on the advice of a physician. Overdoses may be quite harmful. Antihistamines, cortico-steroids, epinephrine, antibiotics, and adrenalin are some of the products used for various allergies. They do not cure the allergy but help minimize the symptoms and prevent complications.

Abscesses in the body, such as an infected tooth, seemingly can provoke allergic attacks in some people. In general, a person in good health who eats a well-balanced diet seems to be less prone to allergy.

If someone in your family has an allergy, by all means help him to overcome it. But don't pamper him to such extremes that you cause emotional strain throughout the whole family. Blanket restrictions on diet or on the choice of a vacation spot because of one asthmatic person in the family, for example, can build up feelings of resentment among the other children. Have a family conference, and use a little diplomacy in such matters.

The allergic person needs some assurance that he can live a fairly normal life. He might take a lesson from the golf star Billy Casper, who had allergies that would have kept a man with less determination at home. Among his problems were reactions to pesticides that had been sprayed on golf courses weeks before his arrival; inability to sleep in a hotel room that had been recently painted or was not heated by electricity; reactions to cigarette smoke; and the need for a special diet while on tour. Yet he kept on playing golf and winning tournaments.

If you cannot eliminate your allergy, you can usually learn how to live with it.

Alopecia. Loss of hair from any cause is known medically as alopecia. (*See* BALDNESS.)

Altitude Sickness. Some people become ill at high altitudes—for example, when climbing mountains or flying in a plane. Altitude sickness is the result of an insufficient amount of oxygen in the blood for the body's needs. Its symptoms are fatigue, shortness of breath, dizziness, headache, nausea, and faulty judgment.

The average person is accustomed to living at altitudes under 5,000 feet. Some people, such as the Tibetans and the Indians of Peru and Bolivia, have become well adapted to very high altitudes. At 17,000 feet they can perform hard labor, whereas the newcomer to that region would find it difficult to take even one step without gasping for breath.

In the past, many pilots lost their lives because they failed to realize the importance of having sufficient oxygen at high altitudes. Modern-day aircraft are equipped with pressurized cabins and oxygen-breathing devices which provide oxygen as it is needed during high altitude flying.

Alum.   Ordinary alum is a crystalline hydrated double sulfate of aluminum and potassium. Alums in general are used in medicines and baking powder, and for water purification and other industrial uses. They may also be found in astringents and styptics which stop the bleeding from cuts.

Aluminosis.   Workers handling alum are subject to a chronic catarrhal affection of the respiratory passages. This inflammation of the mucous membrane of the nose and pharynx is called aluminosis.

Aluminum.   The chemical element aluminum (or aluminium) is one of the most abundant on earth, but it occurs in nature only in the form of compounds with other elements. It was first obtained in the form of metallic beads in 1854, and later as a molten, silvery metal in the 1880's. It is now produced electrically in enormous quantities and is widely used because it is light in weight and conducts both heat and electricity very well. Its oxide and hydroxide are colorless and nontoxic.

Three of its compounds are now much used as antacids in treating various chronic gastric and duodenal diseases: aluminum hydroxide, basic aluminum carbonate, and dihydroxyaluminum aminoacetate; their chief disadvantage is their constipating effect. Alum, a hydrated double sulfate of aluminum and potassium, is astringent and is used in styptic pencils for small cuts. A solution of aluminum acetate, called Burrow's solution, is sometimes used in wet dressings in cases of acute inflammatory eruptions of the skin. Aluminum acetate and certain related compounds have an immediate deodorizing effect when applied as dusting powder on sweating skin-surfaces.

Alveolitis.   This advanced stage of periodontal disease is usually the result of failure to get early dental treatment. (*See* PERIODONTAL DISEASE.) If the accumulation of calculus is not removed from the teeth regularly, the eventual result may be a chronic inflammation of the gum tissues. This inflammation will spread from the gums to the underlying bony tissues which support the teeth. Then the supporting alveolar bone begins to resorb. After this is lost, there is nothing left to hold the tooth in place. No therapy has yet been devised to guarantee the growth of new alveolar bone. However, there is an experimental technique in which the bone is rebuilt through bone grafts from the patient's hip.

Early dental treatment is absolutely necessary to avert such bone loss. If the calculus and what dentists call "oral debris" are removed, the disease will be arrested—until new debris forms and sets the cycle in motion again.

Alveolus.   In anatomy, any basin-like or bowl-shaped structure may be called an alveolus. The sockets in the jaw into which the teeth fit are called alveoli. The roots of teeth extend into these alveoli, and are held in place by connective tissue. (*See* TEETH.)

Each bronchiole in the lungs ends in small, irregular chambers, or air sacs. These are also called alveoli. They are surrounded by blood capillaries that pick up

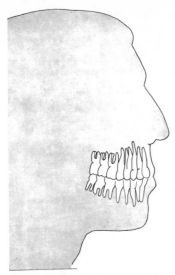

All teeth have deep roots, each in a bony socket called an alveolus. The part of the jaw that contains the teeth is known as the alveolar process.

oxygen and carry the gas to other larger vessels and then throughout the body. There are 700,000,000 or more alveoli in the human lungs. (*See* BREATHING; LUNGS; RESPIRATORY SYSTEM.)

Amaurosis. Blindness occurring when there are no apparent defects of the eye is termed amaurosis. This permanent blindness may come from a disease of the optic nerve, retina, spinal cord, or brain.

Amaurosis sometimes results from renal disease, or is associated with diabetes, or may exist from birth.

A brief episode of blindness, lasting ten minutes or less, is called amaurosis fugax. Sometimes amaurosis is caused by a systemic poison such as alcohol or tobacco. It may be caused by the reflex action of a remote irritation or may occur during an attack of acute gastritis.

Ambidextrous. When a person can use either hand equally well to perform manual tasks, he is said to be ambidextrous. (*See* LEFT-HANDEDNESS.)

Amblyaphia. A dullness or bluntness of the sense of touch is termed amblyaphia. Studies in industrial medicine show that work with vibrating hand tools can cause a temporary decrease in sensitivity of touch.

Amblyopia. When vision becomes dim but no physical change in the affected eye is observable, the condition is called amblyopia. Usually this means amblyopia ex-anopsia, in which the vision in one eye is unconsciously suppressed.

Amblyopia ex-anopsia often occurs when a child has strabismus (cross-eyes). Because the cross-eyed child sees double or otherwise receives a disturbing or unclear image, his brain may automatically suppress the use of one eye. The child then sees in a monocular (one-eyed) manner, avoiding the double image he would see if he used both eyes (binocular vision).

The eye which the child tends to suppress has been termed the "lazy eye." Somehow he must learn to use this eye or its vision may be permanently lost. The ophthalmologist (eye specialist) may have him wear a patch over his better eye. This will force him to use the lazy eye and restore it to use. The doctor may also have him wear the patch over the weaker eye for a short period, since the better eye may need to improve its focusing before being exposed to the binocular (two-eye) image.

"Lazy eye," or amblyopia, in children is often treated by a patch worn over the normal eye. The "lazy eye" is thus forced to be more active. An eyeglass frame may be used to hold the patch in place.

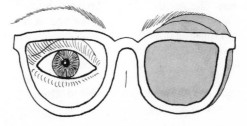

If your child must wear an eye patch for amblyopia, explain to him that the eye is tired and needs a rest. This also is a good explanation for him to give his playmates. Youngsters often tease a child with cross-eyes.

The patch helps the weaker eye regain its sight, but the focus of the two eyes together must also be corrected. This may be accomplished by a combination of techniques including eyeglasses, special exercises (orthoptics), and surgical repair.

These methods, as well as warning signs of strabismus and amblyopia in children, are discussed in the article CROSS-EYES. (*See also* EYE CARE; EYESIGHT.)

Ambulatory Patient. The patient who is no longer confined to bed and is able to walk around unassisted is referred to as an ambulatory patient. After illness, surgery, or other disability this stage of recovery, once reached, indicates a good prognosis. The nursing care and medical complications of the ambulatory patient are minimal.

Since serious complications arising from continued lying in bed can prolong a hospital stay and perhaps take a life, patients are no longer allowed to stay in bed for weeks after surgery or illness. When a patient has had fairly minor surgery, he is often asked to stand beside his bed the night after his operation. The next day he is encouraged to walk. After major surgery, the patient may sometimes remain quiet in bed for two days to a week, but ambulation is encouraged as soon as possible.

Nursing care for a patient confined to bed is time consuming and difficult. Bed baths must be given daily. Sheets must be changed with the patient in the bed. A bedpan must be provided for collection of urine and feces. All these services require time and cost money. Early ambulation of the patient eliminates much of the nursing care and reduces the cost of hospitalization (*See* NURSING CARE.)

Ambulatory patients escape some of the severe disorders which result from confinement in bed. They recover faster, require less hospitalization, and pay a smaller hospital bill. The patient encouraged to leave his bed and walk should realize that his physician is paving the way toward complete recovery.

Amebiasis. This word means invasion of the body by parasitic amebas. When it affects the intestines the disease is also known as amebic dysentery. (*See* AMEBIC DYSENTERY.)

Amebic Dysentery. This disease, also termed amebiasis, is caused by the infiltration of microorganisms called Entamoeba histolytica. They are taken into the human system in foods or liquids that have been contaminated by the ameba.

Amebic dysentery is characterized by diarrhea and abdominal pain. It is to be distinguished from bacillary dysentery, or shigellosis, which is described in the article DYSENTERY.

Carriers of amebic dysentery are believed to be in almost every part of the world. These people have the disease within their system, but have no symptoms. Such a person may pass along the amebic infection through his excrement, just like a patient with an active disease.

The risk of epidemics of dysentery is greatest in countries with poor sanitation. Visitors to these nations take a risk when they eat and drink the same food and water as the natives do.

The tiny amebic organisms concentrate in the lower intestines as they multiply within the body. Small abscesses appear, which later turn into shallow ulcers. Tumors, called amebic granulomas or amebomas, sometimes grow in the large intestine.

SYMPTOMS. The diarrhea may contain specks of bloody mucus. In severe cases there may be large quantities of blood and mucus in the feces. The feces are brown, semi-fluid, and malodorous. The sufferer has a fever and a lack of appetite.

The symptoms may disappear within a few days, then reappear, unless the microorganisms are destroyed. During the periods of remission (disappearance of symptoms) and flare-ups, the patient may lose weight and feel weak. The symptoms tend to recur in some patients when they are tired, become emotionally tense, or drink too much alcohol.

Amebas may migrate from the intestines to the stomach, where they may perforate the walls of the organ, or to the liver, where they can cause hepatitis (hepatic amebiasis) and abscesses. Treatment with antibiotics, sulfonamides, chloroquine, and amebicides (agents to kill ameba) is varied, depending upon the parts of the body affected and the severity of the disease.

When people who carry this disease are identified, they also are treated. Particular attention is paid to preventing the spread of cases in institutions where amebic dysentery has occurred. Even a very slight contamination of food with the encysted forms of the ameba, carried by fingertips or flies, may spread the disease.

Persons who have had amebic dysentery and have apparently been cured should be reexamined within a year to be sure all the amebas have been destroyed. Carriers may be persons who once had the disease actively or persons who have the disease in their system, but show no outward signs.

Diagnosis is made by microscopic examination of the feces or by examination of the lower intestines with a sigmoidoscope. Using this illuminated, flexible device the physician may look inside the sigmoid colon—the lower end of the intestinal tract.

Amebic dysentery may be fatal, especially to debilitated (weakened by disease) persons, or when treatment is delayed. With prompt treatment most patients recover, some comparatively quickly and others after a number of remissions.

Some types of ameba can cause a separate disease called amebic meningoencephalitis, which affects the brain and other parts of the central nervous system. This uncommon disease has been known to be passed through contaminated water in swimming pools.

Amenorrhea. When a girl or a woman has no menstrual flow for three months or longer, this condition is termed amenorrhea. Amenorrhea is a symptom, not a disease in itself. (*See* MENSTRUAL FAILURE.)

Amentia. This word, used more in Europe than in the United States, means mental deficiency. It usually refers to those born with a mental deficiency. (If mental deficiency appears later in life, it is called dementia.)

The word amentia is also sometimes used to mean a mental disorder characterized by mental confusion of varying degrees—sometimes so severe that the patient is in a stupor. This condition can be caused by malnutrition, poisons, or infections.

Amino Acids. These are the basic building-blocks of protein; all proteins can be broken down into amino acids. They have similar structures, and can join together to form the giant molecules of proteins.

Like the proteins they make up, amino acids contain carbon, hydrogen, oxygen, and nitrogen; some also contain other elements.

We obtain amino acids from the protein foods we eat, from animals and plants. However, proteins from foods cannot be used directly by our bodies. When these proteins are digested, they are hydrolyzed into amino acids. Then our cells put these amino acids together again in different ways to form the proteins of our bodies. Foods rich in proteins are meats, fish, milk, eggs, and cereals.

The breakdown of proteins into amino acids is accomplished by enzymes in the digestive tract. These tiny amino acids are able to pass through the walls of the intestines and are then distributed within the body as they are needed.

About twenty-one amino acids are commonly found in foods. Many of them can be made in the body, but there are eight essential amino acids that must be supplied in the foods we eat: tryptophan, phenylalanine, lysine, threonine, valine, methionine, leucine, and isoleucine. Your body needs a proper balance of these essential amino acids in order to maintain proper protein nutrition. A well-balanced diet, rich in protein foods, will provide all of them. (*See* DIETS; NUTRITION.)

Aminopterin. This compound is used to combat the effects of folic acid (a member of the vitamin B_2 complex) in certain diseases, and is widely used in the treatment of leukemia and other neoplastic diseases. It is known to chemists as 4-amino-pteroyl-glutamic acid.

Ammonia. Known by several names, ammonia is a gaseous compound, NH_3, produced by the combination of nitrogen and hydrogen gases. It is used chiefly in refrigeration and the manufacture of chemicals. It dissolves in water to form strongly alkaline ammonia water, which can be fatal when swallowed. (*See* POISONING.)

The gas is extremely irritating and can cause chemical pneumonitis if inhaled. Aromatic spirits of ammonia, a pleasantly scented alcoholic solution, is used in treating stings and removing irritants from the skin, and as a stimulant in "smelling salts."

Amnesia. When a person loses his memory for past events, either totally or partially, he is suffering from amnesia.

Amnesia may result from organic causes, such as disease, injury, or deterioration of the brain. Or it may be psychogenic in origin, when a person's memory is inhibited

because he needs a defense against unbearably painful or anxiety-producing experiences. If the anxiety is severe, the victim may lose not only his memory of past experiences but his identity. This escape supplies the patient, without awareness on his part, with a seeming solution for his difficulties.

Another more frequent form of psychogenic amnesia is "forgetting" to keep an appointment or perform a task that is unpleasant or represents a conflict of wishes or interests. Thus a person can "forget" a dental appointment if he is offered tickets to a play.

Anterograde amnesia extends forward to cover a period after the patient has apparently regained contact with his environment. This is seen in boxers who receive a severe blow on the head yet keep on fighting in what seems to be a normal manner. Later they report that they have no memory of continuing the fight after the injury.

The person with retrograde amnesia has a loss of memory that extends back to a time before the onset occurred. This too can happen after an injury to the head, with loss of consciousness. The person will be unable to remember events that happened over a period before he was hurt.

Recovery from retrograde amnesia is chronological; that is, those memories nearest the time of the injury are the last to return. This type of amnesia can be of psychogenic origin; the painful experience that has been blotted out can be recalled only through association of ideas.

If a patient's consciousness has not been disturbed nor his intellectual function impaired, his amnesia is probably psychogenic in origin. When the amnesia is selective—that is, only inconvenient events are forgotten—it is probably also the psychogenic type.

A fragmentary type of amnesia with a scattered loss of memory for unrelated experiences is of organic origin. A generalized failure of memory for both recent and remote events indicates an organic degenerative disease of the brain.

A sudden and complete recovery of memory is common in cases of psychogenic amnesia but does not occur if the cause is organic. Any recovery of memory in the organic type comes gradually and is not always complete.

Amniocentesis. The process of probing the amniotic fluid surrounding a developing infant in the womb is called amniocentesis. The procedure consists in inserting a small needle through the abdominal wall and withdrawing a small amount of amniotic fluid.

This process can provide valuable clues regarding the developing infant. By examining fetal cells from the fluid, an investigator can often determine the child's sex. In addition, he can sometimes tell whether the child may have an inherited disease. For instance, it is possible to determine whether an infant will be born with Down's syndrome (mongolism). Early diagnosis of various conditions can lead to therapeutic abortion.

Amniocentesis is especially valuable when a woman carries a high risk for certain conditions.

Amnion. The balloon-like fluid-filled sac which surrounds the developing infant during pregnancy is called the amnion, and the liquid it holds is called the amniotic fluid. For further information see BAG OF WATERS.

Amphetamine. Commonly known as "speed" in illicit drug circles, amphetamine is one of a group of antidepressant drugs used to stimulate the central nervous system and produce confidence, energy, a sense of peace, alertness, and endurance. The drugs most commonly used are amphetamine, dextroamphetamine, and methamphetamine. Taken in small doses under a doctor's care, these drugs are useful against mild, temporary depression, though they can also have unfavorable side effects such as heart palpitations, emotional instability, and headaches.

Large overdoses of "speed" and "pep pills" can be not only habit-forming but highly dangerous to the users. ("Pep pills" can produce a mental condition indistinguishable from schizophrenia.) Some authorities on drug addiction are concerned about the ease with which these and other amphetamines can be obtained through prescriptions. They have proposed that the supply be limited at the source by legislation curtailing the number of tablets manufactured each year. (*See* ADDICTION; DRUG ABUSE.)

Amputation. The removal of part or all of a limb, of a projecting part such as an ear, or of an organ is amputation. Amputations are usually done surgically, although they may also be due to injury (acquired amputations). Congenital amputations are the result of nondevelopment of a part of the body in a fetus.

Surgical amputations are done in the case of a malignant or benign tumor, or an injury that is beyond repair, or an extensive infection that will not heal by medication only, or various forms of vascular disease. The majority of all amputations on persons over the age of fifty are done for vascular reasons, the most common being diabetic gangrene and arteriosclerotic gangrene. (*See* ARTERIOSCLEROSIS; DIABETES MELLITUS.) These are usually done on the leg. Amputations of the arm are usually done because of injury. Cancerous tumors require that more tissue be amputated than just the part containing the tumor. Amputations on young people are usually done because of tumor or injury.

Leg amputations are divided into two general groups based on the site of amputation. "AK amputations" are above the knee: "BK amputations" are below the knee. In the same way, arm amputations

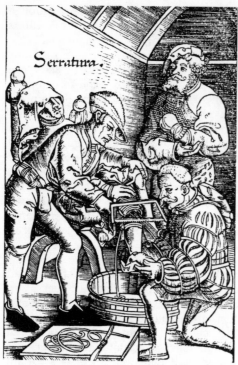

National Library of Medicine

Early physicians recognized that it was sometimes necessary to amputate a patient's limb rather than risk losing his life. This surgery of removal of the lower leg is shown in a 1517 woodcut from H. von Gersdorff's *Feldtbuch der Wundtartzney*.

even. The nerves are stretched, then cut, so they will later retract and not cause a neuroma (see below). The skin is left longer to supply flaps that will cover the incision. The muscles are tied together across the end of the bone, and the skin flaps are sutured closed. Myodesis amputations are done like conventional amputations except that holes are drilled near the end of the bone; the muscles are then sutured to the holes, which enables them to function better. Guillotine amputations are seldom performed. They are used only in cases of emergency or if the physician is not sure the stump will heal and wants to leave it open to drain. The limb is cut straight across and

After long hours spent in physical therapy building up his sound leg, an amputee must learn the "amputee gait" by practicing with his prosthesis. The parallel bars help support him during training.

VA Hospital, Hines, Illinois

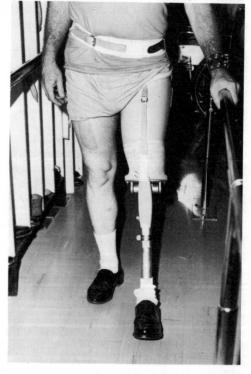

are divided into AE (above the elbow) and BE (below the elbow). In all amputations, the surgeon tries to save as much length as possible, because more length gives better function. This is especially true of the joints: BK and BE amputees generally are less disabled than AK and AE amputees. The surgeon also plans to leave as little scar tissue as possible on the stump, as well as adequate padding over bony areas.

There are three general types of amputations: standard, or conventional; osteomyoplastic, or myodesis; and provisional, or guillotine. In conventional amputations the muscles, blood vessels, and bone are cut the wound left open. The skin is then placed in traction until it stretches enough to cover the wound. This type of amputation leaves a larger scar than the other two.

After surgery, the stump is placed in a firm dressing—generally a plaster cast or an elastic bandage—to prevent swelling. There may be tubes in place to drain the wound. The patient is instructed, usually by a physical therapist, in proper positioning to prevent contractures and in exercises to strengthen the stump. (*See* CONTRACTURE.) He is then fitted with an artificial limb (prosthesis). Most devices require the stump to heal first. However, there is a newer type which is attached to the rigid plaster dressing immediately after surgery. This is called an "immediate postsurgical fitting," abbreviated to IPSF. With such a limb the amputee may begin to walk as early as twenty-four hours after his surgery.

Artificial limbs can be made to fit almost any amputee. The artificial legs usually look quite natural, and a person can learn to walk very well with them. The arms do not look so natural because they terminate with a hook to replace the hand. Artificial hands, both functional and cosmetic only, are available, but these do not give the dexterity of the hook. Often an amputee will have an interchangeable hook and hand, for daily use and for dress occasions.

Complications can follow amputations. The wound can heal poorly or may break open after it has healed. A nerve can grow until it hits something which stops its forward growth; it then becomes curled back on itself to form a neuroma, which is very painful when pressure is put on it.

It is very normal for an amputee to have a "phantom sensation"—that is, to feel that the amputated part is still present. This feeling may last only for a few weeks or for years. It usually subsides after about two years. "Phantom pain" is different from phantom sensation, and is not normal because the person feels actual pain in the amputated part. In most cases the cause is unknown, but sometimes the pain is due to a pinched nerve.

Amyloidosis. Sometimes, following a long-standing infectious or suppurative (pus-producing) disease, there may be a disorder of the body's utilization (metabolism) of protein. The result is tumor-like deposits of a protein substance, amyloid, in the body tissues of such organs as the liver, kidneys, spleen, adrenal glands, and larynx.

Sometimes amyloidosis may develop in a person who has no infectious disease, but it more commonly follows conditions like cavitary tuberculosis, osteomyelitis, ulcerative colitis, and others that produce a debilitating (weakening) response in the system.

The use of newer antibiotics and other germ-killing drugs for the underlying infection has greatly reduced the incidence of amyloidosis. But the so-called primary amyloidosis, of unknown cause, is unaffected by any known drugs.

The disorder is often associated with multiple myeloma, a serious and often fatal disease in which there is an abnormal increase in certain cells of the bone marrow. (*See* MYELOMA, MULTIPLE.)

Analgesia. The absence of sensitivity to pain—analgesia—can be produced by medications given for the relief of pain and can also occur in some physical and emotional disorders. It is not the same thing as anesthesia, which is an absence of all sensation.

Analgesic drugs act on the central nervous system to reduce the body's ability to feel pain. The most widely used are aspirin and related compounds, which provide fast, cheap, and effective relief for many everyday aches and pains, like minor headaches, colds, and hangovers. (Aspirin is also used to treat rheumatoid arthritis and gout.) In addition to relieving pain, aspirin and its relatives combat fever and reduce the inflammation and swelling which can cause pain. These drugs are not addictive, but in some people they can irritate the lining of the digestive tract. And some people have an allergic reaction to aspirin.

For severe pain, morphine and chemically related drugs provide potent relief. In addition, they give a feeling of freedom from anxiety, which reduces the psychological reaction to pain. The drugs in this group, however, generally have two disadvantages: they depress breathing, and they create drug dependence, or addiction.

Analgesia may occur as a disease state when disorders such as tabes dorsalis affect the pain pathways on the spinal cord. In the nerves, the fibers for pain, pressure, touch, and temperature are usually combined. When they reach the spinal cord, the fibers are separated. But since pain and temperature are nearly always in the same pathway, both senses can be lost at the same time. Inability to feel pain may also occur in hysteria. (*See* PAIN; TABES DORSALIS.)

Analgesic. A drug or some other agent that relieves pain without causing loss of consciousness is called an analgesic. The most widely used analgesic drugs are aspirin and its related compounds, which give fast and effective relief for minor aches and pains. More powerful analgesics—morphine and similar drugs—are used for severe pain. (*See* ANALGESIA.)

Anaphylaxis. Anaphylaxis consists of a violent adverse physiological response to an antigen to which a person is sensitized. This anaphylactic sensitization is usually created artificially (e.g., by drugs, such as penicillin), but it may also result from some unusual exposure to an antigen (e.g., a bee sting), or from the administration of serum from a different species (as by immunization with a substance containing horse serum), or from eating antigenic foods (such as fish or eggs).

The reaction is uncommon in children. However, it may be that children who become sensitized will, as adults, manifest the severe reactions of anaphylaxis.

The anaphylactic state is characterized by respiratory and circulatory collapse and must be treated immediately as an emergency. (*See* ALLERGY.)

Anastomosis. A passage formed either by surgical means or by a disease process that connects two vessels or cavities in the body is called an anastomosis. Common vessels and cavities which may be involved include arteries, veins, ureters, and intestines.

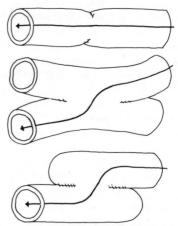

Anastomosis is a joining of tubelike parts of the body by surgery. The connecting of the two portions of the intestines in the top illustration is by an end-to-end method; in the center by a side-to-side technique; and at bottom by a procedure called isoperistaltic, a term referring to identical (iso) muscular movements (peristalsis) of the two parts of the intestines as they move food material and wastes in the direction of the arrow.

Various disease processes can erode the wall of a body cavity or vessel and cause perforation. This often happens when a disease results in a puncture of the wall of the bowel as well as the wall of a nearby organ (bladder, uterus, vagina). (*See* CANCER; DIVERTICULITIS; ULCERATIVE COLITIS.)

This produces an abnormal communication between the bowel and the other organ.

Surgically, anastomoses are made therapeutically in many disease states. After cutting out a section of bowel, the surgeon must connect the remaining bowel so that it functions normally. This connection of bowel to bowel is one frequently used type of anastomosis. Another type is done in cases when the urinary bladder has to be removed, for various reasons, so that the ureters which normally drain urine into the bladder have no place to drain. In such cases the ureters are anastomosed to the bowel or to the skin where they empty outside the body (ureterostomy).

Before a patient is put on an artificial kidney machine he must undergo a small surgical procedure by which an anastomosis is made between an artery and a vein in his arm. This channel is then used to connect the patient to the kidney machine, thus allowing his blood to be "cleaned." (*See* DIALYSIS.)

Anatomy. The scientific study of the location, structure, and relationships of the various body organs and tissues is called anatomy. The word is derived from the Greek and means "to cut up," and the study of human anatomy involves the cutting up (dissection) of the human body.

In order to diagnose and treat diseased organs the physician must know exactly where the organs are, what vessels and nerves supply them, and what organs are nearby. In medical school the young physician studies every organ (brain, lungs, heart, intestines, kidneys, etc.) and thoroughly examines every region of the body. Hence anatomy is the foundation of the physician's knowledge and the prerequisite for surgical therapy.

Androgens. Internal secretions of the testes and, to a limited extent, the adrenal glands, which help to determine male sexual characteristics are termed androgens.

(*See* MALE HORMONES; MALE SEX ACT; SPERMATOGENESIS; TESTES.)

Anemia. When there are not enough red cells (erythrocytes) in the circulating blood, the result is anemia. One of the problems is that too few red cells mean too little hemoglobin, an important pigmented substance that carries oxygen from the lungs to the tissues of the body. When there is not enough hemoglobin, there is therefore not enough oxygen, and widespread complications result.

Anemia may occur even when there is a plentiful supply of red cells in the blood—if hemoglobin within the cells is deficient.

There are a number of types of anemia, but all involve difficulty in transporting oxygen to nourish the body. The circulatory system responds by pumping blood faster than usual.

In fact, some anemic persons, while at rest, do get enough oxygen to meet the needs of cells throughout the body. Even though the number of red cells is reduced, they still move fast enough to deliver the same total volume of oxygen as the normal complement of cells did before the patient became anemic.

When these same persons are active, however, the body needs more oxygen, and the heart will pump even harder in an effort to fill the need. A person with severe anemia, especially when he also has a weak heart, risks heart failure under these conditions.

Thus, in all cases of anemia, it is wise for the patient to avoid overexertion until his red blood count or hemoglobin level improves.

TYPES OF ANEMIA. In general, there are four classes of anemia. One results from loss of blood. Another is caused by defects in the blood cells which do not permit them to mature fast enough, if at all. (This is the case in pernicious anemia.) A third class is due to aplasia of the bone marrow, where the cells are produced. This means that the bone marrow is not functioning sufficiently to develop enough normal red cells to meet the demands of the body. This is a critical condition, as red cells have a normal life span of only some 120 days and must constantly be replaced by new cells (erythropoiesis).

Hemolysis—the dissolving of cells for one reason or another—determines the fourth basic class of anemia. This occurs in sickle-cell anemia, of which the tendency is inherited.

Anemic persons are usually pale, have little energy for even normal daily tasks, and complain of fatigue. Some, depending on the extent and nature of the anemia, may have jaundice (yellowing of the skin), difficulty in breathing, an enlarged spleen, intestinal troubles, aches and pains, nausea, fever, a sore tongue, rashes, and other complications.

The reason for such a wide range of symptoms is that the human body is highly dependent on a normal blood content, not only for transporting oxygen but also for supplying many other basic needs of tissues and organs.

A portion of the hemoglobin is protein, but the rest contains iron, a mineral very important to the body. It is the iron portion of the hemoglobin that transports oxygen. So when a person has anemia, he also lacks iron. About 65 percent of the body's total iron is contained in the hemoglobin.

Iron-deficiency anemia is often produced by a loss of blood, through physical injury or internal bleeding disorders. Some women may acquire it in menstrual periods when the blood discharge is excessive, but a normal loss of blood will not cause anemia unless the woman already has a low red blood count. (*See* HYPOTHYROIDISM; MENSTRUATION IRREGULARITIES.)

For persons with uncomplicated iron-deficiency anemia, doctors prescribe oral doses of iron, as well as correcting the basic problem, such as bleeding.

Sometimes, if a person has a shortage of vitamin B_{12}, a nutrient necessary for all cell growth, the red cells may fail to develop or progress to maturity. Or he may have sufficient vitamin B_{12} for his normal needs, but a problem of body chemistry may not permit B_{12} to be utilized properly in red cell development. In either case the result is anemia.

A substance that is absolutely essential to the body's use of vitamin B_{12} is called intrinsic factor, found in gastric (stomach) juice. If the amount of this intrinsic factor is reduced—say, by surgery to remove all or part of the stomach—there will be a vitamin B_{12} insufficiency. Indeed this condition is one cause of pernicious anemia. Patients with this problem must have repeated injections of extra vitamin B_{12}, sometimes for the rest of their lives.

Also necessary for red cell development, and related to the utilization of vitamin B_{12}, is folic acid. If insufficient for any reason it too may cause anemia, which must be corrected with added folic acid.

NUTRITIONAL ANEMIA. Nutritional anemia is a disease of people whose regular diet is lacking in iron, vitamin B_{12}, folic acid, and other blood cell essentials. Many of these people live in countries where food supplies are inadequate, but it afflicts some pregnant women throughout the world, as well as alcoholics suffering from malnutrition.

A pregnant woman may develop nutritional anemia because her unborn child needs so many minerals and vitamins that she does not have enough left to provide for her own proper red cell development. This is one reason why pregnant women must have highly nutritious diets.

Folic acid and other dietary supplements are prescribed for the treatment of nutritional anemia.

APLASTIC ANEMIA. Bone marrow inadequacy (aplasia), which results in too few or immature red cells, may be caused by cancer of the bone, by poisoning from benzene and similar chemicals or drugs, or by excessive X-ray or other radiation treatments. In the case of radiation, if it has not been severe enough to damage the bone marrow permanently, patients may gradually recover their capacity to produce normal red cells.

HEMOLYTIC ANEMIA. Some patients acquire hemolytic anemia from reactions to a variety of drugs, including large doses of penicillin. The complications from this type of anemia can be severe, with pain in the abdominal area, shock, and growth of gallstones. The patients are treated by stopping the offending medication and administering steroid drugs.

Probably the most widely known type of hemolytic anemia comes from an inherited defect called the sickle-cell trait. Patients with this defect have hemoglobin SS instead of the normal type, hemoglobin AA; this results in sickle- or crescent-shaped immature blood cells which lack the elasticity they need to squeeze through small blood vessels. If these persons have hemoglobin SS, they may have recurrent attacks of sickle-cell anemia, accompanied by abdominal pain, aching in bones and joints, fever, and jaundice. The sickle-cell hereditary trait is largely confined to Negroes.

Another type of anemia, thalassemia, in which a person has hemoglobin F instead of the normal type, is found among the natives of the countries of the Mediterranean basin.

Destruction of red cells by hemolysis with resultant anemia may also occur during allergic reactions to transfused blood, and as a complication of infective diseases such as malaria and syphilis.

A severe anemia in which there is massive destruction of red cells occurs in erythroblastosis fetalis, or Rh factor disease, in which the blood of the fetus reacts against elements in the blood of the mother. (*See* RH FACTOR.)

OTHER ANEMIAS. There are many variations of all these anemias, some due to specific hemoglobin disorders, poisons such as lead, allergies, and many systemic (wide-

spread) or limited diseases of the body. (*See* BLOOD CELLS.)

Anesthesia. This term, which means loss of feeling or sensation, applies to the loss of any of our senses but especially to the loss of pain. The relatively recent development of drugs and techniques which cause a state of anesthesia has paved the way for modern surgery. (*See* ANESTHETIC.)

When surgery or any other painful procedure becomes necessary the patient is given a variety of drugs (anesthetics) which will eliminate his sensation of pain. Several options are open to the person giving the anesthetic (the anesthesiologist) regarding the way the drug is given. An anesthetic agent may be injected into the immediate area being worked upon, altering the nerves in that area so that they are unable to carry the pain impulse. This is local anesthesia, used in small operations and in sewing up minor cuts.

Or the anesthesiologist may decide to inject the anesthetic drug into the region of a large nerve which supplies the area being operated upon. For example, the nerves which supply the hand and arm pass through the tissues of the armpit (axilla). An anesthetic drug can be injected into this armpit region, thereby causing these nerves not to function. The result is that all sensation from the hand and arm is stopped. This method is regional anesthesia.

Another alternative is to inject the anesthetic into one of the spaces which surround the spinal cord. In this region the anesthetic can affect the nerves as they enter the spinal cord, so that they cannot pass the pain impulse to the spinal cord and brain. This method is spinal anesthesia. The anesthetic agents used in local, regional, and spinal anesthesia are generally similar to the procaine used by dentists. (*See* ANESTHETIC.)

Major surgery usually requires that the patient be asleep in addition to being in a

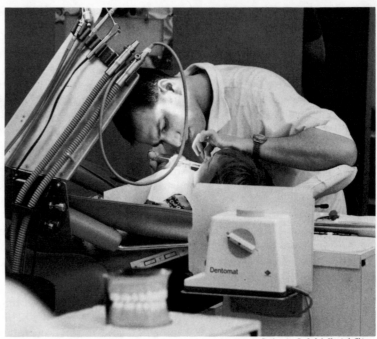

Presbyterian St. Luke's Hospital, Chicago

A local anesthetic, such as Novocaine, is given to induce temporary loss of sensation in a specific area. Local anesthesia permits pain-free medical and dental attention to diseased or infected parts of the body.

state of anesthesia. In these cases, anesthetic agents are given intravenously (into the vein) or are inhaled by the patient. Once the anesthetic is inhaled it is absorbed along with oxygen by the blood. The blood then carries the drug to the brain where it can act. The exact changes in the brain cells which result from contact with an anesthetic remain unclear. Somehow the anesthetic temporarily alters the cells in the patient's brain so that pain impulses do not register and he feels no pain. This method of eliminating pain is general anesthesia.

In addition to causing anesthesia, these general anesthetic agents induce sleep, eliminate the body's reflexes, and cause the muscles to relax. While this makes the surgeon's work easier, it puts a great deal of responsibility on the anesthesiologist. (*See* ANESTHESIOLOGIST.)

Anesthesiologist. A physician who is specially trained to administer anesthetic agents is called an anesthesiologist. (*See* ANESTHETIC.) After receiving an M.D. degree and completing an internship a doctor may decide to take three years of additional training in anesthesiology. During this time he learns how to induce safely a state of anesthesia for surgical patients. (*See* ANESTHESIA.) After this training period the physician may take a qualifying examination and, if he passes, be certified by the American Board of Anesthesiologists.

Patients under general anesthesia are unconscious, have no sensations or reflexes, and are without muscular responses. The anesthesiologist's great responsibility is to take over these functions for his patients. He is the guardian of the surgical patient as well as the chief of the surgical team.

Anesthetic. A drug used to bring about the state of painlessness termed anesthesia is called an anesthetic. (*See* ANESTHESIA.) Two main groups of anesthetics are used today—local and general.

The local anesthetics are usually chemical relatives of procaine, which dentists use to "deaden" a tooth before they repair it. Local anesthetics block conduction in the nerves in a certain area and keep them from carrying the pain impulse to the spinal cord and brain. These local anesthetics can be injected with a needle and syringe directly into the skin and underlying tissues to "deaden" the region. (*See* INJECTION; SYRINGE.) Then minor surgery or repair of a cut can be performed painlessly.

Similarly, the local anesthetic can be injected near a large nerve which supplies a given area (usually arm or leg), or into the space around the spinal cord.

General anesthetic agents, given through a vein (intravenously) or inhaled by the patient, cause the patient to lose consciousness. There are many such agents, all acting on the cells of the brain, brain stem, and spinal cord. The end result is that the patient goes to sleep and does not feel pain.

The most commonly used intravenous general anesthetic is thiopental, known commercially as Pentothal, one of the class of drugs called barbiturates. Usually the patient is given a small amount of thiopental to rapidly put him to sleep. Then a different drug is given by mask for inhalation to maintain the degree of anesthesia.

The first general anesthetic to be used was ether (1842). Since then many others have been developed. Because anesthetics can have side effects, and because some of them may be harmful to persons who have had certain diseases, it is fortunate that a whole spectrum of anesthetics is available. Every patient's case and medical history must be reviewed and the proper anesthetic selected.

Among the more commonly used general inhalation anesthetics are ethyl ether, nitrous oxide, cyclopropane, halothane, and methoxyflurane. Each of these has a different set of characteristics and advantages but all are widely used.

Anesthetist. People specially trained to administer anesthetic drugs are called anesthetists. (*See* ANESTHETIC.) Usually they are registered nurses who have completed a special training program in anesthesia, and are qualified to give anesthetics and monitor patients during surgery. Anesthetists usually handle the less complicated surgical cases, leaving the more difficult ones to the anesthesiologists. (*See* ANESTHESIOLOGIST.)

Aneurysm. An abnormal bubble-like or balloon-like bulging (dilation) of a blood vessel is an aneurysm (also spelled aneurism). It usually results from a weakening of the vessel wall due to a deteriorating disease of the blood vessels, such as arteriosclerosis or a systemic disease like syphilis. (*See* ARTERIOSCLEROSIS; SYPHILIS.)

High blood pressure (hypertension) commonly plays a part in forcing the weakened vessel wall outward. The aneurysm may become quite large, pushing against various organs of the body. Or it may break open and result in internal hemorrhage, a very serious consequence when a large blood vessel is involved.

One of the most severe aneurysms is that of the aorta, the large artery leaving the heart; it brings marked pain in the chest, back, abdomen, and elsewhere. Other common sites of aneurysms are the blood vessels of the lungs, kidneys, and legs. In the brain, an aneurysm may result in a stroke. (*See* STROKES.)

Drugs to reduce blood pressure are given to relieve the symptoms of aneurysm. Later the damaged blood vessels may be repaired by surgery or replaced by artificial vessels.

The patient who has a large aneurysm in the chest or abdominal area, particularly if it is ruptured, often spits up blood (hemoptysis), coughs, and sometimes suffers paralysis of the legs or feet (due to pressure on spinal nerves).

The passage of blood at the site of aneurysms may be further blocked by the formation of clots. (*See* EMBOLISM; THROMBOSIS.)

Anger. All of us, at times, have strong emotions of displeasure and belligerence against frustration or injustice, along with a desire to retaliate. What we feel is anger.

The expression of anger is probably an infant's first outward response to internal or external frustration. He may thrash around, try to strike something or somebody, or cry or scream. Even a three-month-old baby can show his anger unmistakably.

As a child matures, his expressions of anger become more specific and more varied. He may bully other children, or taunt them, in addition to employing the age-old physical expressions, like slapping, hitting, and kicking.

Our ways of expressing anger have to be modified and changed as we mature and adapt to our culture. We learn that in some situations we cannot express our anger outwardly, so we have to manage to discharge it through energetic activities or in some other relatively harmless fashion. The person who "bottles up" his anger, however, can become highly neurotic, even develop a psychosomatic reaction such as ulcer.

Psychiatrists advise people who get angry easily to try to hold back their impulses for a while and to do something constructive with the pent-up energy—such as cleaning house, playing tennis, or taking a long walk. Working the anger out of his system and letting it cool for a day or two will leave the angry person much better prepared to handle his problems and emotions. (*See* MENTAL HEALTH; TEMPER TANTRUMS.)

Angina Pectoris. A certain type of discomfort in the chest is called angina pectoris. The term is used to describe a symptom that might be related to other heart problems, or to identify a disorder in which the main symptom is typical angina discomfort.

Angina pectoris is not a sharp pain, but rather a sensation of pressure, squeezing, or tightness. It usually starts in the center of the chest under the breastbone (sternum) and radiates to the throat area.

Pains along the inside of the left arm, part of the wrist, a few fingers, and the shoulder are called "referred pain"—false messages sent to the brain accidentally by nerve pathways next to the nerves from the actual trouble area.

The symptoms of angina are usually due to the fact that the muscle fibers of the heart are not getting enough blood through the coronary arteries to nourish them. This condition, known as myocardial ischemia, is part of the problem of coronary heart disease. (*See* CORONARY HEART DISEASE; ISCHEMIA.)

The ischemia is usually the result of the narrowing of blood vessels by atherosclerosis. It may also be related to heart failure, other heart conditions, blood deficiency diseases such as anemia, or circulatory problems such as hypotension (low blood pressure). (*See* ATHEROSCLEROSIS; HYPOTENSION.)

Skillful diagnosis of the symptom by a physician is necessary. Most chest pains and discomfort are not angina, but are caused by emotional tension, strain of the chest muscles, neuritis, referred pain from a spinal disk disorder, ulcers, indigestion, lung problems, hernia, or other disease not directly related to the heart.

The typical angina symptom appears when a person exerts himself, and disappears when he rests. Most attacks last for only two or three minutes, but if they are set off by anger or other emotional tension and the patient cannot relax, they may last ten minutes or more.

The standard remedy for an attack is immediate rest and a tablet of nitroglycerin (also called glyceryl trinitrate) dissolved under the tongue. This drug is often taken as a preventive measure, if the person subject to angina attacks is going through a period of stress or unusual physical activity.

Amyl nitrite is also sometimes used. It is supplied in ampoules that must be crushed, and the contents then inhaled. When neither of these is available, one or two ounces of whisky or brandy may help.

Persons with angina pectoris should learn what conditions precede attacks and should avoid them. Reduction of animal fats in the diet (believed related to atherosclerosis), weight reduction to normal levels, taking sedatives when emotionally disturbed, and eliminating or reducing smoking are advisable. Tobacco may provoke an angina attack because it tends to speed up the heartbeat (tachycardia), constrict blood vessels, and raise the blood pressure.

Persons with angina pectoris have a shorter average life expectancy than others, but many can live almost normally if they avoid sudden strenuous activity and restrict their exertions to just below the degree that could cause an attack.

The first time a person has uncomplicated angina pectoris, he may fear that he is having a fatal attack. He needs to be assured that he has little to fear if he rests physically and mentally. (*See* HEART ATTACK; HEART CARE; HEART FAILURE.)

Angiography.   The taking of X-ray pictures of blood vessels is called angiography. Pictures of blood vessels near organs can tell doctors much about the organs themselves. Opaque material in the renal arteries, for example, can help the physician determine if the kidney is pinched, if it is functioning properly, or if it is damaged. Angiograms of the head can show evidences of stroke. And the condition of blood vessels around a tumor or cancer can help radiologists and surgeons decide on the best method of treating it.

Blood clots are also shown on angiograms. In a new form of angiography, called lymphangiography, opaque iodine compounds are seeped into the lymphatic system. Because some cancers may send their seeds through the lymph vessels, X-ray pictures of the lymphatic system can show whether an existing cancer has spread or not and, if so, where and to what extent.

With the help of opaque solutions, angiograms can show the fine network of blood vessels that feeds the brain, helping physicians to look at arteries that have been shoved aside by growths or clots suffered during injury, and at arteries that have burst or are pinched. In the skull there are also natural chambers which hold fluids. When these chambers are emptied and air is pushed in, the air becomes a contrast medium, just like the air in the lungs. With air around the brain and under it, growths and enlargements that would be otherwise invisible can be seen by X ray. (*See* RADIATION; X RAY.)

Angioma.   Benign lesions originating in either blood vessels or lymphatic channels are termed angiomas. If the tissue of origin is a blood vessel, the tumor is called a hemangioma. (*See* TUMORS.) If the tissue of origin is lymphatic, the term lymphangioma is used.

These angiomas are usually present at birth and increase in size as the child grows. Sometimes, when the child reaches maturity, the tumor stops growing and becomes dormant. Hemangiomas can occur almost anywhere but are commonly seen on the face and arms. Lymphangiomas are often found in the head and neck region. One form of lymphangioma called a cystic hygroma occurs in the neck (and sometimes armpit) and can grow to a large size, causing compression of the arteries, trachea, and esophagus.

Animal Bites.   Puncture wounds and lacerations caused by bites of pets or stray animals can cause serious infections, even occasionally death. Because of the infectious organisms present in the saliva of both infected and healthy animals, immediate medical attention is necessary. (*See* DOG BITES; RABIES; RAT-BITE FEVER.)

Any animal bite should first be thoroughly washed with strong soap. If the wound is a puncture, encourage it to bleed while rinsing it under warm tap water. Careful rinsing will remove most of the infectious organisms.

Bandage the wound with a sterile dressing, and do not permit the victim to move the injured area. Take him immediately to the hospital or to a doctor, report the bite to police or health authorities.

Animal Research. The use of animals for experimental study takes place in all allied medical fields (dentistry, pharmacology, medicine, veterinary medicine, and other biological sciences).

Animal research is also valuable for education and training in these sciences. It furthers the development of surgical skill, is used to test vaccines, toxoids, antiserums, antitoxins, and antivenins; and is used in the standardization of drugs.

In the medical sciences all forms of animal life, ranging from microscopic cells to apes, are studied. Those most frequently used are frogs, mice, rats, sheep, goats, cats, dogs, pigs, and monkeys.

Many new medicines and surgical techniques have been discovered through research on dogs. It has benefited bone, brain, and abdominal surgery. It has aided in the prevention and control of shock and in the safe transfusion of blood plasma substitutes and whole blood. Diabetes sufferers benefit daily from the role the dog has played in research on their behalf.

Animal research helps both men and animals to achieve good health and longer life. This cow is providing detailed information on her water intake, body wastes, and amount of air breathed.

U.S. Department of Agriculture

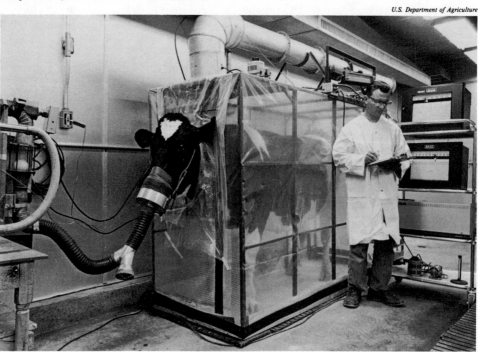

Smaller laboratory animals have played a part in the testing of food spoilage, the processing and distribution of drugs, and the nutritive quality of food and vitamins. New drugs are tested on several species of animals. If the test results are positive, the product is considered safe for human consumption. Rabbits, for example, have been used to test new birth control pills. They are also injected with new antibiotics to make sure these contain no ingredients which will produce human fever. Mice receive injections from each batch of a new drug to eliminate the possibility of a toxic (poison) factor. Such widespread practices reduce the threat of harm or death to human consumers.

Not all research animals are subjected to physical pain, trauma, or death. The use of animals for such purposes is regulated by animal experimentation laws. Antivivisection societies are actively involved in protecting all research animals. (*See* VIVISECTION.)

Animal research is accepted by common law in most countries. In the United States, bills against animal experimentation have been introduced into, and vetoed by, the Congress since 1897. In 1945, the National Society for Medical Research (N.S.M.R.) was founded. Supported by donations and panmedical schools, it began to inform the public about animal experimentation. Within several years, more research centers were established. Many cities passed legislation making stray or unclaimed animals available to approved research institutions.

Working with humane societies are those people known as antivivisectionists. This group believes that no man has the right to inflict pain or suffering upon helpless animals; it is man's duty to protect them.

In the middle of the nineteenth century, in England, the antivivisectionists formed the future National Antivivisection Society. After the Cruelty to Animals Act of 1871, many of these societies were founded in England. The American Antivivisection Society was founded in 1883. Today there are over 200 societies, including five nationals.

Ankle. The joint between the leg and the foot, the ankle, is a hinge joint. Only two motions are allowed, plantar flexion and dorsiflexion. Plantar flexion is the motion of the top of the foot away from the leg, as if to stand on tiptoe; dorsiflexion is just the opposite.

The ankle is formed by the medial malleolus (of the tibia), the lateral malleolus (of the fibula), and the talus (one of the tarsal bones). (*See* FOOT; LEG.) The talus is dome shaped. It fits into the mortise (cavity) formed by the two malleoli. The talus cannot be felt from the outside, but the malleoli form the bony knobs on either side of the ankle.

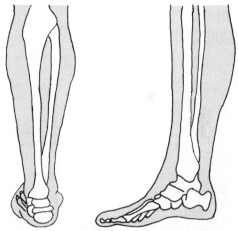

Relationship of the bones of the ankle, lower leg, and foot.

Ankle injuries are usually caused by athletic accidents, but any fall or sudden twist may cause more force than the ligaments and malleoli can withstand. The ankle joint is surrounded by a capsule. (*See* JOINT.) There are strong collateral ligaments on the medial and lateral sides of the foot. These can be sprained or torn completely by forceful adduction (pointing the toes inward) or abduction (pointing the toes outward) of the foot. (*See* SPRAINS.)

Osteoarthritis of the ankle is usually the result of an earlier injury. Occasionally, arthrodesis (fusion) is performed surgically to relieve arthritic pain by preventing motion. This involves the removal of joint surfaces and bone grafting to immobilize the ankle in a functional position. The position is usually with the foot at a right angle to the leg or in slight plantar flexion to allow for shoe height.

Anomaly. A noticeable deviation from a normal standard is referred to as an anomaly. The word is used in regard to anatomical defects, blood cells, hereditary disorders, and in other areas of medicine. (*See* ANATOMY; BIRTH DEFECTS; BLOOD; BLOOD CELLS; BLOOD DISEASES; CONGENITAL DEFECTS; GENETIC DEFECTS; HEREDITY.)

Anorexia. A person with a complete lack of appetite, who never becomes hungry even when using up energy, is said to have anorexia. Anorexiants are drugs that suppress appetite. (*See* APPETITE.)

Anosmia. The inability to smell is called anosmia. It can occur when the air passages of the nose are obstructed by polyps or tumors, or by displacement of the septum, the cartilage that divides the space inside the nose. It can also occur when the olfactory (smelling) nerve is damaged by a head injury or a tumor. Sometimes anosmia develops after a severe cold or influenza; the loss may be temporary or permanent. (*See* SMELLING.)

Anoxemia. When the amount of oxygen in the bloodstream falls below normal, the condition is called anoxemia. When this happens, the blood cannot supply enough oxygen to body tissues, such as those of the brain. (*See* ANOXIA; CYANOSIS; DIZZINESS; SYNCOPE.)

Anoxemia can occur in a number of

ways. There may not be enough oxygen in the air a person breathes, for instance, as happens at high altitudes. There may not be enough oxygen passing from the lungs into the bloodstream, as in such disorders as pneumonia, asthma, or emphysema. The oxygen-carrying capacity of the blood may also be impaired, as it is in various anemias.

Anoxia. When the level of oxygen in the body tissues is so low that it interferes markedly with the chemical processes of the body, the condition is called anoxia. It is caused by a number of things: insufficient oxygen in the blood; impaired blood circulation; or a problem in the cells—such as cyanide poisoning—which impairs the intake of oxygen from the blood. The term hypoxia is used to describe similar, but not so severe, deficiencies of oxygen in tissue cells. (*See* BLOOD CIRCULATION; OXYGEN.)

Antabuse. The medication used to help alcohol addicts is a chemical compound (disulfiram) called Antabuse. It makes an alcoholic vomit when he takes a drink. (*See* ALCOHOLISM.)

Antacid. Antacids are substances which counteract or neutralize acidity within the body. Mild alkalis used as antacids are taken orally to reduce hyperacidity of the stomach. Among them are sodium bicarbonate (baking soda) and magnesium oxide (milk of magnesia). Others contain compounds of aluminum hydroxide, magnesium hydroxide, and calcium carbonate.

When the stomach functions normally, it produces pepsin and hydrochloric acid. Sometimes, however, too much acid is produced. Antacids temporarily neutralize—but do not stop—this secretion of the acid in the stomach.

Many persons take antacid tablets, available in drugstores and at candy counters, when they become uncomfortable after eating or drinking too much. Antacids can also relieve the pain of ulcers, although there is little evidence that they influence either the

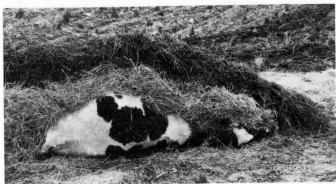

The carcass of a heifer dead of anthrax, ready to be cremated. The animal may be disposed of in this manner or by digging a trench in which the carcass is burned.

U.S. Department of Agriculture

rate of ulcer healing or the frequency of relapses.

When a patient needs to take an antacid repeatedly or over a prolonged period of time, he should consult a physician for examination and diagnosis.

Anthracosis. "Black lung" is the layman's term for anthracosis, a condition caused by inhalation of coal dust. The lungs become discolored and function improperly because of the dust deposits. Coal miners are most subject to the disease. It has no known cure, and further damage to the lungs can be averted only by preventing the entry of more dust.

Anthracosis is a form of pneumoconiosis. (*See* BLACK LUNG DISEASE; PNEUMOCONIOSIS.)

Anthrax. One of the most deadly diseases affecting livestock and man, anthrax, is caused by a bacterium which strikes suddenly and kills quickly. It is primarily an infectious disease of animals, but man may contract it directly by handling infected animals or indirectly by handling by-products of such animals. (*See* ZOONOSES.)

Epidemics of anthrax have taken a toll of human and animal losses in most countries of the world. The disease is caused by *Bacillus anthracis,* found mostly in low-lying marshy areas and where land is periodically flooded. In these soils, which are rich in animal and vegetable remains, the germs live. They can survive for long periods because they form resistant spores. They are microscopic in size while in the soil but once in the body they multiply, invade the bloodstream, and cause a fatal blood infection. (*See* SEPTICEMIA.) In man, the disease sometimes takes the form of a local infection in the lungs or intestines or on the skin. The carbuncle form affecting the skin is the most common. (*See* SKIN.) If this is allowed to go untreated, the skin lesion may result in a generalized blood infection.

The form that affects the lungs, known as woolsorter's disease, is caused by inhaling the spores while the hair and wool of the infected animal are being processed. This form of anthrax is usually fatal.

The spores may also infect man indirectly. Before the U.S. Public Health Service required that all interstate shipments and imports of hair and bristles used in brush manufacture be sterilized, the disease was more common. Shaving brushes, furs, and leather goods, plus other animal by-products, are now required to be sterilized.

Early treatment is of the utmost importance in combating the disease. Excellent results are obtained with penicillin, antianthrax serum, antibiotics, and many other drugs.

Anti-. Many words begin with this prefix from the Greek language which means against, opposite of, or opposed to. The prefix anti- is combined with a word to give the opposite meaning of the word used alone. Examples: antihistamine, anticoagulant, anticonvulsive.

Antibiotic.

Antibiotics are for the most part natural substances produced during the culture of specific fungi. These substances, when administered to persons infected with certain bacteria, inhibit the growth of the bacteria or destroy them, thus producing a cure of the infection. Penicillin, obtained from a green penicillium mold, was the first safe antibiotic (1946). This was followed by streptomycin and then by the several tetracyclines.

Most antibiotics cannot be synthesized chemically. Chloromycetin is an exception. Penicillin has been modified chemically into a number of new antibiotics effective against certain bacteria which penicillin does not touch.

Some antibiotics, like Neomycin, Bactracin, and Polymycin, are too toxic to be given internally, but are useful in skin infections.

Certain antibiotics, used without medical supervision, cause the patient to develop rashes, swellings, and other symptoms of severe allergic reactions. Excessive doses damage the kidneys; in the case of streptomycin, they have sometimes caused complete and permanent deafness. In every case, the appropriateness, choice, and dosage of antibiotic must be decided by the physician.

Antibody.

The human body develops antibodies to help fight off invasion by foreign substances (antigens). Most antibodies consist of molecules of a protein substance known as gamma globulin.

The antibodies are usually quite specific—that is, a particular type of antibody is created to oppose a specific antigen. It may attack the antigen in various ways, such as by dissolving the antigen (lysis) or by weakening the antigen (opsonization) so that it may be more easily digested by phagocytes, cells which literally eat other material.

Other methods by which the antibodies block the damaging effects of antigens is by making them insoluble (precipitation), by neutralizing them, or by clumping and isolating them in masses (agglutination).

Once an antigen provokes the development of antibodies, the latter tend to keep developing in the body for some time even after the antigen disappears. This is the basis for immunity.

A person who has a certain virus disease, for example, develops antibodies. After he becomes well, he may never get the disease again, even when exposed years later, because he still has a supply of the antibodies in his system or can make them more rapidly.

Vaccination, in which small quantities of an antigen are introduced through the skin, has the same effect of developing antibodies to protect the individual against diseases for varying lengths of time, depending largely on the nature of the specific disease. (*See* IMMUNIZATION; VACCINATION.)

For reasons not yet quite understood, the body sometimes overreacts to antigens and produces an apparent oversupply of antibodies and toxic (poisonous) by-products. The result is an allergic reaction, which can take many forms. Antigens which cause allergy are called allergens. (*See* ALLERGEN; ALLERGY.)

There are two general groups of antibodies. The first group are released into the blood and other body fluids by the lymph nodes—the lymphlike (lymphoid) tissue of the stomach and intestines, the spleen, the liver, or marrow of the bones.

The second group appear to develop in the tissues of the body, do not release into body fluids, and apparently give longer lasting immunity to disease than that given by the antibodies which flow into the bloodstream.

Anticoagulant. This is a substance that prevents the clotting of blood and blood-related fluids in or on the body.

Medications used to prevent coagulation in the body are called *intravascular anticoagulants.* They are used in heart disease and diseases of the blood vessels to prevent the formation of internal clots, called *thrombi.* Anticoagulants are used in surgery to prevent unwanted clotting during and after operations. These include heparin, coumarin, and preparations related to coumarin, such as Tromexan.

Chemicals also are added to fluid blood and plasma used in transfusions and research to prevent them from coagulating. Among these are the citrates, oxalates, and fluorides of sodium and potassium.

The intravascular anticoagulants are of two types; each works in different ways. One is fast and short lasting; the other is slower and longer lasting.

Heparin, the first type, is an anti-clotting agent that the body produces naturally. The medicinal type is extracted from animal lungs and liver. Given by injection, it prevents coagulation by interfering with the normal chemical processes that produce clots. Heparin was first produced for medicinal use in 1918.

The clot-preventive effect of heparin is fast, but its action lasts only a short time. In emergencies it is the best anticoagulant to use, but it must be injected more than once in twenty-four hours.

Coumarin anticoagulants, such as Dicumarol, are much slower, needing about twenty-four hours to have any effect at all. They prevent coagulation by interrupting the action of vitamin K, which is used by liver enzymes in synthesizing prothrombin, a necessary substance in clot formation. (*See* CLOT; COAGULATION.) Coumarin can be prepared from green forage crops, such as clover, or from synthetic sources. Chemically it is bishydroxycoumarin—which is much harder to take than the preparation itself. The Dicumarol anticoagulants can be taken orally, in tablet form. The first coumarin-based anticoagulant was produced in 1939.

Intravascular anticoagulants are used in the long-range treatment of heart disease and thromboembolic (clot-producing) diseases of the circulatory system.

In myocardial infarction they are given to prevent further clotting in the coronary arteries and hence further infarction in the heart itself. In many other conditions of the heart valves, arteries, and veins they are used to lessen the possibility of clot formation. Also, about twenty-four hours before operating time, coumarin anticoagulants are given to some patients awaiting abdominal surgery. And they may be given after surgery, too, to guard against clot formation in the bloodstream.

Medical men hold different opinions about whether coronary and myocardial patients who are working and leading normal lives should use anticoagulants for a long period. The lack of medical supervision is their major cause of concern. On the other hand, there is more agreement about using anticoagulants for short periods in the hospital.

Statistics show that anticoagulants are effective. Indeed, their use has reduced deaths from clot-related diseases by one-third.

Anticonvulsives. To prevent or control convulsive epileptic seizures or convulsions which occur in some childhood diseases, drugs are given to quiet the patient and affect his central nervous system. Phenobarbital and diphenylhydantoin sodium prevent excessively rapid brain waves in the treatment of grand mal seizures. Oxazolidine compounds and amphetamine sulfate control the slow electrical rhythms of petit mal epilepsy.

Many anticonvulsant drugs are now known. Since each has its characteristic advantages and disadvantages, the choice often depends on precise diagnosis of the disorder and constant watchfulness to guard against side effects. The list includes various barbiturates related to phenobarbital, hydantoins related to diphenylhydantoin, and many others like primidone and methsuximide.

Antidotes. Agents used to counteract the action of a poison are called antidotes. There are three basic kinds: chemical, mechanical, and physiological. Chemical antidotes react directly with the poison (usually in the stomach), producing a harmless compound. Mechanical antidotes prevent the absorption of a poison from the intestinal tract. Physiological antidotes produce changes in the body which counteract the effect of the poison.

Antidotes are available for poisoning by mercury, arsenic, snake venom, acids, alkalies, and alkaloids. A mixture of activated charcoal, magnesium oxide, tannic acid, and water, formerly referred to as the universal antidote, is no longer considered effective. (*See* POISONS.)

Antigen. Any substance which, when injected into a living animal, can provoke the formation of antibodies, and can react with these antibodies in some way, is called an antigen. Most antigens are either proteins or protein-sugar complexes. (*See* PROTEINS.) Upon entering the body these antigens stimulate certain lymphoid tissues to produce blood proteins called antibodies. This stimulation of antibody formation is referred to as immunization. (*See* ANTIBODY; IMMUNIZATION.)

When some bacteria acting as antigens combine with their specific antibodies the result is the disintegration of the bacteria. Other bacteria may combine with their antibodies and form a precipitate, or they may clump together.

Antibodies are formed by the body to protect it against foreign invaders. These invaders (bacteria, transplanted organ, etc.), the antigens, bring about their own destruction by inducing antibody formation.

Antihistamines. Products which help prevent histamine from causing ill effects are called antihistamines. They are often used in remedies for allergic conditions, since histamine is a common by-product of the antigen-antibody reaction. (*See* ALLERGY; ANTIBODY.)

Antihistamines must be taken with caution. They may cause various side effects, particularly drowsiness or dizziness. If you have taken an antihistamine, consult your doctor before driving a car, operating machinery, or engaging in tasks which can cause injury if you are not completely alert. Reactions vary with the specific drug and with the individual.

While antihistamines block the effects of histamine, other drugs such as epinephrine and ephedrine produce similar results in a different fashion. They are not strictly antihistamines, but nullify some of the effects of histamine by opposite action.

While histamine will dilate (expand) blood vessels and constrict the bronchioles of the lungs, epinephrine and ephedrine tighten the blood vessels and enlarge the bronchioles. (*See* HISTAMINE.)

Antipyretic. An agent which relieves or reduces fever is called an antipyretic. A common antipyretic is aspirin. (*See* ASPIRIN.)

Antisocial Behavior. People who lack the capacity to form attachments or loyalties to other persons, groups, or codes of living are said to be chronically antisocial. They have no sensitivity to others, have no sense of responsibility, and, like children, insist on immediate gratification of their wishes. They lack social judgment and even though their actions may be offensive, they convince themselves that what they have done is reasonable and right. No matter how much they are punished and humiliated, their personalities are not likely to change.

The antisocial person, though intellectually normal or above normal, is emotionally deficient. Typically, this person lacks feelings of affection for others, is selfish, ungrateful, narcissistic, and egocentric. He demands much and gives little. He shows few feelings of guilt, anxiety, or remorse for his hostile acts. He is often plausible and talkative but completely unreliable. Frequently the only environment he can adjust to is one he can dominate. If things go wrong, he blames others.

His behavior ranges from what is thought of as slightly odd all the way to criminality. Between those extremes are the people often referred to as cranks, eccentrics, habitual delinquents, pathological liars, swindlers, and misfits.

Antisocial individuals appear to lack ambition and foresight. It is difficult for them to stick to a job and be efficient at it. They may be irritable, arrogant, and rarely feel remorse. They lack a sense of honor or of shame, and when frustrated may become dangerous. Changes in mood are sudden and often without apparent cause. Often they are rebellious toward authority and society.

Those whose antisocial behavior reaches the criminal stage are involved in theft, embezzlement, forgery, robbery, brutal sex attacks, and other acts of violence. Many are pleased by their struggle with the law and feel pride in their defiance of it. Unfortunately, they regard punishment as expressions of society's injustice, so that imprisonment has no deterrent effect on their behavior.

Although the exact causes underlying the antisocial personality are unknown, it often develops in a child who is not wanted or loved. The mother transmits her negative feelings to the child and both parents may display violent anger toward him, or physically abuse him. If only one child in a family develops an antisocial personality, he may have had particularly disturbing early emotional or social experiences in the family.

These children are emotionally immature and never seem to learn acceptable social behavior. They may be given to tantrums or outbursts of rage if their needs are not satisfied. They may steal, run away, and be defiant, deceitful, and erratic. And when they reach adolescence, the tendencies become more apparent. (*See* ANGER; MENTAL HEALTH.)

When antisocial behavior is caused by environmental influences, treatment must first consist in placing the individual in another more favorable environment—a home where he can experience affection and interest and learn to trust other human beings. For instance, an adolescent delinquent may be placed in a family with a strong authoritative father figure who is a warm person and with whom the adolescent can identify. An older antisocial person will have a more difficult time, since his basic distrust of other people is much more ingrained, and treatment may be almost impossible.

When these antisocial personalities are treated by an individual psychiatrist or in a group, they must be handled with firm authority. Specific goals and standards for acceptable behavior are set for them. If they fail to live up to the expectations of the psychiatrist or the group, loss of privileges must be part of their treatment.

If a child or adolescent exhibits antisocial behavior caused by a disturbing family situation, he should be separated from the family during treatment, and his parents should undergo therapy at the same time.

Sometimes the pattern of behavior is so fixed that it cannot be changed by any treatment. The patient shows only hostility toward the therapist, with no desire to change his behavior. Fortunately, many of these do improve significantly. Indeed the antisocial person whose behavior becomes criminal might well benefit more from psychotherapy than from imprisonment, but society and the law do not as yet make this distinction.

Antitoxin. When a specific toxin irritates or threatens to harm the body, a substance called antitoxin is produced to fight the toxin. Antitoxins may also be developed by the blood of an animal which has been injected with a specific toxin.

There is a specific antitoxin for each type of infection. If a bacterium enters the body and causes disease, its toxin can be annulled only by the antitoxin effective against that particular bacterium. For example, an antitoxin effective against the toxin of diphtheria would not be potent against the toxins of botulism, scarlet fever, tetanus, staphylococcal infections, or snakebite. (*See* IMMUNIZATION.)

Antitoxins against many infections are no longer used, having been replaced by penicillin and the sulfonamide drugs. These drugs are powerful chemicals, but not antitoxins.

Anuria. This word means a total absence of urine secretion. Anuria may be either a symptom of another disturbance or a difficulty in itself. Renal anuria is the failure of urinary secretion by the kidney, even though the glomeruli and most other renal aspects are adequate.

Anuria may be brought on by an obstruction of the ureters, a blockage in the kidney itself, or by a deterioration of the kidney. It is one of the symptoms that appear during acute glomerulonephritis. (*See* KIDNEY; KIDNEY FAILURE; URINE.)

Anus. The opening at the lower end of the intestines through which one defecates (releases waste matter) is called the anus. The passage extending upward from it

about one inch (2.5 cm.) is the anal canal.

Rings of muscle, called the external and internal anal sphincters, contract and remain closed except during defecation. Normally, the sphincters may be relaxed consciously when the person chooses his own time for a bowel movement.

If the muscles cannot be so controlled, the problem is known as fecal incontinence. This may be the result of muscular tearing due to complications of childbirth, injury (trauma), or bouts of diarrhea. In the last case the difficulty will clear up when the intestinal disturbance is corrected, but muscular injury can usually be repaired only with surgery.

Neurological (nervous system) problems also may cause incontinence, particularly in elderly persons. These cases can be corrected only by treating the basic disease.

A baby is necessarily incontinent until its brain, spinal cord, and autonomic nervous system are mature enough to control the complicated processes of defecation. It is doubtful whether any kind of "training" can greatly hasten the child's maturation.

Hemorrhoids, also called piles, are the most common disorder of the anus. These are enlarged veins which may bleed, resulting in irritation. (*See* HEMORRHOIDS.)

Infections of the anal canal are common. They include abscesses (pockets of fluid or pus), cryptitis (inflammation of pouches or crypts in the membranes of the passage wall), and papillitis (inflammation of papillae, elevated and elongated normal extensions of the anal wall). These infections often respond to simple measures such as correction of constipation or other sources of irritation, application of ointments, or medication in the form of suppositories. A standard treatment is for the patient to take a sitz bath, which simply means that he sits in warm or lukewarm water covering his hips.

Massage of the anal canal helps in certain conditions. This is done with the finger of a rubber-gloved hand and petroleum jelly or some other lubricant. It is performed by the physician or the patient, following specific instructions.

Fissures—cracks in the anal lining—may be the result of straining during bowel movements. They may bleed and become infected. Fistulas of the anal canal (fistula-in-ano) are abnormal openings that extend outward from the anal canal through the skin or sometimes through the vagina of the female. (*See also* VAGINA.) Fistulas usually are preceded by abscesses that weaken the tissue.

Condylomas are enlarged papillae, believed to be caused by a virus.

Narrowing of the anal passage (variously termed stenosis, contracture, or stricture) may be due to a birth defect or an injury.

Most of the above problems also respond to treatment by suppositories, massage, relief of constipation, improved sanitation, and sitz baths. If you have any of these disorders, be very careful to avoid straining during bowel movements.

Sometimes the anal problems must be corrected by surgery. This is usually comparatively simple, with excellent results.

Carcinoma (cancer) is not common in the anus, although it often occurs higher in the intestinal tract. (*See* CANCER.)

The rectum, the part of the colon just above the anal canal, is often subject to problems similar to those of the anus, and also may be involved in general problems of the colon. (*See* COLITIS; INTESTINES.)

The excrement is also termed stercus or feces, and the bulk of feces discharged at any one time is the stool. If you find any traces of blood, large quantities of mucus, or other unfamiliar matter in your feces, a medical examination should be made. The physician uses a sigmoidoscope, an illuminated instrument for looking into the anal canal and other parts of the lower intestines.

Finally, you should remember that problems of the anus and evacuation of feces often are related to larger problems of the intestines and body generally. (*See* BOWELS; CONSTIPATION; DIARRHEA; ENTERITIS; INDIGESTION.)

Anxiety. A persistent feeling of dread, apprehension, and impending disaster, known as anxiety, is the most prevalent of all neurotic reactions. It is the result of unconsciously repressed feelings which are striving to come to the surface of the conscious mind.

When a normal person becomes fearful and anxious, he knows what is causing the problem and faces it realistically. But the neurotic person is not aware of the buried source of his anxiety. In psychiatry the word is applied only to neurotic feelings of painful tension and apprehension.

Since a neurotic person does not really know the reason for his anxiety, he tries to find some plausible source for it. He may complain about many things that could be the source of his unpleasant feeling. He is liable to criticize, be bored, and be irritated by people and situations.

When anxiety is not attached to any specific idea, it is called free-floating anxiety, in which a person's fear jumps from one thing to another.

Anxiety can become more and more deeply disturbing. When this happens, the anxious person may show such symptoms as depression, sleeplessness, and restlessness, and may even be unable to make simple decisions. Psychosomatic difficulties may appear—outbursts of weeping, a sense of inadequacy and inferiority, feelings of being persecuted. He may be chronically tired and have trouble concentrating. He may say he is afraid of losing his mind.

People with chronic anxiety that they are able to keep under control are usually tense and timid, overly sensitive to the opinions of others, and afraid of making mistakes. And of course they worry a great deal.

Often an anxiety-ridden patient will complain of feeling that he has a band around his head, or a quivering stomach, or that his mind is in a constant daze. He is afraid to be alone but does not particularly want sociable conversation. He continually seeks a physical explanation for the symptoms caused by his mental state.

Occasionally a neurotic patient may be subject to very acute anxiety attacks lasting from a few moments to an hour. During these episodes, he will experience a feeling of panic—with rapid heartbeat, palpitations, stomach distress, nausea, diarrhea, a desire to urinate, difficulty in breathing, and a sense of choking or suffocation. His face becomes flushed, and he will be dizzy and may even faint. Death, to him, is not far off, and he needs assurance that he is not having a heart attack.

Anxiety may often be controlled by the patient's own defenses, but it can still give rise to serious personality disorders. Indeed, it is one of the most important factors in abnormal personalities, psychoneuroses, psychoses, and psychosomatic disease.

Psychotherapy is usually advised, so that the patient may discover, and deal with, the cause of his anxiety. (*See* MENTAL HEALTH.)

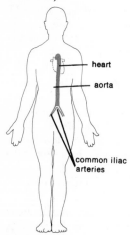

heart

aorta

common iliac arteries

Aorta. Largest of the arteries and the largest of all the blood vessels in the human body is the aorta. In the truest sense the aorta is the main pipeline of life, the main route for carrying nourishment from the heart to the body. (*See* BLOOD CIRCULATION.)

This great vessel carries oxygenated blood from the left ventricle of the heart, passing upward from the heart and then down through the aortic arch. It runs down vertically through the thorax, through the abdomen, and at the fourth lumbar vertebra is forked, dividing into two somewhat smaller vessels. These are the common iliac arteries. They carry the needed large supplies of blood to the legs.

Diseases or other abnormalities affecting the aorta may cause further malfunctioning of the circulatory system. The telltale sound of this occurrence is a click sound, heard by the physician as he listens to the heart action.

A possible aortic symptom more noticeable to the patient is cramps in the legs and gradually decreasing ability to walk distances or to use the legs normally in other ways. The cause of this condition is an obstruction in the aorta. The treatment is removal of the constricted segment and replacement with a human transplant or artificial tubing.

The aortic valve too may be seriously affected by disease. For example, the aorta alone may be the site of infection in the third stage of syphilis, ten or twenty years after the primary stage of the disease. Or this tertiary-stage infection may spread to the valve. Like all cardiovascular syphilis, this infection of the aorta is quite serious and often fatal.

In most cases of syphilis that affect the heart, the main seat of the infection is in the aorta where it passes through the thorax. (*See* SYPHILIS.)

Apathy. When a person seems emotionally dull, detached, and indifferent to what is happening around him, he is said to be suffering from apathy. He shows no sensitivity or reaction to experiences which normally would give him either pleasure or pain. He has no drive or interest in activities that may have previously appealed to him. His face is empty of expression.

Since he does not respond emotionally, the patient seems to be out of touch with reality. His apathy may be a defense against something too painful to face. (*See* MENTAL HEALTH.)

Aphagia. The refusal to take food is known as aphagia. This term should not be confused with anorexia, which means absence of appetite. (*See* ANOREXIA.)

Aphasia. A loss or impairment of the brain's ability to handle the symbols of language is called aphasia. The term comes from the Greek and means lack of speech.

Aphasia is caused by brain damage. This could happen at birth or result from an illness such as a stroke, or from a severe head injury (as in an automobile accident). The aphasic may have difficulty understanding words he sees or hears, or may have trouble speaking or writing. The speech problem can range from a loss of the grammatical parts of speech, leaving a telegraphic style—"You . . . radio . . . on" —to a meaningless jargon or an almost total loss of speech. Many aphasics can regain their speech with professional speech therapy. (*See* SPEECH DIFFICULTIES.)

Aphonia. When a person loses his voice, the condition is called aphonia. There are many causes. Aphonia may be due to a sore throat, hysteria, paralysis, muscle spasm, or disease of the nerves of the larynx. (*See* LARYNGITIS; LARYNX; SPEECH; SPEECH DIFFICULTIES; THROAT.)

Aphrodisiac. Many   drugs,   foods, sights, and smells have been used to arouse sexual desire. The word *aphrodisia* means sexual desire or sexual intercourse, and an aphrodisiac is therefore anything which arouses or increases that desire. Both words derive from Aphrodite, the ancient Greek goddess of love and beauty.

Because desire is mostly mental, drugs which release inhibitions are sometimes called aphrodisiacs. Certain substances have an irritating effect when excreted from the body and thus stimulate the congestion of the sex organs. (*See* CANTHARIDES.) Certain drugs, such as marijuana, are said to be real aphrodisiacs, leading to sexual desire by depressing the body's center of inhibition. In the case of marijuana, however, this claim is still a matter of controversy.

Cantharides and yohimbine are also considered aphrodisiacs. Yohimbine, a substance from the bark of the yohimbé tree of central Africa, has been used for centuries by Africans to increase their sexual powers. Clinical study has shown that when this drug is taken in safe amounts, the ensuing sexual desire is probably due to suggestion. When the drug is taken in large amounts, which are toxic (poisonous), there is sexual stimulation.

Also listed in the internal aphrodisiac group are various foods, alcoholic drinks, love potions, and medical preparations. Much importance has been placed upon this group, as the preparation of erotic foods has been noted throughout history. But there is little evidence to prove that foods increase sexual desire. None of the fish, oysters, vegetables, or spices named as aphrodisiacs contain any chemical agents to affect the urinary or genital tracts.

If foods cannot act chemically on the body to produce sexual desire, why are they called aphrodisiacs? Centuries ago, before scientific study came into being, certain foods and spices won reputations as being sexually stimulating. In those times, any plant that looked like a part of the human genital area was called an aphrodisiac. People thought that the plant had sexual characteristics and therefore sexual powers. An example of this visual identification of plants is the name of vanilla given to the podlike plant we use for vanilla extract. The word originally meant vagina.

One explanation of the aphrodisiac qualities of food has to do with mental suggestion. It is called a psychophysiological reaction, implying a close interrelationship between the mind and the body; and indeed the partaking of food has often been a prelude to sex.

Aplastic Anemia.   A form of anemia in which no new red blood cells, white blood cells, or platelets develop is called aplastic anemia. (*See* ANEMIA; BLOOD; BLOOD CELLS; BLOOD DISEASES.)

Apocrine Glands.   A specialized type of sweat gland located only in certain parts of the body is responsible for many of the body odors that man finds offensive. This is the apocrine gland, found mainly in the armpits, around the nipple of the breast, and in the pubic and anal areas.

These glands secrete a milky, somewhat oily fluid, containing minute particles of cells. They contrast with the common, or eccrine, sweat glands, which are distributed over most of the body and secrete a more watery fluid. Apocrine glands open into hair follicles, while eccrine sweat glands generally have pores directly to the skin surface.

The secretion from the apocrine glands does not usually have an odor, but it produces a smell when it ferments on contact with bacteria on the skin. Eating garlic and some other foods may cause the secretion itself to smell. The amount of secretion varies with the temperature and humidity, systemic problems of the body, and emotional tension.

For problems of excess sweating and body odor, *see* DEODORANTS AND ANTIPERSPIRANTS; SKIN CARE; SWEAT.

One of the problems of the eccrine glands, prickly heat (or miliaria), has a counterpart in the apocrine glands. This condition is called Fox-Fordyce disease. As in prickly heat, the sweat pores become blocked, and lesions occur on the skin. In Fox-Fordyce disease there is itching, some-

times intense, in the areas where apocrine glands are common. Papules (small rounded lumps) may appear. The disease is noted in some women after they have attained puberty, and may abate during pregnancy. Topical corticosteroid and oral contraceptives have been found effective in some cases, but many women have the disease until the menopause, when it usually disappears.

Apoplexy.   When there is bleeding (hemorrhage) from blood vessels in the brain, the result is called apoplexy. It is one form of cerebrovascular (brain and blood vessel) accident, commonly termed a stroke.

Arteriosclerosis (a disease in which the blood vessels deteriorate) and hypertension (high blood pressure) often combine to cause a vessel in the brain to rupture. The blood vessels may also have been weakened by syphilis, encephalitis, other infective diseases, or by poisons or overdoses of drugs.

The outward symptoms of apoplexy and treatment for it are similar to those of strokes due to other causes. (*See* STROKES.)

Appendectomy.   One of the most familiar operations is removal of the appendix, or appendectomy. When performed promptly after diagnosis of appendicitis, it is also one of the safest. A large incision (cut) is not needed, and the time required for hospitalization and convalescence is fairly short. If the operation is delayed, however, there is always the possibility that the appendix will burst. Infected material then spills into the abdominal cavity, causing peritonitis—a condition that still has a high death rate.

An appendectomy is sometimes done during other operations, such as removal of the gallbladder, as insurance against future trouble. (*See* APPENDICITIS; APPENDIX; PERITONITIS.)

Appendicitis.   When the appendix, a short dead-end extension from the cecum,

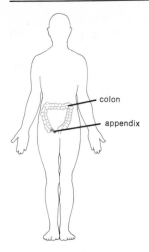

colon

appendix

becomes infected, the critical emergency of appendicitis occurs. (*See* APPENDIX.)

If the inflamed appendix is not removed promptly, there is a high risk that it will rupture into the abdominal cavity. The result—inflammation of the peritoneum, a membrane that lines the abdomen—is a problem difficult to clear up. (*See* APPENDECTOMY; PERITONITIS.)

An obstruction of the opening (lumen) of the appendix will cause appendicitis. The blocking may be by a foreign body in the intestinal tract, a tumor, or a fecalith (hard mass of waste material).

Pain usually starts near the umbilicus (navel or "belly button"), but within a matter of hours moves directly to the site of the appendix, the lower-right abdomen. The area will be quite sore to the touch or when the person coughs or walks.

With the pain comes a general sick feeling, loss of appetite (anorexia), fever, sometimes vomiting and constipation, occasionally diarrhea. The pain may radiate to the rectum.

Appendicitis may occur at any age, but is most common in males from the age of ten to the early thirties. When it occurs among infants, as happens rarely, it may be severe and can result in a ruptured appendix before diagnosis is complete.

If a person has much fat on his abdomen, it may be difficult to rapidly locate the source of pain and identify the disease.

Most patients have excellent chances for full recovery, if the appendicitis is diagnosed early and the appendix promptly removed. However, the incidence of severe complications or death is high if surgery is delayed.

Appendix.   The vermiform appendix, to use the full technical name for this body part, is aptly termed. Vermiform means worm-like and appendix means something hung on. The appendix is a curved addition to the cecum, part of the upper intestine. It is about three inches (7.5 cm.) long.

Presumably the appendix has a function, but it has not as yet been discovered. One theory is that it is a remnant of some organ of the body eliminated in the process of evolution.

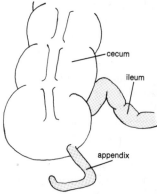

cecum

ileum

appendix

The appendix is a small, dead-end extension from the cecum near the junction with the ileum. The appendix appears to be a useless part of the body and often is the site of inflammation, or appendicitis.

The appendix lacks good drainage and has a small blood supply, which makes it poorly equipped to fight off bacterial invasion. Infection is common and requires surgery. (*See* APPENDECTOMY; APPENDICITIS.)

Appetite. When a person becomes aware of an interest in food or a desire for food, he has an appetite. The difference between appetite and hunger depends on how long the individual has been without food and how much energy he has used.

A newborn baby does not have an appetite, but cries when he is hungry. He knows he is hungry when the walls of his stomach begin to contract. He also knows that he is hungry when his brain (hypothalamus) receives a message that his sugar level has fallen to a low level.

When an infant's taste buds develop, so does his appetite. Food with taste appeal causes salivary and stomach secretions to appear. But the sight or smell of something distasteful to him may stop these secretions. The result may be nausea and vomiting.

Appetite is a rhythmic activity that usually occurs at fairly regular intervals throughout the day. But this activity may vary, depending on the controlling centers in the brain. Appetite may be changed by many factors, such as the absence of food in the stomach. An empty stomach contracts and sends a hunger message to the brain.

Our brain centers are sensitive to the temperature of our blood. To keep warm, we need to eat. That is why we often feel hungry when we are cold. On a very hot day our appetites may not be as large as on cooler days.

Appetite is aroused by the blending of different appeals to the senses, including the scent, sight, and taste of food, even the sound of a sizzling steak on the broiler. The texture of a delicious hors d'oeuvre can also stimulate appetite.

Surroundings are important, too. Mealtimes should be pleasant occasions. To heighten appetite, the table setting should be as attractive as possible. With cheerful touches, the anticipation and enjoyment of a meal are increased.

Memory may have a great deal to do with appetite. A person may tend to feel that certain foods are more appetizing than others, simply because he has eaten them before. We often establish food likes and dislikes in our early years, and these patterns may remain through adult life.

We tend to regulate our appetite over a period of years. If we did not, obesity would be even more common than it is. Some, but not all, of the daily normal variation in body weight is due to variation in the water content in the body. Regulation of body weight by appetite does not operate on an hourly or even a daily basis, but on a time scale of several days or even weeks. We may desire more food for several days and then less food for several days, but on the average we maintain our body weight. If an increased appetite persists for a long time, we may gain weight, while if we lose our appetite over a long period we may lose weight.

ANOREXIA. The most frequent reasons for loss of appetite are continued offerings of personally distasteful foods, poor cooking, or some type of emotional or behavior problem.

We may lose our appetite because of chewing difficulties, which may arise from toothache, ill-fitting dentures, or sore gums. Or nasal stuffiness or a sore throat may make it hard to swallow food.

With a serious infection or fever, the patient usually loses his appetite. He may only want to drink fluids, which are of low caloric value and will not meet his nutritional needs. This can have serious consequences in an already malnourished patient, especially a child.

POLYPHAGIA. Excessive or voracious appetite and eating is called polyphagia. It occurs in diabetes when much sugar is lost in the urine, and in hyperthyroidism when the energy output is increased. It may also be seen in certain involvements of the hypothalamus.

PICA. Pica is an appetite disorder which causes a person—usually a child—to eat crayons, chalk, paint flakes, plaster, and other materials. It may be caused by a nervous or mental disturbance and should be investigated by a physician, since persistent pica may cause lead poisoning.

Apraxia.   When a person lacks the ability to carry out a movement or make proper use of an object without a physical reason, such as paralysis, the condition is referred to as apraxia. The cause may be slight brain damage. A common form of apraxia may be an inability to perform a coordinated, purposeful act, such as moving a spoon toward one's mouth. (*See* ATAXIA; LOCOMOTOR ATAXIA.)

Arches.   There are three curves along the bottom of the foot, called arches. Two of these run from front to back, one on the inner side and one on the outer side of the foot. These are the longitudinal arches. The third arch—the anterior, transverse, or metatarsal arch—is perpendicular to the first two, and runs from side to side along the metatarsal heads (the "ball" of the foot). This arch becomes flat when weight is put on the foot, while the longitudinal arches do not. The height of the arches varies greatly from person to person.

The arches serve two functions: they make the feet better able to balance the body weight, and they provide spring, or flexibility, when walking. The arches are supported by ligaments, which hold the bones together, and by muscles. Damage to either the ligaments or the muscles can cause the arches to collapse, giving rise to "flatfeet." (*See* FLATFEET.) People who have weak feet or who must stand a lot during the day, may need arch supports —wedges of felt or sponge rubber designed to fit inside the shoe. Although these are readily available commercially, a doctor should decide which ones, if any, are necessary. In addition to arch supports, he will often prescribe exercises.

While permanent damage to the ligaments or muscles of the foot may result

from injury or paralysis, temporary damage, known as foot strain, can also occur. Foot strain is caused by poorly fitting shoes which do not let the feet expand and function properly; or by overweight; or by too much unaccustomed exercise, such as a long walk or shopping trip or a game of tennis in flexible shoes that do not support the feet. Soaking the feet in warm water or in alternating hot and cold water can relieve the discomfort. Massaging the feet and staying off them as much as possible will also help. In any event the situation causing foot strain should be found and corrected before permanent damage is done. (*See* FOOT.)

Areola.   The pigmented area surrounding the nipple of the breast is known as the areola. During pregnancy this area often becomes darker because of chemical changes in the woman's body.

Argyrol.   For treating a mucous membrane infection, physicians often prescribe a silver oxide compound containing proteins. It is called argyrol and is a nonirritating antiseptic.

Arm.   The upper limb, or upper extremity, of the body is commonly called the arm. Although the common term arm includes everything from the shoulder to the wrist, doctors use "arm" to include only the upper part of the extremity, between the shoulder and the elbow. The part from the elbow to the wrist is called the forearm.

The motions of the upper arm take place at the shoulder joint. They are flexion, extension, abduction, adduction, internal rotation, and external rotation. (*See* SHOULDER.) The elbow joint allows flexion and extension. Pronation and supination of the forearm take place near the elbow. (*See* ELBOW.)

The primary muscles which attach along the upper arm are the biceps and the triceps. The biceps muscle flexes the elbow.

(*See* BICEPS.) The triceps muscle extends the elbow. The muscles in the forearm perform four movements: There are muscles which flex (bend) the fingers and wrist. These are found on the flexor, or inner, surface of the forearm, the same side as the palm of the hand. Qn the opposite side are the extensor muscles of the hand and wrist. Pronators of the forearm turn the palm down and are on the flexor surface. The supinator muscle turns the palm up and is on the extensor surface. The biceps also helps supinate the forearm as it flexes it. (*See* MUSCLES.)

The humerus, the bone of the upper arm, is the longest and largest bone of the upper extremity. There are two bones in the forearm, the ulna and the radius. The ulna is on the side of the little finger, and the radius is on the side of the thumb.

The main nerves of the arm are the musculocutaneous nerve, which goes to the biceps and the skin over it; and the radial nerve, which goes to the triceps and the skin over it. The radial nerve continues into the forearm, to innervate the extensor surface. The flexor muscles and the skin over them are supplied by two nerves, the median and the ulnar. (*See* NERVES.)

The primary arterial supply to the arm takes the shape of the letter Y, with many small branches leading off. The single stem of the Y is the brachial artery in the upper arm. This forks at the elbow to form the radial and ulnar arteries of the forearm. The radial artery, near the thumb, is the most frequently used spot for counting a person's pulse rate.

The arm can be the site of various diseases and injuries. Arthritis can affect any joint of the body, including the shoulder, elbow, and wrist. Bursitis can occur around the shoulder and elbow—there are no bursae in the wrist. (*See* ARTHRITIS; BURSITIS; ELBOW; SHOULDER; WRIST.)

Paralysis affecting the arm can be flaccid or spastic. Flaccid paralysis is the result of injury to the brachial plexus or the ulnar, median, or radial nerves or can be caused

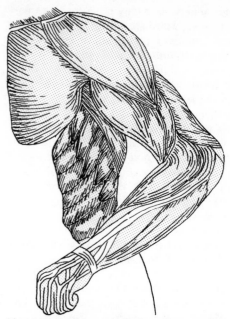

Muscles of the arm. Note how they overlap with those of the shoulder and chest. The brain and nervous system coordinate these muscles for maximum strength and efficiency.

by certain diseases such as poliomyelitis. Spastic paralysis accompanies hemiplegia. (*See* BRACHIAL PLEXUS; HEMIPLEGIA.)

The shoulder-arm-hand pain syndrome occurs after a heart attack. Briefly, it consists of pain and stiffness in the shoulder and hand; the elbow is seldom involved. (*See* SHOULDER-ARM-HAND PAIN.)

A variety of fractures can occur in the arm. (*See* FRACTURES.)

Armpit. The axilla, or underarm area, is popularly known as the armpit. Careful attention should be paid to cleanliness of this area, as it is one of the primary sources of body odor because of the presence of apocrine sweat glands. (*See* BODY ODOR; DEODORANTS AND ANTIPERSPIRANTS.)

Arrhythmia. Any variation from the normal rate of heartbeat is called an arrhythmia. A great many irregularities are of no consequence and happen to most healthy persons. Many others are the result of tension, fear, and other emotions. But some are clues to various heart diseases.

An arrhythmia occurs when the pacemaking or timekeeping nervous system of the heart lacks its normal precision. Usually the impulse centers (nodes) located in the heart tissue send out weak electrical impulses in a very exact manner to stimulate the muscles which regularly contract or relax the various chambers of the heart and so indirectly control the opening and closing of valves.

An irregular heartbeat may be noticed by the person himself, who may feel an unusual sensation in his heart. Or it may be detected by a stethoscope, which amplifies the heart sound and sends it through a tube to the physician's ear.

The most precise determination of arrhythmias, however, is made by electrically detecting and recording heartbeats on a long paper tape, or electrocardiogram. (*See* ELECTROCARDIOGRAPHY.)

Among the various types of arrhythmias are flutter, fibrillation (rapid twitching), premature beats, tachycardia (fast beats), and bradycardia (slow beats).

Among the most common chronic (recurring) arrhythmias is that called atrial fibrillation. This is a malfunctioning of the nerves which control the expansion and contraction of the atria, two of the heart chambers. The problem may be due to an infection, consumption of too much alcohol, a heart injury, surgery, or poison in the system. Thyrotoxicosis, which results from an overactive thyroid, also may cause atrial fibrillation. (*See* HYPERTHYROIDISM.)

Treatment includes correction of the underlying problem with drugs—digitalis, quinidine sulfate, or propranolol—for slowing the heartbeat, and electrical devices called defibrillators.

Devices called pacemakers may be implanted under the skin, or attached on the surface, to substitute an artificial electrical stimulation for the natural weak currents which control heartbeats and valves. These have been highly successful. With them many people are going about their daily tasks instead of being handicapped by their arrhythmias. (*See* PACEMAKER.)

The artificial pacemakers are likewise very useful when there are serious disorders in conducting the natural pacemaking electrical impulses through the tissues of the heart. These disorders are called heart blocks. The two sets of pumping chambers of the heart, the atria and the ventricles, may beat without coordination, seriously upsetting the ability of the heart to keep blood circulating properly.

In heart block, impulses from the atrial area may be delayed in, or prevented from, reaching the ventricles. This atrioventricular (or AV) block is often a complication of coronary disorders or rheumatic fever. (*See* CORONARY HEART DISEASE; RHEUMATIC FEVER.)

Arsenic. Soil, air, water, plants, and animals all normally contain trace amounts of arsenic, but the highest levels are found in seafood. The effects of trace amounts of this element in human beings are uncertain, but scientists have found that small amounts of it promote growth in poultry.

Larger amounts of arsenic, however, are highly poisonous, acting as corrosives in the human system. For the symptoms of arsenic poisoning and first aid treatment, see the chart accompanying the article POISONING. Even moderate amounts of arsenic, when taken in to the system, can be strongly toxic because of their cumulative effect.

Arsenic-containing insecticides and herbicides are now seldom used, but organic arsenicals are used for parasite control, for growth stimulation, and as antibiotic agents in farm animals. In our environment arsenic most often occurs in the pentavalent form, which is far less toxic than trivalent arsenic compounds.

Arsenic has been accused of being carcinogenic (promoting cancer), but rats receiving small amounts of arsenites have been found actually to have a significantly lower incidence of spontaneous tumors. The real culprit may be selenium, an element that often occurs with arsenic. (*See* TRACE ELEMENTS.)

Arteries. The vessels which carry blood away from the heart are called arteries. They have many branches ranging in size from the aorta, or great artery, which leaves the heart, to small units called arterioles and even tinier ones called arterial capillaries. (*See* ARTERIOLES; ARTERIOSCLEROSIS; BLOOD CIRCULATION; CAPILLARIES; VEINS.)

Arteriolar Sclerosis. When the arterioles, tiny branches of the arteries, become

hardened and narrowed by deposits of fats and calcium, they are said to have arteriolar sclerosis. This condition can occur in the arterioles of muscles or of any organ; it is especially frequent in the eye. and kidneys. (*See* EYE.) It is most common in persons with high blood pressure. Indeed it is the hypertension, over a long period of time, which causes the thickening of the arteriolar walls, with degenerative changes in the arterioles and in the organs they supply.

Arterioles. At the outer end of the arterial system, that is, the part of the system connecting with the capillaries, are the smallest of the arteries, the arterioles, also called arteriolae. On the venous side of the circulatory system, the link between the capillaries and veins is the venule, roughly

The X-ray picture at the left shows a complication of hardening of the arteries. The arrow indicates a deposit of fatlike material (arterial plug, or occlusion) near the knee. At right, an occlusion in the main artery of the thigh resulted in loss of blood flow, requiring amputation of the lower leg below the knee.

Dr. Geza de Takats, Presbyterian St. Luke's Hospital, Chicago

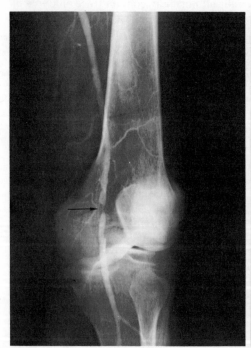
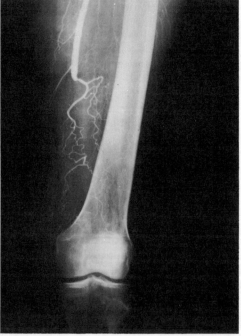

the counterpart of the arteriole on the arterial side. (*See* BLOOD CIRCULATION.)

Blood-pressure control is the main job of the arterioles. The body might live and breathe without them—but not in the same way it lives and breathes with them. The arterioles make it possible for the body to be at rest one moment, up running or working the next moment, then sitting down eating the next. They control the way the blood is supplied to the body at every instant.

To meet all the varied needs of the body, the heart and arteries must feed blood at high pressure into the circulatory system. Otherwise it would never get to the ends of the fingers and toes to keep the body warm and nourished, or into the large muscles to keep it moving. The problem, though, is that blood cannot be sent at *arterial* pressure into hands, feet, biceps, and so on. Its pressure is too high. It would explode the small, delicate capillaries and veins. At the same time, the arteries and heart would be damaged if there were not a way to balance the amount of blood leaving them at the outer end against the amount they were pumping in at the beginning of the system.

The arterioles protect the arterial system (at one end) against pressure damage. And they are the main control of blood-flow rate through all the tissues of the body. The arterioles can do this because they have walls of involuntary muscle that are quite strong. These walls expand and contract, as needed.

About half of all the pressure control in the entire circulatory system is the resistance of the arterioles. The pressure throughout the arterial system can be kept at the necessary normal minimal 100 millimeters of mercury (mm.Hg) because the arterioles are regulating the system so that the same amount of blood is pumped into and out of the system simultaneously. Blood pressure throughout all arteries is the same up to the arterioles. There it drops quickly from a systolic pressure of (typically) 120 mm.Hg to just the right pressure to get it into and through the capillaries and into the veins—about 32 mm.Hg.

At most times the involuntary muscle walls of the arterioles are somewhat tensed or semiconstricted. They are regulated by impulses from the central nervous system, squeezing them smaller to shut off blood or letting them expand to pass much larger amounts.

As nervous sensations signal the arteriole walls, they can change diameter as much as three to five times larger or smaller. This means, however, that much more than three to five times more or less blood can pass through an arteriole tensed or expanded in this way. In fact, the arterioles can change their resistance to blood flow by hundreds of times or even a thousand times.

Two kinds of nervous impulses control arteriole blood flow. First, the local needs for nourishment in each tissue area are controlled by a nervous function called autoregulation. Second, the amount or degree of contraction and expansion is controlled by a type of nervous impulse called sympathetic impulses.

During exercise, for example, the adrenal glands release hormones which put blood where it is needed most. They constrict the arterioles that feed blood to the skin and expand those feeding the large muscles of the arms, legs, and trunk. And during digestion they also constrict those to the skin and expand the arterioles feeding blood to the digestive tract.

Arteriosclerosis. Hardening (sclerosis) of the arteries is known as arteriosclerosis. However, the term is confusing, due to the fact that medical science is learning more about diseases of the circulation.

It is known, for example, that most of the disorders classed in the past simply as hardening of the arteries really were the result of deposits of fatty-like material (atheromas) on the artery walls, and thus more properly should be called atherosclerosis. (*See* ATHEROSCLEROSIS.)

Whatever the primary cause of these problems, if they block the passage of blood the effect on the heart and other parts of the body will be similar. Articles in general magazines commonly use the words *arteriosclerosis* and *atherosclerosis* as though they meant the same thing, and even the medical profession is vague about the distinction between them.

With age, the blood vessels of most people will widen (dilate) and lengthen somewhat, sometimes with deposits of calcium (calcification) in the *tunica intima*, the inner lining of the vessels (intimal sclerosis). The changes may extend deeper, through the intima, into the *tunica media* (medial sclerosis).

In hypertension (high blood pressure), a type of arteriosclerosis called arteriolar sclerosis often hardens and narrows the arterioles (smaller arteries) of the kidney and other organs. (*See* ARTERIOLAR SCLEROSIS.) Which comes first, the high blood pressure or the arteriosclerosis? It is probably the hypertension. But arteriosclerosis of the kidneys induced by hypertension may sometimes bring about an increased hypertension severe enough to lead rapidly to death. The vicious circle is called malignant hypertension. (*See* HYPERTENSION.)

Other disorders, such as diabetes and kidney malfunctions, may increase an individual's tendency toward arteriosclerotic disease. Resentment, jealousy, frustration, and other types of stress seem to help set the stage, at least in some persons, for arteriosclerotic problems. These emotional factors can quicken the heartbeat and stimulate the release into the blood of chemicals intended for "fight or flight"; instead, the chemicals cause reactions of the blood vessels that lead to disease.

Arteriosclerosis seldom affects all the arteries at the same time. It may be confined, for example, to the aorta or the iliac arteries, which are the larger of the blood vessels, or, if confined to the legs, the condition takes the form of arteriosclerosis obliterans. Critical blocking of the large blood vessels and subsequent damage to the heart usually involve atherosclerosis and is discussed in the article on that subject.

ARTERY CHANGES. In senility, the hardened, calcified, so-called pipe-stem arteries of the extremities produce little trouble. The smaller arteries with diminished lumens (passages) produce ischemic changes (decreased blood nourishment). These changes cause intermittent cramplike leg pains and at times gangrene. In the brain, they may lead to hemorrhage or thrombosis which produces strokes. In the heart, they lead to thrombosis and coronary infarction. In the kidneys, they lead to shrinkage in size and function.

The treatment for arteriosclerosis, in its milder form, is often directed at the most important symptom, hypertension. Severe arteriosclerosis invariably includes the formation of atheromas, for which treatment is identical to that for atherosclerosis.

Treatment for arteriosclerosis obliterans is aimed at maintaining circulation in the legs, and is similar to that for Buerger's disease. In both diseases there is danger that mild tissue death will progress to gangrene, requiring subsequent amputation of the limb. (*See* BUERGER'S DISEASE.)

For related information on arteries and their diseases, *see* ARTERITIS; BLOOD CIRCULATION; RAYNAUD'S DISEASE.

Arteritis. Any inflammation of an artery is called arteritis. This may be a symptom of a number of different problems, particularly infective diseases such as tuberculosis or syphilis.

There are many different types of arteritis. Polyarteritis is one, meaning inflammation of many arteries. *Polyarteritis nodosa,* also called periarteritis nodosa, is characterized by the formation of nodes, or tumor-like tissue, about the arteries. *Temporal arteritis* is a type that usually occurs in persons over fifty-five. *Idiopathic arteritis,* also called Takayusu's disease or pulseless disease, is found among young women in the Orient.

Polyarteritis nodosa, like many other types of arteritis, occurs for no clear reason. No infection has been found as a cause. The nodes, with other deteriorations of the arteries, develop into granulomas (grainy tumors).

This trouble may occur in various parts of the body, such as the arteries of muscles, the stomach and intestines, the kidney and heart. One or more body organs may be involved.

The patient may feel weak, run a fever, have aches and pains, lose weight, and have other complications due to the malfunctioning of the affected organs. Often his blood pressure will rise. Corticosteroid drugs are helpful in treatment.

The person with temporal arteritis may have a fever, fatigue, loss of weight, headaches, and loss of vision in one or both eyes (due to deterioration of the retinal artery). The eye problem is the most serious consequence. Both the cause of temporal arteritis and the reasons for its eventual disappearance are unknown. Patients are given corticosteroid drugs and are advised not to smoke, since tobacco is known to affect the blood vessels adversely. (*See* BUERGER'S DISEASE.)

In the so-called pulseless disease of the Orient, the patient has impairment and blocking of the larger arteries, along with dizziness; sometimes blindness, paralysis, and other severe complications can develop.

Cranial arteritis refers to problems of the arteries within the head. The symptoms may be mental confusion, delirium, or only mild ones such as headache, poor appetite (anorexia), and aching muscles. It may be a part of the problem of temporal arteritis. (*See* ANEURYSM; ARTERIOSCLEROSIS; ATHEROSCLEROSIS; BLOOD CIRCULATION; EMBOLISM.)

Arthritis. The name arthritis is applied to a variety of conditions, for it means inflammation of a joint, and many factors can cause such inflammation.

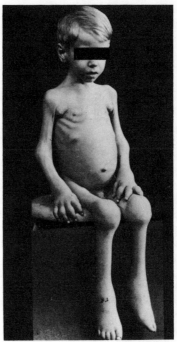

Dr. Edward F. Rosenberg

A ten-year-old boy with congenital (present at birth) crippling arthritis.

When we speak of arthritis, however, we usually mean one of two very common diseases: *rheumatoid arthritis,* which involves not only the joints but frequently other connective tissue, and *osteoarthritis,* a less serious problem, which four out of five persons will have in some form during their lifetimes.

RHEUMATOID ARTHRITIS. Often the rheumatoid type of arthritis begins with inflammation of the synovial membrane, a thin part of the joint that encloses the synovial fluid, a lubricating substance. The fluid then begins to thicken and accumulate, contributing to the swelling. From the temporary inflammation of the synovial membrane comes the growth of permanent granular tissue called pannus.

As the disease advances, the cartilage (soft, flexible extensions of bone at the joints) deteriorates, and may even disappear entirely. Then the cartilage is replaced with a growth of fibrous tissue that can eventually become hard and bonelike, fusing the joint together so it cannot bend.

Most cases of rheumatoid arthritis, however, do not advance this far. The typical arthritic patient will have some swelling at the joints and limitation of movement, but not to the extent of crippling.

Along with the typical symptoms of joint pain and stiffness, rheumatoid arthritis may also produce one or more of a variety of symptoms: fatigue, weight loss, anemia, fever, sweating, weakness in the muscles, cold hands and feet, enlarged lymph glands and spleen.

Most people with arthritis suffer most in the morning just after they get out of bed. The muscles feel stiff and may hurt. Joints may be painful. The patient may be unable to move about freely until he has "loosened up."

Another common symptom is tingling of the hands and feet, the two parts of the body most often involved in arthritis. Sometimes the tissue of body organs, such as the heart and kidney, may be affected.

Small lumps (rheumatoid nodules) appear in the joints in about one of five persons with rheumatoid arthritis. The joint may stiffen as a result of abnormal joining (fusing) of the bones (bony ankylosis) or of scarring or fiber growth (fibrous ankylosis).

Rheumatoid arthritis tends to abate and flare up from time to time. Often each new episode is worse than the one before. The pattern varies with the individual. No one knows why for certain. About 20 percent of patients have full remission—in other words, they fully recover from the pain and other outward signs of the disease. When the cartilage is eroded and scarred, however, these changes will remain, even though the disease may seemingly disappear.

Treatment of Rheumatoid Arthritis. The cause of rheumatoid arthritis is still unknown, although there are many theories. Treatments have been developed on a trial-and-error basis, and give relief or retard the development of the disease rather than curing it.

Some unauthorized treatments are promoted by quacks as miraculous cures. The only effect of these treatments is a depletion of the victim's pocketbook. (*See* QUACKERY.)

Aspirin and other forms of salicylate are the most common and effective drugs to relieve pain and reduce inflammation in arthritis. Cortisone and other corticosteroids have had dramatic success in reducing inflammation and pain, but their use is limited because of side effects. Narcotics, gold salts, hormones, and the so-called antimalarials are other drug agents used to lessen pain and inflammation. Among the newer drugs are phenylbutazone and indomethacin.

Bed rest, warm baths, hot packs, heat lamps, and application of hot paraffin are helpful in reducing joint pain. Exercise is very important to the arthritic, as it helps keep the joints from stiffening. (This is not to suggest that the exercise should be strenuous; far from it.) In most cases, the physician can prescribe exercises that the patient can perform by himself, but the patient with an advanced case may need help with exercising. The Arthritis Foundation, with headquarters in New York City, and its many local chapters distribute some excellent material on exercises for arthritics.

Arthritic patients should have well-balanced, nutritious meals (just as everyone should). Special diets and vitamin supplements have been tried, but in general have proved to be ineffective.

Many persons with arthritis say they feel much better in warm, dry climates, but medical science doubts that climate is a factor in causing or curing the disease. It is known, however, that arthritic patients do feel worse when the humidity is high and the barometric pressure low.

In severe rheumatoid arthritis, surgery to remove abnormal synovial tissue has been helpful in restoring function to the joints of the hands and other joints. Splints, braces, and casts may also be needed, but these must be designed, or occasionally removed, to allow for simple exercises to prevent permanent loss of movement.

Good posture habits and correctly fitted shoes also help the person with arthritis.

The Search for the Cause. Much research has been done in an effort to determine the cause of rheumatoid arthritis. One theory is that an infection starts the disease process. Years ago, physicians placed great emphasis on locating a focus of infection, such as an abscessed tooth. No proof has been found that such an infection causes arthritis, but it is still a good idea to eliminate any infection. (If it doesn't cause arthritis, it may make you sick in other ways.)

A popular modern theory is that rheumatoid arthritis is related to an autoimmune reaction. In other words, it involves the body's development of antibodies to fight certain abnormal substances or chemicals developed by the body itself. Somehow the antibodies may start a cycle of events that could lead to arthritis. Lending some support to this theory is the fact that antibodies are known to create many other abnormal problems and conditions. (*See* ALLERGY; ANTIBODY.)

A specific protein called the "rheumatoid factor" has been found in the blood serum of many rheumatoid arthritis patients, but its relation to the disease is still the subject of controversy and research. Rheumatoid arthritis is usually a disease of persons over twenty years old, and is most common among those from forty to fifty-five. It is found in women more often than in men. A juvenile form of the disease, relatively uncommon, may start with stiffness of the knees and occasionally a high fever and rash. If it is not treated promptly, the eyes and internal organs may be affected, and normal development retarded.

OSTEOARTHRITIS. The disease called osteoarthritis involves deterioration of the flexible ends (cartilage) of bones at the joints. The cartilage loses its elasticity and gradually wears away, stiffening the joints, limiting movement, and causing pain.

Projections of new growth of bone (spurs) may appear and press against tendons and ligaments. (*See* SPUR.) Sometimes the entire cartilage may erode away, leaving the hard ends of the bones to rub against each other.

Cysts may also form in the joints, and pieces of cartilage break off and remain within the joint spaces. Unlike the rheumatoid type, osteoarthritis seldom causes much swelling.

The disease seems to be related to wear and tear on the joints from movement over the years. Usually it strikes those joints that not only bear much body weight, but are also much used, such as the hips, spine, and knees. The joints of fingers and toes are other common sites, and some patients get osteoarthritis of the jaw. Osteoarthritis may become seated in nearly any joint of the body, however, particularly if the joint has had hard use. Trouble may develop, for example, in the elbows of professional baseball pitchers, or in the knees of women who do a great deal of floor scrubbing by hand.

Many cases of osteoarthritis are mild, often without pain. In severe cases the patient's posture may be affected. The abnormal joints may also prevent the patient from getting about or carrying out daily tasks without stiff, jerky movements.

While rheumatoid arthritis may involve the body's system generally and involve some internal organs, osteoarthritis is confined to the joints. Some unusual symptoms may develop, however, as a result of pressure on nerves by spurs or other joint abnormalities. The pressure can cause the phenomenon of "referred pain," or the appearance of pain along the line of the nerve at some distance from the actual site of the disease or injury.

In some persons osteoarthritis manifests itself in hard, bonelike enlargements of the finger joints closest to the nails. These are called Heberden's nodes. When the nodes occur on other joints of the fingers, they are

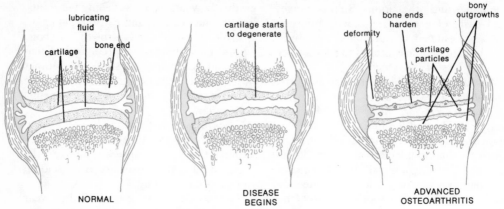

NORMAL   DISEASE BEGINS   ADVANCED OSTEOARTHRITIS

In osteoarthritis there often are marked physical and mechanical changes in body joints. At left is a normal joint. In the center drawing we see some signs of the disease. At right is the late stage, with hardening of bone ends; abnormal bony growths; breaking off of particles of cartilage; disappearance of cartilage; swelling, deformity, pain, and restriction of movement.

called Bouchard's nodes. Both types seem to run in families, but may develop as a result of injuries.

Osteoarthritis is classified as either primary or secondary. The primary type occurs for no apparent reason, usually in persons between the ages of thirty and forty, and involves the smaller joints. The secondary type appears in larger joints or in smaller ones that have been injured or subjected to hard use. It is associated with aging.

Osteoarthritis is treated with drugs identical or similar to those used for the rheumatoid variety. Application of heat and mild exercise help to keep the joints limber and free from pain. Whenever the joints become tired, the patient should rest. Obese persons with osteoarthritis should lose weight.

The crippling seen in some cases of rheumatoid arthritis is not common in osteoarthritis unless the patient has a combination of both forms of the disease. Osteoarthritis usually remains with the patient for life and worsens with advancing years. It is also called degenerative joint disease.

OTHER TYPES OF ARTHRITIS. The term *infectious* or *pyogenic arthritis* refers to an inflammation of the joints caused by the invasion of bacteria or other microorganisms. This type of arthritis comes on suddenly, and may be accompanied by chills, fever, and other systemic symptoms, as well as by joint pain. Gonococcus, staphylococcus, pneumococcus, streptococcus, and meningococcus are among the organisms responsible for this type of arthritis, which may be a complication of venereal disease. Antibiotics suitable to the specific infection are used in treatment.

Arthritis also may appear as a complication of the skin disease psoriasis, or of colitis, enteritis, and other diseases of the intestines. *Tuberculous arthritis* may appear as the tuberculosis germs spread to the joints from lymph nodes or other parts of the body.

Ankylosing spondylitis, or *rheumatoid arthritis of the spine,* is characterized by pain and stiffness in the back. (*See* ANKYLOSING; SPONDYLITIS.) *Gout,* or *gouty arthritis,* is a rheumatic condition caused by urate crystal deposits in joints, bones, and tissue. (*See* GOUT.)

Rheumatic fever, a disease of children, has many manifestations, including problems of the heart and polyarthritis (inflammation of many joints). (*See* RHEUMATIC FEVER.)

Reiter's syndrome is a combination of arthritis with inflammation of the urethra and the eye. (*See* REITER'S SYNDROME.)

Artificial Body Parts. When various parts of the body are lost or cease to function, due to injury or disease, doctors may sometimes replace them with artificial body parts. Their biggest advantage is that, because they are not living tissue, they are not likely to be rejected by the body. (*See* TRANSPLANTS.)

The earliest kinds of artificial body parts were hooks to replace lost hands and wooden pegs to take the place of legs (as

Former March of Dimes National Poster Boy, Marty Mack, was born without arms and with a hip defect which left his right leg three inches longer than his left. He has learned to type, print, and play softball and soccer.

March of Dimes

readers of *Treasure Island* will remember). Today's more sophisticated replacements are made of metal and nylon, operate on batteries, and function nearly like the original part. Other external replacement parts, used primarily for cosmetic purposes, include ears, noses, breasts, and even eyes. Such external parts are called prostheses. (*See* AMPUTATION.)

Thanks to advances in surgical techniques and developments made by biomedical engineers, many parts inside the body may be replaced by artificial ones. Nylon structures can temporarily take over the function of the aorta, and electronic pacemakers replace nature's own. (*See* HEART.) Some doctors think that in the future, transplants will mostly be artificial, since they do not pose the problem of rejection. The major difficulty at the moment is that of size. For example, a machine that does the job of the kidney is as large as a console television set—and that is the smallest one yet built. (*See* DIALYSIS.)

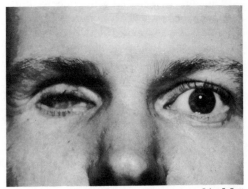

Robert B. Scott

Before and after the fitting of an artificial eye.

Artificial Eyes. Many persons who have lost an eyeball or are blind are more comfortable in public if their blindness is not obvious. To improve the appearance of these persons, eye specialists have recommended replacing the natural eye with an artificial eye.

In recent years, the techniques used in making prosthetic (artificial) eyes have been so refined that an artificial eye can be mobile and can follow the movements of the other eye. A number of standard shapes are available, so that any patient may have a comfortably fitting device, made of plastic or glass. Because of the wide variety of designs, the iris can be in its correct position relative to the eyelids. Coloring of the artificial eye can be matched to the natural eye color and even veins are included to add to the natural appearance.

Because artificial eyes may be expensive, some social and governmental agencies for the blind offer assistance to persons who need them. (*See* EYE; PROSTHESES.)

Artificial Insemination. Depositing semen obtained from a male into a female's reproductive tract for the purpose of initiating pregnancy is termed artificial insemination. Often the procedure is used with couples who have been unable to have children because of the husband's infertility.

The ability or inability to conceive children depends on a great number of factors. (*See* FEMALE SEX ACT; INFERTILITY; MALE SEX ACT; SPERM.) For conception to occur, a viable sperm must reach and fertilize a healthy egg in the female tract. But a number of problems may occur. The semen may not contain enough sperm, the sperm may be abnormal, or the sperm may be unable to reach the egg. In the latter instance, either the male or female may be at fault. The female tract may be hostile to sperm, in that the path the semen must travel may be excessively acid or alkaline. Or the sperm may not be able to travel the distance, sometimes because of slight abnormalities in the male genitalia or problems in ejaculation. (*See* EJACULATION.)

If a couple has been childless and desires offspring, the cause of the infertility must be determined by a physician. If the problem is one described above, they may decide to initiate a pregnancy through artificial insemination.

One of two methods may be utilized. If the husband's sperm are adequate and viable, they may be used for the insemination. If not, donor sperm—that is, sperm from another male—can be utilized. In either case, once the sperm have been obtained, the procedure is the same.

The sperm are collected through masturbation, placed in a ten-cubic-centimeter syringe, and then squirted either directly into the uterus or near the uterine entrance. Most physicians avoid direct transmission, since infections are more common that way. The female lies on a treatment table about twenty minutes after insemination and afterward may go about her normal activities. The procedure is done at a time when the woman is most likely to be fertile, but if pregnancy does not occur, it is repeated.

For psychological reasons, donors are generally determined by the physician rather than the couple. Selections are made on the basis of physical and mental similarities to the wife and husband, especially the husband. Most couples want a child like the one they would have had if normal pregnancy were possible.

In some instances, the husband's semen may contain too few sperm cells to succeed in fertilization. Physicians may then collect a number of ejaculates and separate out the sperm, collect them, and artificially inseminate the entire amount at once. The ability to store the sperm by freezing has developed an interesting concept. If a man decides to render himself infertile by vasectomy when the couple has enough children, he may first store some semen containing his sperm. Then if the couple decide later to have another child, the sperm may be inseminated artificially.

In all cases of insemination by donor, the donor remains anonymous, and does not know who has been given his sperm. Only the couple and the physician know of the procedure. Although there are no legal complications, a consent form must be filed by both husband and wife.

Of course, there are arguments pro and con concerning the procedure. Artificial insemination by a donor allows the child to be at least 50 percent the couple's own, which an adopted baby would not be. The woman's desire to become pregnant and to nurse and rear her child is satisfied. But emotional problems may enter the picture, especially if the husband becomes insecure. For such reasons, the physician questions and interviews the prospective couple extensively to make certain they really want the procedure to be done. There may also be religious ramifications, since some people believe that artificial insemination with a donor's sperm constitutes adultery. This is something which the couple must determine for themselves.

In the United States, 20,000 babies are born by artificial insemination each year, out of a total of several hundred thousand births. The procedure actually began centuries ago in animal husbandry, and is in many cases the prime method used to inseminate animals of particularly high value.

Artificial insemination in humans can also prevent some pregnancy difficulties, especially that of the Rh factor.

Artificial Respiration.
Victims of electric shock, drowning, gas poisoning, or choking have difficulty breathing, and may stop breathing altogether. Artificial respiration could save their lives. It keeps oxygen flowing in and out of the victim's lungs at regular intervals—just like regular breathing—until his body has had a chance to recover and resume natural breathing.

Since most people will die within six minutes after they stop breathing, artificial respiration should begin as soon as possible after the breathing difficulty is noticed.

Basically, there are three methods of artificial respiration. Experts agree that the most practical method is the mouth-to-mouth, or mouth-to-nose, method. The others are the chest pressure–arm lift (Silvester) method and the back pressure–arm lift (Holger-Nielsen) method.

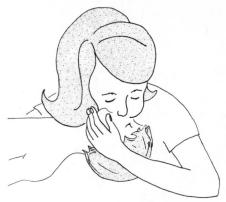

If you need to use artificial respiration (rescue breathing) on a young child or baby, cover his mouth and nose with your mouth in such a way as to prevent leakage of air, and let out shallow puffs of air from your lungs into the child's mouth and nose. Breathe in this manner at about twenty times per minute. Place your free hand just below the child's ribs to put pressure on the stomach and prevent it from filling with air.
Parents can best learn this technique by attending a demonstration by a qualified first aid instructor, using a dummy to simulate a live child.

Here are directions for administering artificial respiration, as outlined by The American National Red Cross.

MOUTH-TO-MOUTH (MOUTH-TO-NOSE). If foreign matter is visible in the victim's mouth, wipe it out quickly with your fingers or a cloth wrapped around your fingers.

1. Tilt the head back so the chin is pointing upward. The victim should be flat on his back. Pull or push the jaw into a jutting-out position. This should relieve obstruction of the airway by moving the base of the tongue away from the back of the throat.

2. Open your mouth wide and place it tightly over the victim's mouth. At the same time pinch the victim's nostrils shut or close the nostrils with your cheek. Or close the victim's mouth and place your mouth over the nose. Blow into the victim's mouth or nose. (Air may be blown through the victim's teeth, even if they are clenched.)

The first blowing efforts should deter-

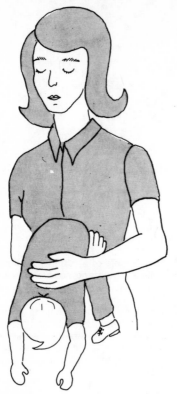

If the air passages of a child or infant are blocked, the child should be inverted over one arm and given two or three sharp pats between the shoulder blades in the hope of dislodging obstructing matter.

mine whether or not obstruction exists.

3. Remove your mouth, turn your head to the side, and listen for the return rush of air that indicates air exchange. Repeat the blowing effort.

For an adult, blow vigorously at the rate of about twelve breaths per minute. For a child, take relatively shallow breaths appropriate for the child's size, at the rate of about twenty per minute.

4. If the victim is not breathing out the air that you blew in, recheck the head and jaw position. If you still do not get air exchange, quickly turn the victim on his side and hit him sharply between the shoulder blades several times in the hope of dislodg-

ing foreign matter. Again, sweep your fingers through the victim's mouth to remove foreign matter.

If you do not wish to come in direct contact with the person, you may hold a cloth over the victim's mouth or nose and breathe through it. The cloth does not greatly affect the exchange of air.

MOUTH-TO-MOUTH FOR INFANTS AND SMALL CHILDREN. If foreign matter is visible in the mouth, clean it out quickly with your fingers or a cloth wrapped around your fingers.

1. Place the child on his back and use the fingers of both hands to lift the lower jaw from beneath and behind, so that it juts out.

2. Place your mouth over the child's mouth *and* nose, making a relatively leak-proof seal, and breathe into the child, using shallow puffs of air. The breathing rate should be about twenty per minute.

If you meet resistance in your blowing efforts, recheck the position of the jaw. If the air passages are still blocked, the child should be suspended momentarily by the ankles or inverted over one arm and given two or three sharp pats between the shoulder blades, in the hope of dislodging obstructing matter.

CHEST PRESSURE–ARM LIFT. If there is foreign matter visible in the mouth, wipe it out quickly with your fingers or a cloth wrapped around your fingers.

1. Place the victim in a face-up position and put something under his shoulders to raise them and allow the head to drop backward.

2. Kneel at the victim's head, grasp his arms at the wrist, cross them, and press them over the lower chest. This should cause air to flow out.

3. Immediately release this pressure and pull the arms outward and upward over his head and backward as far as possible. This should cause air to rush in.

4. Repeat this cycle about twelve times per minute, checking the mouth frequently for obstructions.

When the victim is in a face-up position, there is always danger that the victim will choke on vomitus, blood, or blood clots. This hazard can be reduced by keeping the head extended and turned to one side. If possible, the head should be a little lower than the rest of the body. If a second rescuer is available, have him hold the victim's head so that the jaw is jutting out. The helper should be alert to detect the presence of any stomach contents in the mouth and keep the mouth as clean as possible at all times.

BACK PRESSURE–ARM LIFT. If there is any foreign matter visible in the mouth, wipe it out quickly with your fingers or a cloth wrapped around your fingers.

1. Place the victim face down, bend his elbows, and place his hands one upon the other, turn his head slightly to one side and extend it as far as possible, making sure that the chin is jutting out.

2. Kneel at the head of the victim. Place your hands on the flat of the victim's back so that the palms lie just below an imaginary line running between the armpits.

3. Rock forward until the arms are approximately vertical and allow the weight of the upper part of your body to exert steady, even pressure downward upon the hands.

4. Immediately draw his arms upward and toward you, applying enough lift to feel resistance and tension at his shoulders. Then lower the arms to the ground. Repeat this cycle about twelve times per minute, checking the mouth frequently for obstruction.

If a second rescuer is available, have him hold the victim's head so that the jaw continues to jut out. The helper should be alert to detect any stomach contents in the mouth and keep the mouth as clean as possible at all times.

FOR ALL METHODS. Continue artificial respiration until the victim begins to breathe for himself, or until a physician pronounces the victim dead, or until the person appears to be dead beyond any doubt.

If the victim should vomit, turn him on his side, wipe out his mouth, and then put him in position to continue artificial respiration.

If the victim begins to breathe for himself, time your respiration movements to coincide with his breathing.

Keep the victim as quiet as possible, and cover him so he does not become chilled.

In most cases, the victim should recover quickly. However, in cases of electric shock, drug poisoning, or carbon monoxide poisoning, artificial respiration must be continued for a long period because the nerves and muscles that control breathing are paralyzed or slowed down greatly.

Call a doctor. Even after a victim begins to breathe on his own, a doctor should check him to make sure that no respiratory problems develop. (*See* EMERGENCY CARE; FIRST AID.)

Artificial Sweeteners. Often artificial sweeteners are used to sweeten food in place of sugar. The three types of artificial sweeteners are saccharin, sodium and calcium cyclamate, and cyclamic acid.

For many years diabetics, who have to restrict their intake of sugar, have been using saccharin. Saccharin is three hundred times sweeter than an equal amount of sugar. It is available in powdered form and also is packaged in tablet form for handy table use.

The U. S. Food and Drug Administration used to classify saccharin as GRAS (generally recognized as safe). Recently, however, it was removed from the GRAS list, pending study and investigation of its effects in the body.

Cyclamates are thirty times sweeter than an equal amount of sugar. Recent research has revealed that when large amounts of cyclamates are fed to rats, certain tumors develop. The use of cyclamates as food additives was discontinued because part of the federal Food Additive Law prohibits the use of any substance which can cause cancer in man or in other animals.

At present, there is no evidence that cyclamates cause cancer in man. Their only known effect on man is a softening of the feces when extremely high amounts of cyclamates are taken.

The discontinuance of cyclamates as artificial sweeteners and food additives was required by law, but was not considered an emergency. Cyclamates and foods containing cyclamates are now classed by the Food and Drug Administration as drugs and continue to be available, as drugs, for those who benefit from them.

Asbestosis. Inhalation of asbestos fibers results in a disease called asbestosis. It belongs to the general class of lung disease known as pneumoconioses, which means disorders due to inhaling dust particles.

The disease begins with a cough and difficulty in breathing. The bronchioles (small lung passages) become obstructed with the asbestos particles. The tiny air sacs, or alveoli, of the lungs may collapse. Fibrosis—abnormal development of fibrous tissue—may also occur in the lung. Like other pneumoconioses, asbestosis has no cure.

The disease is found among workers engaged in the mining or processing of asbestos (magnesium silicate). In recent years asbestos-like particles, from building construction and other sources, have been found in the lungs of large cross-sections of the general public. This raises the question whether asbestos may be a major air pollutant. (*See* PNEUMOCONIOSIS; POLLUTION.)

Ascariasis. When one is infected with a particular type of roundworm, the condition is known as ascariasis. (*See* ROUNDWORMS; WORMS.)

Ascites. An excess accumulation of fluid in the abdominal cavity is known as ascites. It is sometimes referred to as abdominal dropsy, or hydroperitoneum. Ascites is often associated with cardiac failure, cirrhosis of the liver, and renal deficiency. (*See* EDEMA; PERITONEUM.)

Ascorbic Acid. Known also as vitamin C, ascorbic acid is necessary for maintaining our body cells and connective tissues. The average minimum daily requirement is 40 milligrams for children and 60 milligrams for adults.

Because the body does not store vitamin C in excess of the amount needed to keep tissues saturated, a daily supply is needed.

A lack of ascorbic acid may cause a disease known as scurvy. However, a diet may contain enough vitamin C to prevent scurvy, but not enough to prevent ill health. Even a slight deficiency may cause a decrease in a person's general body tone and lessen his resistance to disease. He may become irritable, lack vitality, and lose weight.

In scurvy, the tissues become depleted of vitamin C, the intercellular material does not form, and tissue structure is disorganized. The victim's gums are sore and bleeding, his teeth crumble easily and are loose. The deterioration of his body structures makes his joints sore and stiff. The ends of growing bone enlarge, there are capillary hemorrhages in joints and muscle tissue, as well as possible enlargement of the heart.

Fresh foods are the best source of vitamin C, because slight amounts of it may be lost during storage and cooking. However, when orange juice is properly stored in a closed plastic, wax, or glass container in the refrigerator, it loses very little vitamin C content.

Citrus fruits, tomatoes, strawberries, and other fruits are outstanding sources of ascorbic acid. Good sources are melons, berries, broccoli, brussels sprouts, cabbage, asparagus, and cauliflower. One serving each day of any one of these foods will provide all the vitamin C the average person needs.

Infants are often given vitamin C, usually in the form of orange juice, as soon as artificial bottle feeding begins. (*See* VITAMINS.)

Pineapple contains less vitamin C than do citrus fruits, but it, too, is a good source. An average serving of pineapple provides children with one-half and adults with one-third of the recommended daily vitamin C intake. Three ounces of fresh pineapple contain about 20 milligrams of vitamin C. There are about three milligrams of vitamin C in a fluid ounce of pineapple juice.

One of the richest sources of vitamin C is acerola, a fruit related to the cherry that grows in the West Indies. A little less than one-half cup of acerola juice contains 1,494 milligrams of vitamin C, nearly thirty times the vitamin C present in the same amount of orange juice. Some baby-food manufacturers use acerola juice to increase the vitamin C content of their fruits and juices. So parents need not be puzzled if this ingredient is noted on the label.

Ascorbic acid may be in food preservation, particularly in the freeze-packing of fruits and vegetables. It prevents color and oxidative changes, and is especially effective in preserving the color of peaches. Standard cookbooks usually give information on the quantity to use in home canning fruits. Pure ascorbic acid may be purchased at pharmacies.

In recent years vitamin C has achieved great popularity as a possible preventive or cure for the common cold. While this idea is supported by some scientific leaders, there has as yet been no real evidence that vitamin C is more helpful than any other vitamin in preventing or curing colds.

Asian Flu.   Known since the early twelfth century, influenza, or flu, was first thought to be caused by the influence of the planets in our solar system. It was and still is one of the diseases most puzzling to medicine. (*See* INFLUENZA.)

Despite many deadly outbreaks of influenza through the centuries, the three related virus types (A, B, and C) which are suspect were not discovered until after 1930. The A influenza virus, now known to cause Asian flu, is believed to come from a virus reservoir in central Asia. Because many large epidemics start there, a majority of scientists are convinced that such a reservoir exists. The virus is spread by high-speed modern transportation, which can cause an epidemic to break out anywhere in the world.

Influenza may start like a cold or some other respiratory infection, but is soon characterized by severe prostration, a high temperature, aching muscles, sore throat, and a hacking cough. The symptoms usually last five days and may be followed by weeks of convalescence. Fatalities from Asian flu occur when staphylococci bacteria complicate the normal course of the illness.

Before contracting the disease, a person may receive a vaccination helpful against type A virus. However, once influenza sets in, there is no medication to eliminate or alleviate it. Antibiotics are usually given, but they are used only to prevent secondary bacterial infection and the threat of pneumonia. Victims should remain in bed, drink fluids, and stay isolated from others, as the disease is highly contagious.

Asphyxiation.   When there is too little oxygen and too much carbon dioxide in a person's blood, he will lose consciousness and his condition is known as asphyxia. Carbon monoxide is the gas usually responsible for asphyxiation. It is a colorless, odorless gas that forms whenever there is incomplete combustion of materials such as coal, wood, gas, paper, or charcoal. In the home, it is usually produced by faulty heating equipment.

A person may also be asphyxiated by manufactured gases that leak from appliances, by carbon tetrachloride fumes and fumes from other chemicals, by the fumes from fires in the home, or by the fumes produced by an automobile with its engine left running in a closed garage.

A person who has been overcome by gas, or asphyxiated, should receive fresh air immediately. Either move the victim to another room or open all the doors and windows and shut off the source of the poisonous gas. Begin artificial respiration immediately; the asphyxiation victim is in serious need of oxygen. (*See* ARTIFICIAL RESPIRATION.) Call a doctor.

In 1970, about 1,600 persons died from poisoning by gases and vapors, according to the National Safety Council. Of these deaths, 1,200 occurred in and around the home. To prevent asphyxiation in your home, take these steps: Have your heater checked and cleaned each year. Make sure space heaters are properly vented. Avoid using carbon tetrachloride for cleaning clothes indoors. Don't inhale too strong a concentration of paint, varnish, or chemical fumes. Never use a charcoal barbecue grill inside the house. Never keep an automobile engine running in a closed garage.

Aspirate. This is a broad term used to describe any action of drawing in fluids or gases. Thus when one breathes air into the lungs, this is aspiration, though the more common term is inhalation. When gases form, say in the stomach, the physician may decide to remove the pressure by aspiration through a tube. However, the word is most often used to describe removal of fluids. A dentist uses an aspirator to suck out saliva and blood when working in the mouth. Surgeons also use devices to withdraw pools of blood in the incision during an operation.

Aspirin. The most widely prescribed pain reliever for headaches, arthritic pain, and colds is aspirin, also called acetylsalicylic acid. One of a group of salicylates, aspirin will relieve pain without becoming an addictive drug or influencing the development of a disease.

Some aspirin users find that it creates gastric distress, characterized by abdominal pain and gas. Others are hypersensitive to it and develop skin rashes and anaphylaxis (increased susceptibility to a foreign substance resulting from previous exposure or use). (*See* ANAPHYLAXIS.)

Salicylate poisoning from overdoses of aspirin occurs primarily in children. Although warnings and protective covers are placed on children's aspirin, the rate of salicylate poisoning keeps increasing. Because the drug is flavored, many children think of aspirin as candy. Youngsters from one to four years of age have the highest mortality rate.

Aspirin poisoning, like all forms of salicylate poisoning, has definite characteristics. At the beginning of the cycle, symptoms may not be evident until twelve to twenty-four hours after the overdose has been consumed. If, in treating an illness, a person unwisely overdoses a child—or himself—at regular intervals over a period of time, the symptoms may take longer to appear.

The first sign is rapid breathing, with indications of difficulty in catching a breath of air. If treatment is not begun at the onset of this sign, further complications develop. The clotting time of the blood is lengthened, thereby causing hemorrhaging in tissues and organs. Vomiting with dark clots of blood may occur along with bleeding from the nose and gums. The skin is pale, fever is usually present, and severe stomach pains develop. Immediate medical treatment should be sought *before* these symptoms develop. (*See* ACETYLSALICYLIC ACID.)

Assimilation. The process that transforms food into living tissue is called assimilation. (*See* DIGESTION.)

Asthenia. Weakness, or lack of strength or energy, is sometimes called asthenia. It may be caused by disease—a severe infection, a high fever, or anemia, for instance.

It can also result from lack of exercise—as when a patient must remain in bed for a long time.

The term is also used in combination words which describe special kinds of weakness. Neurasthenia, for example, is a psychoneurotic condition also called nervous prostration or nervous exhaustion. Myasthenia is a muscle weakness which occurs in disorders such as myasthenia gravis, a condition that brings increasing paralysis of muscles, usually of the face and neck. (*See* MYASTHENIA GRAVIS; NEURASTHENIA.)

Asthma.   Millions of people suffer from bronchial asthma all over the world—but it is particularly common on the American continent and in Europe.

The disease is marked by extreme discomfort. The patient has trouble breathing, wheezes and coughs, and spits up phlegm. In mild cases these symptoms come and go, depending upon the patient's exposure to the specific irritants that bring on attacks and upon his emotional reactions.

Often the episodes of discomfort get more frequent over a long period of years, until the asthma becomes a condition the patient must live with for the rest of his life. On the other hand, perhaps one quarter of the cases that begin in childhood will clear up in middle or late adolescence. The reasons for such a wide variance in the course of the disease among individuals are not clearly understood.

The causes of asthma have long been debated. However, there is general agreement today that bronchial (as distinguished from cardiac) asthma is an allergic disease. In other words, the asthmatic is particularly sensitive to certain substances in his environment. These irritants, called allergens, may be any number of things. Those that most commonly provoke asthmatic attacks are plant pollens (such as ragweed), house dust, feathers, foods, and various natural and manmade air pollutants. Close

to one-third of persons with hay fever, another allergic disease, eventually develop asthma. (*See* ALLERGEN; ALLERGY; HAY FEVER.)

Some asthma patients can simply walk through the front door of a home and realize at once that a cat is somewhere inside. Danders—dandruff-like scales from hairy animals like dogs and cats—become airborne and reach the nostrils of the allergic person, provoking sneezing and other asthmatic symptoms.

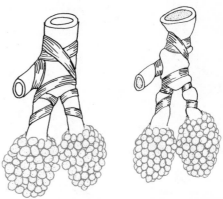

Asthma. In a normal section of the lungs, here greatly enlarged, the bronchioles (small air passages) would appear as in the drawing at left. In asthma (*right*), the bands of muscles of the bronchioles constrict (tighten). At the same time, mucus forms in the passages. The result is a restricted flow of air to the alveoli, or tiny air cells.

Sometimes asthma develops after a patient has had a long history of respiratory infections, such as the common cold or bronchitis. It is suspected that some of these people may have become allergic to the bacteria or virus causing the infection, or to by-products of the infection.

The emotional stress and frustrations common to modern society can trigger an attack of asthma. They are not considered causes of the disease, but rather factors that reduce the patient's resistance or increase his sensitivity to the allergens to which he reacts.

Questions and Answers About Asthma

Q. *What is asthma?*

A. It is a disease of the bronchial tubes of the lungs, resulting in a chronic sickness marked by attacks of difficult breathing. It is not contagious.

Q. *What is an asthma attack like?*

A. The victim seems to be suffocating. The skin turns pale and bluish, he perspires and appears to be using all his strength to draw a breath. The attack occurs because the bronchial tubes tend to close during an attack, due to a bronchial muscle spasm, swelling of the mucous membrane, or the formation of phlegm in the bronchial tubes.

Q. *Are there different causes of bronchial asthma?*

A. Yes, most of them allergic. Approximately 75 percent of sufferers are allergic to foreign substances which enter their bodies. These include animal hair, fur, or feathers, dust, pollen, face powder, foods, and many other substances. Some sufferers are sensitive to conditions and substances within their own bodies, as in bacterial infections of the respiratory tract.

Q. *What should a person with asthma-like symptoms do?*

A. See a doctor. Tests can be made to identify the irritant. Emotional as well as physical conditions may also aggravate the patient's condition.

Q. *Is asthma curable?*

A. In many cases it is. In other cases, a doctor can provide relief. Sometimes a change in climate can end symptoms which have failed to yield to ordinary treatment.

In asthma, the bronchioles (small air passages) of the lungs become obstructed, involuntary muscle fibers surrounding the bronchioles go into spasms, and the linings of the air passages swell and cause further blocking of air. The mucous membranes lining the windpipe react by secreting abnormal amounts of mucus, a sticky, watery fluid. The coughing of the asthmatic is an effort to free the passages of this mucus.

ASTHMA IN CHILDREN. Unfortunately, many parents bank heavily on the hope that their child's asthma will go away by itself, but their optimism can subject the child to serious risks. If attention is not given to the problem, asthma at any age not only can get much more severe, but may progress into emphysema, cor pulmonale (a heart problem resulting from lung obstruction), atelectasis (lung collapse), and other complications. (*See* ATELECTASIS; EMPHYSEMA; PULMONARY HEART DISEASE.)

Asthma is not passed directly from parent to child, but a tendency toward it is found in families. If both parents, for example, have a history of some kind of allergy, the chances are about three out of four that their child will develop asthma or another allergic condition. Most cases of asthma develop before the age of twenty or twenty-one, though many cases do start later in life.

The first step in caring for an asthma patient is to try to determine the allergen and either remove it or move the patient away from it. You can use air conditioners with filters in the home, and travel in an air-conditioned car to avoid exposure to ragweed, if that is the allergen. Or give away the cat, if that is the cause of the problem. Or, if all else fails, escape a local allergen by moving to an area where the specific pollen or air pollutant does not exist.

Drastic measures that entail uprooting an entire family for the sake of one asthmatic member may not be practical or advisable. A more common solution today is desensitization. In this procedure, the patient is injected repeatedly with minute quantities of the allergen so that he may gradually develop defensive antibodies. (*See* ANTIBODY.)

Asthmatic persons also tend to breathe improperly, using the upper part of the chest instead of the diaphragm. For exercises to develop diaphragmatic breathing, see the article BREATHING. The method of breathing illustrated there not only will help avoid chest deformities, but also can reduce the severity of asthma attacks. The exercises are especially important for asthmatic children.

Tobacco smoke should be avoided by the asthmatic person. It is certainly not helpful, and it can provoke attacks and cause complications. Good nutrition, adequate rest, and avoidance of emotional strain will help the patient, too.

Persons with asthma often are sensitive to drugs that do not bother nonallergic persons. Antitetanus injections prepared from horse serum, for example, may provoke severe attacks.

Infections of the respiratory tract must be treated carefully, as they may complicate the asthma, or the patient may be sensitive to antibiotics normally given for the infections. Exposure to rapid temperature changes, or extremes of hot or cold, should be avoided, as they can bring on asthmatic symptoms.

RELIEF FROM ATTACKS. Bronchodilator drugs, which dilate or open up the air passages of the lungs, can give the asthmatic

The shape of the chest of a person with asthma, as shown in these views of a twelve-year-old boy, may be abnormal due to labored breathing patterns. But usually the doctor can make a diagnosis of asthma only after having observed the patient during an attack—noting breathing sounds in the chest and the nature of the patient's efforts to breathe—as well as by examining spit-up material (sputum), and determining the patient's background. Often a tendency toward the disease runs in the family.

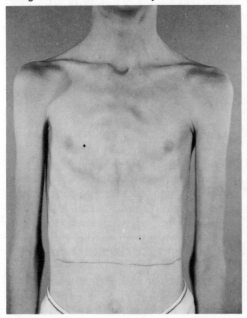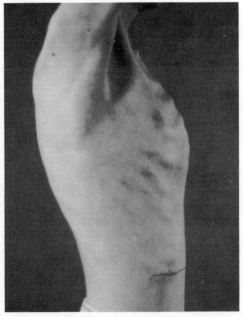

quick relief. Two of these are epinephrine and isoproterenol, which are available in aerosol sprays. Drugs taken by mouth, such as ephedrine or theophylline, also help. They do not act as fast as the aerosols, but usually give longer lasting relief.

Drugs in the form of rectal suppositories or enemas work well in relieving asthma, particularly when quick results are needed and the patient has not responded to other treatments.

Expectorants—products that help you release and spit up phlegm—help the asthmatic person get his breathing back under control during or after an attack. Pressing the hands against the diaphragm aids in releasing air from the lungs. Sedatives are sometimes used to relax the patient.

Steroids and hormones may be prescribed for long-term therapy—among them cortisone, ACTH (corticotrophin), and prednisone. Some are given in injections, others by nasal aerosol or by mouth. During the term of treatment, the physician must be ever alert for possible side effects from these products.

STATUS ASTHMATICUS. An attack may last for minutes or much longer. If it persists for days and does not improve with the usual treatment, it is called status asthmaticus and requires emergency measures, since the patient will fight for air, and his face may turn bluish.

Oxygen administration may be necessary, even mechanical respirators. Rarely, surgery to clear air passages is needed.

Compared with the high number of persons with asthma, deaths from the disease are not common. Even if you have mild asthma, you should consult your physician regularly. Following his instructions can help you ward off many of the complications of asthma and live a happy, well-adjusted life. (*See* BRONCHITIS.)

Astigmatism. If the cornea, the most forward part of the eye, is curved abnormally, it will bend the incoming light rays improperly. This condition, known as astigmatism, and the visual problems it creates can usually be corrected by eyeglasses. (*See* CONTACT LENSES; EYEGLASSES; EYESIGHT.)

Astringent. A drug that has a binding or constricting effect is an astringent. Some astringents coagulate blood when applied to wounds or mucous surfaces. Astringents protect, heal, and stop bleeding. Most astringents are salts of metals such as aluminum, iron, and zinc. An astringent enema is one given to contract intestinal tissue and provide subsequent evacuation of worms. (*See* COAGULATION.)

Ataxia. A lack or loss of muscular coordination is called ataxia. Common symptoms of this condition are a staggering walk and difficulty in completing movements like touching the tip of the nose with the tip of one finger. Ataxia is the result of disturbance in, or damage to, the cerebellum, that section of the brain which plays an important part in controlling movement. The problem has many causes.

Intoxication with alcohol, barbiturates, and some other drugs can produce the uncoordinated movements of ataxia. The cerebellum can also be affected by a head injury, a tumor, or a number of diseases which attack the central nervous system—among them cerebral palsy, multiple sclerosis, poliomyelitis, St. Louis encephalitis, and syphilis. A syphilitic infection results in a painful form of ataxia called *tabes dorsalis,* or locomotor ataxia.

Acute cerebellar ataxia of childhood strikes children between one and twelve years old, sometimes after infections such as chickenpox, measles, and scarlet fever, and sometimes when the child seems to be in good health. The disorder usually runs its course in a period of weeks.

Ataxia also occurs in a number of hereditary diseases, such as Friedreich's ataxia. (*See* ALCOHOLISM; CEREBRAL PALSY; MULtiple sclerosis; st. louis encephalitis; syphilis; tabes dorsalis.)

Atelectasis. The collapse of a lung or portions of a lung, called atelectasis, may be caused by obstruction of the bronchial air passages, which accompanies lung diseases such as pneumonia, or by pneumothorax. In pneumothorax air enters the pleura, the membrane surrounding the lungs, and presses back on the lungs, making them collapse.

Pneumothorax is the result of a tear in the lung wall which permits air to pass through. The air escapes from the lung, which deflates and collapses. This may occur for obscure reasons, or may be the result of various lung diseases, infections, or a stab wound. In most cases the tear seals itself and the lung can reinflate.

At one time atelectasis was a complication of surgery of the abdomen, but it has become less common with improved methods of handling anesthesia and drainage of the lungs during surgical procedures. Atelectasis is also a grave result of neonatal hyaline membrane disease. (*See* HYALINE MEMBRANE DISEASE.)

In typical cases of acute or spontaneous atelectasis, which occur without complicating diseases, the patient may turn blue from insufficient oxygen in the blood, have trouble breathing, and run a fever. These symptoms clear up rapidly as the lung again inflates with air. If there is an infection, appropriate medication is given.

Chronic (long-lasting or recurrent) atelectasis, with collapse of part of one lung, is usually associated with some other underlying lung disease.

Atherosclerosis. When deposits of fatty-like material, called atheromas, are laid down in the lining (intima) of arteries, the disease called atherosclerosis results.

In North America and other affluent nations, close to half the adult population over the ages of forty or fifty are estimated to

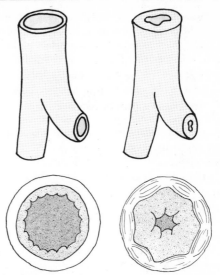

Atherosclerosis. In the normal arteries, as shown in the two drawings at left, the lining (intima) of the vessels is comparatively thin, permitting normal flow of blood. Atherosclerosis occurs when deposits of fatlike material (atheromas) thicken the lining, sometimes almost entirely blocking the blood flow, as in the two drawings at right.

have atherosclerosis in some form or another. In aged persons the rate is even higher. Atherosclerotic heart disease is a very common cause of death.

The word atherosclerosis is often used as though it were identical to arteriosclerosis, which literally means hardening of the arteries. The confusion is due to the fact that most of the cases of disease which were classed as arteriosclerosis in the past apparently really involved atheromas, and thus should more properly have been classed as atherosclerosis.

Also, the results of the restriction of blood flow are often identical, whether due to atherosclerosis or anything else which clogs or narrows the arteries. If the result is a heart crisis, this must be treated as an emergency in itself and little can be gained by quibbling over whether arteriosclerosis or atherosclerosis is at fault. (*See* ARTERIOSCLEROSIS.)

FORMATION OF ATHEROMAS. Prevention is a different story. Knowledge of how atheromas are formed can certainly help you avoid trouble. This is true even though medical scientists are not exactly sure what causes atherosclerosis. The caution flags are up and you will do well to take care.

Statistics show that atherosclerosis is by far more prevalent in the so-called prosperous countries where food is plentiful and man chooses to eat lots of animal fat. It is less common in countries where the diet is low in animal fats.

Full proof seems to escape the researchers as yet, but there is little doubt that too much cholesterol, a substance vital to the body in moderate quantities, is related to atheroma formation.

The level of cholesterol in the bloodstream increases with the consumption of saturated fats, a type found in meat, whole milk, butter, and coconuts. If your diet is altered so that you eat more unsaturated or polyunsaturated fats, found chiefly in vegetables, then your cholesterol level will be lowered. (*See* CHOLESTEROL.)

Corn, peanut, cottonseed, and safflower (sunflower) oils are good sources of unsaturated fats. These are recommended in diets for persons with atherosclerosis or heart disease.

Anyone over the age of forty would do well to cut his consumption of saturated fats and substitute the unsaturated variety. If you prefer to wait for absolute proof of how cholesterol causes atheromas, you will be taking the risk of heart trouble just like the person who waits for absolute data on how smoking is harmful to his health.

Researchers have proved that the first patch, or plaque, which appears in the inner lining (intima) of the arteries in atherosclerosis contains cholesterol, as well as other lipids (fatty materials) and protein. From this start the deposits increase, and calcification (deposit of calcium) hardens the plaque. The blood vessels weaken and lose the elasticity needed for normal function.

The build-up of atheroma often reduces the caliber of the arteries and diminishes blood flow to the region. Hypertension frequently accompanies atherosclerosis, though there is no known causal connection between the two disorders. But the presence of hypertension from other causes increases the risk of hemorrhage, particularly in the brain.

The great danger of atherosclerosis, especially in middle-aged persons, is in the coronary arteries of the heart. Here the damaged lining of the vessels may cause sudden thrombosis, with symptoms and signs of a "heart attack." The mortality in acute coronary occlusion, as it is called, is quite high. (*See* HYPERTENSION.)

When the aorta and other large blood vessels of the body are partially or almost completely blocked by atherosclerotic material, the patient is in grave danger of death. Blocking of arteries in the coronary area (that surrounding the heart) will cause insufficient nourishment of the heart muscles, and the heart may fail. (*See* HEART ATTACK; HEART FAILURE; MYOCARDIAL INFARCTION.)

POSSIBLE CAUSES. The cholesterol theory of atherosclerosis is the most widely researched and discussed, but there are excellent scientific studies which show that other factors may be involved, such as consuming too much sugar, vitamin D, hard water, oral contraceptives, smoking too much, breathing in carbon dioxide, not getting enough exercise, or living under emotional tension.

While we await more conclusive studies, one point becomes quite clear: Moderation in diet, in physical activity, and in your psychological reaction to life seems to be good advice if you would avoid atherosclerosis. Lack of exercise is not moderation, but rather a dangerous excess—of inactivity.

Overweight, as might be expected, increases your chances of developing atherosclerosis and its complications. So do certain diseases like diabetes, thyroid irregularities, and disorders of the kidney. There also may be an inherited tendency to develop atherosclerosis. However, inasmuch as mothers teach their daughters to cook and shape their sons' eating preferences, it may be the family's diet habits rather than its physical inheritance which is at fault.

COMPLICATIONS. In addition to the heart problems noted above, atherosclerosis may lead to many circulatory disorders. There may be intermittent claudication—lameness from time to time, due to insufficient blood flow through the legs. (*See* CLAUDI-CATION.) Or there may be blood clots which can block blood vessels at the site of origin (thrombosis) or travel through the body to block vessels elsewhere (embolism).

Atherosclerosis increases the tendency toward thrombosis or embolism in two ways: First, the fatty deposits can break off or move through the blood while in the process of formation. Second, they are more likely to clog up a passage already narrowed by disease. Cerebral strokes, in which there is blocking of small blood vessels in the brain, are more likely to occur among atherosclerotic individuals. (*See* EMBOLISM; STROKES; THROMBOSIS.)

When a person develops atherosclerosis, he seldom has any signs until the symptoms of a complicating problem, such as hypertension or heart disease, appear. However, many people who have atherosclerosis to some degree may live through life without knowing it or developing obvious complications. Some of the blocking of smaller arteries by atherosclerosis is compensated for by an increased blood flow through other nearby blood vessels, the so-called collateral circulation. (*See* BLOOD CIRCULA-TION.)

Surgery is sometimes necessary to remove the atheromatous deposits, which often tend to form at junctions of blood vessels. Some work has been done with devices which clear the deposits through a reaming action. Anticoagulant medication is useful in preventing complications of the disease.

Athlete's Foot.   Tinea pedis, one of several forms of "athlete's foot," is a ringworm infection of the feet. (*See* RINGWORM.) It is often confused with dermatitis caused by dyes, antioxidants, and other chemicals used in making modern footwear.

Atmospheric Pressure.   The weight of air from the top of the atmosphere presses down on the layers below to cause air pressure. The upper atmosphere, having less air in it, has less pressure than the layers of air below. At sea level, air pressure averages about fifteen pounds on every square inch. The air pressing down on a person's shoulders weighs about a ton. We do not feel this weight because we are supported by an equal pressure of air on all sides of our bodies.

At altitudes over 10,000 feet the light, rarefied air cannot sustain enough oxygen for most of us to breathe easily. Our bodily well-being is affected in various ways. We have to breathe harder and faster to obtain the oxygen we need to maintain body processes. The hemoglobin in our blood increases, along with other systemic adjustments, and any weaknesses in the heart or lungs may become more severe. When the summer Olympics were held in Mexico, at a high altitude, athletes from low-altitude countries had to spend some time "working out" in the mountains before they were ready to participate in the games.

Atomizer.   An instrument which breaks up a liquid into a fine spray is called an atomizer. The purpose of such an instrument is to apply medicines uniformly to a body area. The shape and size of atomizers vary, but they all simply spray a liquid mixed with air.

A drug called phenylephrine is usually packaged in a small plastic squeeze bottle. This drug, when sprayed into the nasal passages, relieves the congestion of a cold. Various drugs in the bronchodilator category are available in atomizers. When inhaled, these drugs spray open the lung passages and help relieve asthma. Topical anesthetics used to numb the skin or throat before various procedures are available in atomizers for the physician's convenience.

Atony. A lack of normal muscular tone or strength is called atony. (*See* CHOREA; MUSCLES; PHYSICAL FITNESS.)

Atresia. When an absence or closure of a normal body orifice or passage occurs, the condition is known as atresia. It can occur in various parts of the body, including the anal area, eye, heart, or ovary. (*See* ANUS; BLOOD CIRCULATION; HEART; OVARY.)

Atrium. When the blood from the systemic veins (superior and inferior vena cava) reaches the heart, it enters an upper chamber called the right atrium. A similar upper chamber on the left side receives blood from the pulmonary veins and is called the left atrium. These two chambers were formerly called the auricles ("little ears") because their outer surfaces have earlike projections that are now called the auricular appendages. The two atria always beat simultaneously. They are synchronized by the pacemaker, a small mass of neuromuscular tissue called the sino-atrial node.

The two lower chambers are the right and left ventricles. Blood from the right atrium passes through the tricuspid valve into the right ventricle, which then discharges the blood into the pulmonary artery for passage through the lungs. Blood

from the left atrium passes through the mitral valve into the left ventricle, which then discharges it into the aorta for distribution to the systemic and coronary arteries. The two ventricles beat simultaneously and are synchronized by impulses from an atrioventricular node.

The two atria are separated from each other by a sheet of muscular tissue called the septum. This partition also separates the two ventricles, so that blood from the right side cannot mix, in the normal adult heart, with the blood on the left. In the normal fetal heart, however, there is a hole (the foramen ovale) in the septum between the two atria. It should close before birth. Failure of the foramen ovale to close is one of the characteristic findings in congenital heart disease, and other imperfections of the septum occur. (*See* BLOOD CIRCULATION.)

Atrophy. The reduction in size of a previously normal body organ or cell is called atrophy. Muscles, bones, nerves, the liver, the heart, and other tissues are subject to atrophy. Atrophy may result as a normal process in the life span of an organ (physiologic atrophy). This occurs to the thymus gland as adulthood is reached, and to the breasts and ovaries as female menopause is reached. Disease processes of many kinds can cause atrophy of an organ (pathologic atrophy). Muscles and other tissues may atrophy simple because they are not used (disuse atrophy). Atrophy should be differentiated from dystrophy, which is abnormal development or degeneration of a given organ or tissue. (*See* DYSTROPHY.)

Disuse atrophy can be forestalled or slowed down by adequate use of the muscles and tissues that may be, or may have been, affected. But this is seldom possible in pathologic atrophy, when nerves are severely damaged or destroyed (as in polio) and their muscles are thereby rendered useless. In such cases, it is sometimes possible for other muscles to take over the functions of those that have been atrophied.

Atropine. This substance, used in many medicinal products, relaxes the involuntary muscle of various organs. It is used in treating acute attacks of bronchial asthma and intestinal colic, and in cathartic pills. It is also used in ophthalmology for dilating the pupil and treating various eye conditions. (*See* ASTHMA; BELLADONNA; CATHARTICS; COLIC; EYE.)

Aura. The feeling or sensation that comes before the beginning of a sudden attack, such as an epileptic attack, is known as the aura. (*See* ASTHMA; EPILEPSY; VERTIGO.)

Aureomycin. Also known as chlortetracycline, this broad-spectrum antibiotic is one of the most popular of the chlortetracycline, oxytetracycline, and streptomycin group.

Originally extracted from molds, the product is now synthesized into a yellow crystalline compound sold under the trade name of Aureomycin. It is active against staphylococci, streptococci, and other microbes which are affected by penicillin. Unlike penicillin and the sulfonamides, which are bactericidal, chlortetracycline is bacteriostatic, meaning that it prohibits the growth and multiplication of, but does not kill, bacteria, viruses, and other microbes.

Auricle. The two upper chambers of the heart, now called the right and left atrium, were formerly called the auricles. (*See* ATRIUM.)

Auscultation. When the physician listens to the patient—not the patient's voice but the many other sounds within the body—he is practicing auscultation. Such listening may be done to the lungs, abdomen, pleura, and other organs. It is used to detect the body sounds of the mother and the fetus during pregnancy. Auscultation is also important in diagnosing the condition of the heart.

Listening may be direct—that is, without the use of an instrument such as a stethoscope—or it may be mediate, using a stethoscope. (*See* STETHOSCOPE.)

Examination of the heart includes a thorough external examination of the chest region; it consists in touching and thumping the heart region and listening to heart sounds. The listening, or auscultation, is most significant in diagnosing heart disease. The physician listens for normal heart sounds, murmurs, and other sounds indicating abnormalities.

Normal heart sounds are two loud noises made by two sets of valves—two inflow, or atrioventricular, valves separating the atria from ventricles, and two outflow, or semilunar, valves separating ventricles from two main arterial trunks. The first sound is the closing of the ventricular valves (systole); the second sound is the closing of the semilunar valves (the beginning of diastole).

In the case of heart disease the physician will often hear third and fourth sounds, indicating abnormalities of valve action, pressure changes in the heart, or too rapid blood flow through the heart.

Autointoxication. The notion that anyone who does not have a daily bowel movement is in danger of self-poisoning, or autointoxication, from retained body wastes has caused much needless anxiety. It has also been worth millions to quacks and to the patent medicine industry. Excrement smells bad, but it is not actively poisonous, in the body or outside it. Furthermore, the normal large intestine absorbs water and food materials digested by helpful intestinal bacteria, but very little else.

In many diseases, toxins (poisonous substances) are actually produced in the body, but the word "autointoxication," as commonly used, refers to an imaginary condition. (*See* CONSTIPATION; INTESTINES.)

Autonomic Nervous System.

While the central nervous system connects with every part of the body and is the main system, a second one exists in the body—the autonomic nervous system. Its function is to provide for automatic control of the vital involuntary internal organs. (*See* NERVOUS SYSTEM.)

The autonomic nervous system has two divisions, the parasympathetic and the sympathetic, which have opposite functions and thereby balance each other.

The sympathetic division starts at the base of the brain and divides to form two parts (right and left sympathetic trunks) which continue down each side of the spinal column. From each trunk, lying on either side of the spine, are many nerves which extend to the glands (salivary, pancreas, liver); to the involuntary muscles found in the blood vessel walls; and to involuntary muscle fibers in the walls of organs like the heart, bladder, and intestines.

The sympathetic division serves to stimulate the heartbeat, dilate the pupils of the eye, constrict blood vessels to raise the blood pressure, and stop glandular secretions.

The parasympathetic system contains two major nerves, the vagus and the pelvic. The vagus nerve starts in the medulla oblongata, at the base of the brain, and branches off into the chest and abdominal area. The pelvic nerve rises from the spinal cord in the hip area and branches off to the organs in the lower half of the body.

Autophobia.

Everyone, at some time or other, does not want to be alone; but a person afflicted with autophobia, the morbid fear of being alone or the fear of oneself, is almost incapable of being alone. (*See* PHOBIAS.)

Autopsy.

The thorough examination of a human body immediately after death is termed an autopsy. Its purpose is to establish the cause of death. During the autopsy the body wall is opened, each major organ is weighed and examined, and specimens are set aside for later microscopic examination. The medical specialist who performs an autopsy and determines the cause of death is a pathologist. (*See* PATHOLOGIST.)

Permission must be obtained from the closest relative before an autopsy can be performed. Although many people are hesitant about granting an autopsy for emotional reasons, the cause of death is, from a medical point of view, almost always valuable to know. The relatives can benefit in the event that the killing disease is found to be genetic or infectious. Medical science and education can frequently benefit by gaining new knowledge from the results of an autopsy.

In the case of a violent or unexplained death, an autopsy can reveal important legal information and is usually demanded by the coroner. (*See* POSTMORTEM EXAMINATION.)

Auto Safety.

For children, an automobile can be almost as dangerous when parked in the driveway as when speeding down the expressway. Children should not be allowed to play in, around, or under parked cars. Even a young child has no difficulty releasing the parking brake, allowing the car to roll down the driveway or a hill.

Never leave a child alone in a car with the engine running, even for as long as it takes you to get out and open the garage door. That's enough time for a child to put his hands on the wheel and step on the accelerator—just as he has seen you do.

For that matter, a child should *never* be left alone in a car. And the danger is increased if you close all the windows but leave the ignition key in the lock.

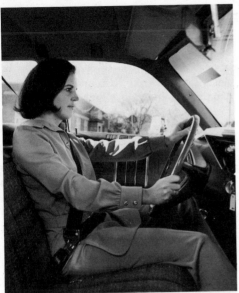

Gateway Industries

Auto safety begins with a protective device to fasten passengers securely in a relaxed but restrained position. The safest device designed thus far is the harness and lap belt combination, required in all new automobiles now sold in the United States. Also being studied is an air-bag device which inflates instantaneously upon collision and provides a cushion between passengers and car.

A child should never be permitted to ride standing up in the car. If he is small, he should have his own car seat where he can be high enough to see what is going on and where he will be secure if the car should stop suddenly. A baby should ride in a bassinette, not on Mother's lap where his chances of surviving an accident are small.

All passengers in a car should wear safety belts, no matter how long or short the trip will be. Children imitate adults, so if parents make it a habit to always wear a safety belt and keep the doors locked, their child is likely to follow their example.

No matter how much of a hurry you are in, watch carefully for children playing when you back out of the driveway or a parking space. And as you drive be alert for children who dart into the street after a ball or ride their bicycles in traffic.

Never drive when you are tired or emotionally upset; that's inviting an accident. On long trips, the American Automobile Association recommends that a refresher break be taken at least every two hours. Get out and stretch, even if you only walk around the car.

Children get restless on long car trips. They too need periodic breaks to run around and work off excess energy. Games are fine to play on long car trips—as long as they don't involve roughhousing to distract the driver. Counting out-of-state license plates makes time pass more quickly; or counting red barns, or blue convertibles, or white horses; or playing memory games or word games, if the children are old enough.

If young children want to bring a favorite toy on an auto trip, make sure that it is soft, with no sharp edges that could turn into a weapon if the car should stop suddenly.

If you want to have a snack on the road, don't eat in the car while it is moving. Pull off to the side and stop. This will give you a good rest break, and eliminates the danger of a child's getting his teeth knocked out on a pop bottle or choking on a piece of food when the car brakes to a sudden halt.

More people are killed and injured each year in motor vehicle accidents than for any other reason. While bad driving accounts for many accidents, mechanical problems are often at fault, too. Auto safety begins with making sure your car is in safe operating condition. Have your car inspected and tuned up periodically.

The American Automobile Association recommends that these items be checked, especially in the fall before winter snows begin:

1. Battery—fully charged.
2. Antifreeze—enough for zero weather.
3. Water hoses—tight and free from leaks.

4. Windshield—wipers and washer working.

5. Tires—front tires with tread, snow tires on rear.

6. Lights—all operating properly.

7. Heater and defroster—operating properly.

8. Brakes—properly adjusted.

9. Exhaust—free from leaks.

And remember, stopping on slick or icy surfaces requires nearly ten times the distance as stopping on dry roads. Lengthen the distance between your car and the car ahead of you in bad weather to give yourself room to stop. Pump the brakes up and down when you stop on slick roads, so that you'll have maximum steering control when the brakes are up and maximum stopping power when the brakes are down. If your car starts to skid, take your foot off the accelerator and steer the front wheels in the same direction as the rear of the car is skidding in. As soon as the car begins to come out of the skid, straighten the front wheels, being careful not to swing it around too far or too abruptly.

Here are some other pointers for pleasant and safe driving from the American Automobile Association:

1. Always signal far enough ahead for other drivers to anticipate your move.

2. Give full time and attention to your driving. Continually size up traffic around you by checking mirrors, and observing cars ahead of and beside you.

3. Always turn from the proper lanes. When moving to another lane, allow yourself plenty of room.

4. Stay in your lane and avoid lane weaving. Never straddle center line or lane markings.

5. Learn to recognize at a glance the meanings of standard traffic control signs, signals, and markings.

6. When driving at night, avoid looking directly at headlights of oncoming cars. Look instead at the right-hand edge of the roadway.

7. Remember that alcohol and driving do not mix; be alert for drivers who may have forgotten this.

8. Be courteous and tolerant to other drivers. If a driver passing you runs out of space, slow down to help him pass so as to avoid an accident in which you might be involved.

9. Watch for pedestrians who might step into your lane. Always yield the right-of-way to pedestrians.

10. Adjust your speed to existing traffic, road, and weather conditions. Reduce speed when visibility is low. Remember that visibility is poorest at dusk.

11. After passing another vehicle, return to your lane only after you can see the passed car in your rear-view mirror.

12. If a tire blows out, don't brake. Let up on the accelerator and grip the steering wheel firmly to keep the car in a straight path. Only when your car is under complete control should you apply the brakes gradually.

13. If you must stop your car, pull completely off the roadway as far away from traffic as possible.

14. On slippery road surfaces, make all maneuvers gradually. Avoid sudden starts, stops, and turns, which may result in skidding.

15. Skidding on curves can be avoided by braking and slowing down before, not after, you enter the curve. With foot on accelerator, maintain constant speed when rounding the curve.

16. If it is necessary to get out of your car on the traffic side, check traffic before opening the door.

17. You may be a safe driver, but to keep out of accidents, you must be on the alert for mistakes of other drivers.

Avitaminosis. When a person has a deficiency of vitamins in his diet, the condition is called avitaminosis. (*See* VITAMIN DEFICIENCIES; VITAMINS.)

Babies. In the United States, medical men use the word "infants" for humans not yet able to walk. However, the British often use the word "babies." (*See* INFANTS.)

Babinski Reflex. When the large toe straightens out upon stimulation or tickling of the sole of the foot, the phenomenon is known as Babinski's reflex. It is also called Babinski's toe sign. (*See* FOOT; TOES.)

Bacillus. Any of a vast number of rod-shaped bacteria are termed bacilli, the plural of bacillus. Such bacteria may be prevented from growing in food by heating the food to a sufficiently high temperature.

Bacteria in the bacillus category are responsible for a great number of diseases and infections, including tuberculosis, typhoid fever, and shigellosis. (*See* BACTERIA.)

Back. The human back is an exceedingly complex unit, but it is made of the same structures as the rest of the body: bones, ligaments, muscles, nerves, and blood vessels. However; it does contain one structure that no other part of the body has, the spinal cord.

The bones of the back are the hip, sacrum, vertebrae, ribs, and scapulae. The hipbones and sacrum unite to form the pelvis, which supports the upper half of the body and connects it to the legs. The vertebrae are the individual bones of the back, joined by ligaments which allow a slight bit of motion between each pair of vertebrae.

Intervertebral disks between the vertebrae also add to the amount of motion permitted, as well as cushioning the vertebrae against jolts and sudden movements. Although only slight motion is permitted at each intervertebral joint, the total amount of motion from the twenty-four joints is considerable. Most of it occurs in the cervi-cal (neck) and lumbar (low back) areas.

The twelve pairs of ribs form the rib cage, one rib coming from each side of the twelve thoracic vertebrae.

The scapulae, or shoulder blades, are triangular flat bones across the back at shoulder level; they form part of the shoulder joint. (*See* HIP; PELVIS; SACRUM; SPINE; VERTEBRA.)

The muscles of the back control the motions of the spine, and keep the spine stable when the arms are being used. These muscles are arranged in layers. Some are flat and broad, others short and thick. The muscles at the base of the back balance the back and provide stability. Paralysis of a muscle causes the back to bend away from that muscle. Spasm or overactivity of a muscle causes the back to bend toward it.

A strong, erect back is necessary to support the abdominal organs and allow them to function at their best. Exercising and gymnastics help to keep the back in good condition.

When the back is in a position of proper posture, it is not straight; rather there are characteristic front-to-back curves. (*See* CURVATURE OF THE SPINE; POSTURE.) Most backs also show some degree of side-to-side asymmetry, which increases with age or poor physical condition. When severe it is called scoliosis.

Because the back is so complex, many things can go wrong with it. Most of these can be prevented or made less severe by proper care. (*See* BACK CARE.) If a person's back is injured in any way, he will almost always have a backache. (*See* BACKACHE.)

Backache. From the time man's ancestors stopped walking on all fours and stood upright, he has had backaches due to a variety of causes. The basic reason, however, was that when man assumed a vertical position, only minor changes took place in his body, and great strain was put on his back.

Backache is a symptom, not a disease in itself. That is, backache always has a cause, usually an organic or mechanical dysfunction. On the other hand, it is second only to headache as a psychosomatic illness. (*See* PSYCHOSOMATIC MEDICINE.)

Because the genuineness of back disorders is often hard to prove or disprove, backache can be a form of malingering (pretending to be sick even after being cured). Because backache is so common, more quackery has been aimed at the back than at any other part of the body.

The cause of backache is often difficult to determine. A back which may appear very diseased, after physical examination and X rays, may produce no symptoms, while a back which appears healthy or only minimally damaged may produce excruciating pain. Thus the amount of pain may not actually indicate the severity of the condition. As we know, sensitivity to pain varies considerably between individuals and even from day to day in a particular person.

Backache can have many causes, from poor body mechanics to ruptured disks and degenerative changes in the spine. Injuries or diseases of the spine can produce both backache and spinal cord injury. The muscle-spasm pain that almost always accompanies injuries or diseases can occur by itself because of chronic anxiety—rather like a tension headache. Diseases of the abdominal organs can also cause pain that is referred to the back.

Poor posture does not just look bad: it puts a strain on the back and can interfere with organ function. (*See* POSTURE.) Overweight, particularly when the abdomen is large and protruding, can also strain the back. The lower part of the back is especially susceptible to mechanical injury from bending, twisting, and lifting. (*See* BACK CARE.)

Degenerative changes are brought about by normal activity or the aging process. Ruptured disks are thought to be a degener-

To avoid backaches, learn to lift correctly. Fig. 1 (*left*) shows the wrong way to lift—back and shoulder muscles may be strained. Fig. 2 (*right*) shows the correct way to lift—the legs bear the weight and push the body up.

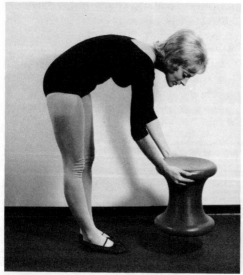 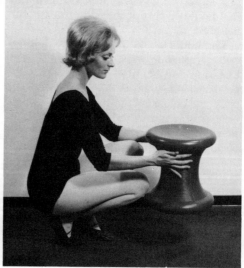

ative change made worse by bending or lifting. (*See* RUPTURED DISK.) They may cause irritation of the spinal cord, backache, and often sciatica. (*See* SCIATICA.) Changes in the bone, such as osteoporosis and Paget's disease, can result in crush or compression fractures of the vertebrae. (*See* OSTEOPOROSIS; PAGET'S DISEASE.) The pain in such a case is made worse by weight-bearing (standing or sitting) and is relieved by rest. Ankylosing spondylitis, gouty arthritis, spondylolisthesis, and spondylolysis can also cause backache. (*See* ANKYLOSING; ARTHRITIS; SPINAL INJURIES; SPONDYLITIS.)

If a person who has previously had no backache feels a sudden snapping or sharp pain when lifting or bending, this usually indicates a tearing of ligaments or muscles or a bit of bone broken off by muscle pull. Arthritis, muscle atrophy, and fatigue can predispose him to such injuries. Muscle spasm occurs immediately and may cause deformity or loss of motion. A pain that comes on gradually indicates some sort of inflammation. If a person's back is stiff after rest but limbers up with exercise, his pain is usually due to a rheumatic disease such as arthritis. If the pain is made worse by exercise and relieved by rest, it is probably due to mechanical injury.

Strains and sprains are a common kind of back injury. Strains are produced by overstretching of muscles, sprains by overstretching or tearing of ligaments. The two often occur together and are treated in the same way. The joints of the lower back are particularly subject to sprain. Certain conditions can predispose a person to strain and sprain: muscle weakness or fatigue, postures that put the muscles and ligaments in poor positions, and diseases such as arthritis.

Backache may also be due to visceral (organ) diseases. The pain is referred to the area of the back that is innervated by the same spinal nerve as the diseased organ. For example, aneurysm (bulging) or embolism (blocking) of the abdominal aortic artery can cause pain in the lumbar area. So can inflammation of the pancreas or prostate gland. Pain from these causes is not usually accompanied by loss of motion.

Backache is treated by medications and physical therapy to relieve the pain. The physical therapy usually begins with some form of heat, such as hot packs or hydrotherapy. (*See* HYDROTHERAPY; PHYSICAL THERAPY.) After the heat, the tense, aching muscles are massaged. (*See* MASSAGE.) This is usually followed by exercise. Strain can be taken off the back by the use of a brace or plaster cast. Of course, the underlying condition causing the backache is also treated.

Back Care. Because the back is such a complex structure, it is easily injured. Many injuries, however, can be prevented or made less serious by proper back care.

The basic principle of back care is to use proper posture at all times—when sitting, standing, or lying down. Proper sitting and standing posture is discussed under POSTURE. As for lying down, the first essential is a firm mattress which allows the shoulders and hips to sink in while the spine remains straight. But firm does not mean rigid. On a rigid mattress, the shoulders and hips cannot sink, so the spine bends. If you have a sagging mattress on your bed, there is no support for your spine, and it will sag too. So put a bed board under your mattress.

The back is particularly liable to injury when the muscles are fatigued, for in this condition, they can no longer support the back properly. You can avoid fatigue by being sure to eat a well-balanced diet and get plenty of rest and sleep. In any physical activity, take frequent breaks or change your position often to relieve the strain on your muscles. Remember that the muscles of the back perform best when they are kept strong and limber through exercise. Exercises should always be started gradually.

Doing too much with back muscles that are not in good condition can cause muscle strain or more serious injury.

High-heeled shoes change the posture of the body and put a great strain on the back. Women should wear them as little as possible. Overweight also places great strain on the back. Keep your back warm in cold weather to prevent muscle tenseness. Wear long jackets, sweaters, and underwear that cover the lower back and are snug enough to protect you from drafts. You may find that if your back and neck are warm, you will require less clothing on your arms and legs.

Regular physical examinations will reveal conditions that can cause back trouble and, if corrected in time, avert the trouble. Back conditions corrected early can prevent much damage. Consult a doctor at the first twinge in your back. Don't wait until the pain is too much to bear.

Many preventable back injuries occur in the home. Falls can be caused by highly polished floors, loose rugs, slippery bathtubs, and scattered items, such as toys and shoes, on stairs—all these hazards can be easily corrected. Ladders and other equipment should be kept in good repair and used properly.

Some household tasks, like vacuuming and bedmaking, are very hard on the back. A housewife should avoid them on days when her back is "acting up"; they will only aggravate the backache. Work surfaces such as kitchen counters should be at a comfortable working height, and should not require stretching or stooping.

Sports activities also contribute their share of back injuries. Pay attention to the safety rules for each particular sport. Follow such basic safety precautions as not diving into shallow water (check the depth), using safety bindings on skis, and not making head-down football tackles. Take lessons in the sport so you can do it properly. Give yourself a warm-up period before beginning active play. The muscular strains required may be more than cold, stiff muscles can handle.

Most back injuries occur when lifting things. A person should always lift with his leg muscles instead of his back. The muscles and bones of the legs are much stronger, and intended for work. The back, by contrast, is much more flexible and intended for mobility. Whenever you pick up anything, even a paper clip, always bend at the waist and knees. *Never* bend from the waist and use the back as if it were a hoist. It just is not made to withstand this sort of strain! Lift and carry objects close to the center of the body. Picking up objects by reaching across barriers is especially hard on the back—for example, opening a window by leaning across a radiator or lifting a bag of groceries out of a car trunk.

More cautions: If possible, stand to the side of the object to be lifted rather than facing it directly. Don't take heavy items such as books and suitcases off high shelves by reaching up over your head. Instead, use a step stool and get at least your head, preferably your shoulders, on a line with the object. Don't attempt to move furniture or other objects that are too heavy for you. When working with a partner, plan in advance how you will do the job, so neither of you gets stuck with an unexpected load.

With proper care, the back can perform all its functions without trouble and aches. Follow the above suggestions to ensure as pain-free a back as possible.

Bacteremia. The presence of bacteria in the bloodstream is called bacteremia. (*See* BACTERIA.) Almost any bacterial infection can seed the blood with bacteria. (*See* INFECTIONS.) Even the bacteria which normally inhabit the mouth can enter the bloodstream when the dentist repairs or pulls a tooth. Frequently an infected organ will spill bacteria into the blood after having been manipulated in some way.

Bacteria are divided into two large groups, depending on what color they are under a microscope after contact with a material called Gram's stain. Those which stain red are called gram-negative; those which stain blue or black are called gram-positive. The offenders in many cases of bacteremia are gram-negative. These organisms are introduced into the blood during urinary tract infections, infections of the bowel, and infections around the site of an intravenous needle. Birth, abortion, and infection of wounds, ulcers, or burns can also precipitate bacteremia. Gram-negative organisms have recently become more prominent since the advent of penicillin, which can usually control gram-positive organisms.

The common gram-negative organism which is often the offender is called *Escherichia coli*. It is a normal inhabitant of the bowel and the number-one cause of urinary tract infection. Gram-negative bacteria referred to as gonococci can cause bacteremia while they infect the female genital tract. Meningitis can be caused by a gram-negative organism called the meningococcus. (*See* MENINGITIS.) The entrance of this organism into the bloodstream (meningococcemia) results in a very serious illness that often ends in death.

Gram-positive bacteria can also enter the blood. A disease of the heart valves called bacterial endocarditis can result when some gram-positive bacteria infest the bloodstream. These bacteria are usually in the streptococcus or staphylococcus group of organisms. Pneumonia is often caused by a gram-positive bacteria, the pneumococcus, which during this type of pneumonia will frequently enter the bloodstream.

When patients with bacteremia show severe symptoms, the condition is called septicemia. The onset is often marked by an episode of shaking chills followed by a fever of 101° to 105° F. At first, the white blood count may be low, but after six to twelve hours it rises to an above-normal level. (*See* TESTS.) Often the blood pressure will fall and even a shocklike state may occur. Small bruises or a rash may sometimes appear.

The real danger of most bacteremia is a condition known as septic shock. Many bacteria (especially gram-negative ones) release powerful chemicals which are toxic to human tissues. These alter the blood vessels to such an extent that the patient's blood pressure drops. If the blood pressure falls so low that the vital organs will be unable to get their blood supply, the result is death. Approximately 40 to 80 percent of patients who go into septic shock die. The key to preventing this is early diagnosis of severe infection and prompt treatment with the proper antibiotic. (*See* ANTIBIOTIC.) If bacteremia is prevented, septic shock will not occur.

Bacteria. Tiny, single-celled plants which can be seen only under a microscope or a magnifying glass are called bacteria. They reproduce by fission; that is, each cell splits in half to form two completely new organisms.

The shape of bacteria varies from round to rod-shaped and they grow in clumps, chains, pairs, or singly. Sometimes they are equipped to move about—i.e., for motility. When grown on an artificial medium they form colonies visible to the naked eye.

There are many, many kinds of bacteria but only a few are dangerous to humans. These, known as pathogens, are responsible for some of our most serious infectious diseases. Tuberculosis, diphtheria, gonorrhea, typhoid fever, pneumonia, and tetanus (lockjaw) are but a few of the systemic infections caused by pathogenic bacteria. Among the numerous bacterial skin infections are syphilis, leprosy, boils, impetigo, folliculitis, erysipelas, and scarlet fever. In addition, secondary bacterial infections may complicate the treatment of other skin diseases.

Bacteria may be classified according to the shape of the cells, and also their pattern of growth. A spherical or elliptical bacterial cell is usually termed a coccus, an example of which is the *Gonococcus* responsible for gonorrhea. The cells of other bacteria are rod-shaped and relatively straight. Such a rod-shaped organism may be called a bacillus. The bacterium responsible for diphtheria, *Corynebacterium diphtheriae,* is a bacillus. Other common bacteria are long and spirally curving, such as *Spirillum.*

The cocci, which are responsible for over 90 percent of all skin infections, are subdivided according to the arrangement and grouping of the bacterial cells. Those which form rows of cells resembling a chain of beads are known as streptococci. When the cells remain in pairs after splitting they are known as diplococci. When the cells remain in irregular masses resembling clusters of grapes, the name used is staphylococcus.

Staphylococci and streptococci are pus-producing bacteria that produce the infections commonly referred to as pyodermas. Among the most common pyodermas are impetigo, folliculitis, furuncles, erysipelas, and ecthyma.

Bacteriologist. Specialists in the field of biology who study the microscopic life forms called bacteria are bacteriologists (*See* BACTERIA), generally holding degrees from a B.S. up to a Ph.D. There are also physicians and veterinarians who later specialize in bacteriology by taking postgraduate work.

A bacteriologist may do research, may teach others in college, or may work in applied bacteriology. In the applied bacteriology field, he may work with disease prevention as a sanitary bacteriologist, or as a pathological bacteriologist, working with bacteria that cause disease in man and animals.

Bad Breath. Unpleasant odors of the mouth, or bad breath, arise from many causes. The general term for bad breath is halitosis. (*See* HALITOSIS.)

Bagassosis. A respiratory disorder caused by inhalation of dust of bagasse during sugar cane or paper manufacturing is called bagassosis. (*See* ALLERGY; DUST; OCCUPATIONAL HEALTH; PNEUMOCONIOSIS; SILICOSIS.)

Bag of Waters. During pregnancy the developing infant (fetus) is protected by membranes (thin layers of tissue) filled with fluid in which he floats and moves. This is popularly called the bag of waters, but in medicine it is known as the amniotic sac. Normally it may hold as much as a pint or quart (500–1,000 cc.) of fluid during pregnancy, but the amount varies widely from one mother to another.

The bag of waters cushions the fetus from possible injury, such as a bump or blow to the mother's abdomen. The effect is much like trying to hit an object which is inside a strong balloon filled with water.

CHORION. The amniotic sac, or amnion, is covered by a second membrane. This outer layer is called the chorion. Its external surface touches the greatly thickened wall of the uterus (womb) itself. By the fourth month of pregnancy the bag of waters is about the size of a large orange and fills the uterus, which has begun to stretch.

AMNIOTIC FLUID. The "water" contained in the amnion is the amniotic fluid, or liquor amnii. The fluid surrounds the developing infant, providing lubrication to give it more freedom of movement than it would have in a dry environment. It also helps keep the fetus at a safe, even temperature.

In addition, the growing fetus drinks some of the amniotic fluid, providing a material to pass through his digestive and urinary tracts during prenatal development. Part of the fluid is also absorbed through his lungs.

In a continuous process, the water in the amniotic fluid is replaced completely every three hours, apparently through the amniotic membranes. The fluid contains the electrolyte minerals sodium and potassium, which also are replaced every three hours. (*See* ELECTROLYTES.)

MEMBRANES IN CHILDBIRTH. During labor, the amniotic and chorionic membranes must break to release the amniotic fluid and aid the birth of the infant. However, it also is possible for them to burst before labor begins.

In some cases, the rupture of the membranes is the first sign that labor has begun. It may be followed by only a few drops of liquid, or by a rush of watery outflow.

Mothers in the late stages of pregnancy should be careful to distinguish this from urinary leakage caused by pressure of the fetal head on the bladder. Any passage of blood should be reported immediately to the doctor.

Most of the time the membranes do not open until after labor has begun, usually in the last stages before the infant is born. In fact, sometimes the membranes remain intact so that the physician must open them to aid delivery of the infant.

Premature Rupture. If the membranes rupture early, labor usually begins soon. When the pregnancy is near term (forty weeks), labor may start within a few hours. If more than twenty-four hours pass there is a greater chance of infection (amnionitis), as bacteria enter through the membrane opening. Extra precautions must be taken to prevent this. The mother should avoid tub baths, douching, and sexual intercourse. If amnionitis should occur, the child must be delivered soon to protect it from the spreading infection. (*See* CESAREAN SECTION; INDUCTION OF LABOR.)

There also is greater likelihood that the umbilical cord may become prolapsed. That is, if the membranes burst before the birth canal is completely blocked by the arriving infant, the gush of fluid may wash part of the cord out past the baby. Later downward pressure or movement of the infant's head or body may pinch the cord and shut off the flow of blood carrying vital nutrients and oxygen. (*See* UMBILICAL CORD.)

Breech birth is more common when the membranes rupture early. The infant may not yet have turned to a head-down position, and may be born with the feet or hips first. If birth can be delayed, the baby may shift naturally into a better position.

When the membranes rupture before the thirty-sixth week of pregnancy (a month or more early), there is more likely to be a premature birth. The baby's chances can be improved if birth can be postponed. (*See* PREMATURE BIRTHS.) The mother is usually kept in bed, precautions are taken to avoid amnionitis, and so on. If necessary, antibiotics may be used to counteract infection.

Physicians used to be more worried than they are now about a so-called "dry birth"—that is, childbirth after the membranes have ruptured and released all the amniotic fluid prematurely. Actually, there is little danger of the infant's becoming "stuck" in a dry amniotic sac. The membranes continue manufacturing about a pint of fluid per hour, which flows around the infant and then out.

Baldness.　When hair falls out and is not replaced by new hair growth, the result is baldness.

The most common type is "male pattern baldness," which accounts for about 95 percent of all cases of baldness in men. This type has a characteristic pattern and course that make it easy to diagnose. It usually begins at the temples with a receding hairline that eventually assumes the shape of the letter M. Sometimes it begins at the crown, forming a bald area known as a "monk's spot." Eventually the receding hairline and balding crown may meet and leave only a thin fringe of hair around the head.

Male pattern baldness may begin early in the twenties—even, in a few cases, the teens. More often it is a condition of middle age, though a few men never lose any hair.

The exact cause of male pattern baldness is not known. Sex, age, and heredity are all involved and there isn't anything we can do about any of them: the baldness is permanent and incurable. Treatments and products that claim to prevent baldness or regrow hair are a waste of money because they are totally ineffective. The only effective treatments are (1) concealing the bald spots with hairpieces and (2) redistributing the remaining hairs through a surgical procedure known as hair transplantation.

While women do not become bald as men do, their hair generally thins with age. The hairline may recede slightly, as in male pattern baldness, with a diffuse thinning over the crown and the front of the scalp. This hair loss is sometimes called "female pattern baldness." However, obvious bald spots do not develop, and most women retain sufficient hair to provide adequate coverage.

Women with female pattern baldness usually have female ancestors with "thinning" hair in their family history. Thus the baldness seems to be related to age and heredity, like male pattern baldness. For women, too, the condition is permanent and incurable.

The most practical remedy for a woman whose hair becomes excessively thin is a wig. Since wigs have become fashionable and are available at modest cost, no one will know that the wig is being worn out of necessity.

Other types of hair loss and baldness occur, but they are usually temporary and are not patterned. Such hair loss may be produced by infections, systemic diseases, some scalp disorders, pregnancy, and certain drugs. Temporary baldness may also be the result of mechanical stress, traction, or friction exerted on the hair for prolonged periods.

Hair loss after pregnancy is not uncommon. It may begin toward the end of pregnancy or immediately after childbirth, but most often several months later. This type of hair loss ordinarily will cease after a few months and normal regrowth will begin.

Infections which may cause temporary baldness include ringworm of the scalp (tinea), bacterial infections, and viral infections such as herpes. Among systemic diseases which can lead to baldness are advanced diabetes, influenza, scarlet fever, syphilis, pituitary disorders, leukemia, and cancer. Drugs used for the treatment of some diseases may cause hair loss as a side effect.

Certain chemicals have a toxic effect on hair and act as depilatories (hair removers). For example, thallium, a chemical found in some insecticides and rat-killers, will cause loss of hair if swallowed by accident. Years ago some cosmetic depilatories contained thallium as the active ingredient, but its use is no longer permitted because it can be absorbed through the skin and cause serious harm.

Certain hair styles which exert prolonged traction on the hair can produce temporary baldness by literally pulling the hairs out by the roots. Girls who wear tight pony tails or braids sometimes develop this type of hair loss.

Babies can develop a temporary bald spot on the back of the head. The friction produced by rubbing the head against bedding causes hairs to break off close to the scalp. Bald spots of this sort also occur in adults whose work gear or rough clothing produces friction.

Perhaps the most unusual, distressing form of baldness is alopecia areata. In this disease bald patches suddenly appear on the scalp and occasionally on other hairy areas such as the beard, underarm regions, eyelashes, and eyebrows. A person may awaken one morning and find small heaps of hair on his pillow and one or more circular bald spots on his scalp. Often other spots form on distant or adjacent parts of the scalp. The cause of alopecia areata is unknown and there is no cure. Fortunately, the hair generally regrows.

The temporary forms of hair loss are either self-correcting or are treated by removing the underlying cause of the baldness (for example, curing ringworm or changing the hair style). Well-advertised hair-restoring preparations and treatments will not be any more effective for these forms of hair loss than they are for male pattern baldness. (*See* HAIR; HAIR CARE.)

Bandages. Any strip of cloth, or other kind of dressing such as gauze, which is used to bind a wound or cover an injury, is a bandage. Bandages help control bleeding and protect against contamination.

A bandage may be as simple as the kind packaged commercially that consists of a strip of tape with a piece of sterile gauze in the center. These are generally adequate for scratches and shallow wounds.

For more serious wounds and burns, however, it is important to know how to devise sterile bandages with supplies that should be available around the house or in the home first-aid kit.

PRESSURE BANDAGE. In cases of severe bleeding, apply a pressure bandage directly to the wound. Hold a sterile gauze pad, or several folds of any available material such as a cloth or a soft piece of clothing, tightly on the injured area. The pressure squeezing the blood vessels against tissue, muscles, or bone should stop the flow of blood. After the bleeding stops, apply a bandage compress, being careful not to make it so tight that it cuts off circulation.

BANDAGE COMPRESS. For burns and for wounds too large or too deep for small adhesive strip bandages, a bandage compress should be used. Sterile bandage compresses come in sizes ranging from two to four inches wide, and may be bought at the drugstore. They consist of a thick gauze pad sewed to a strip of gauze or muslin. A bandage compress may be fashioned at home by putting a gauze pad on the wound and securing the pad with adhesive or a gauze roller bandage.

GAUZE PADS. Perhaps the handiest item in a home first-aid kit is a package of three-inch-square gauze pads. A gauze pad may be used as a pressure bandage to control bleeding, and as a dressing applied over a wound and attached with adhesive strips or a gauze roller bandage.

GAUZE ROLLER BANDAGE. Strips of sterilized gauze, which come in rolls about ten yards long and in widths of one, two, or three inches, are excellent for bandaging wounds on extremities. The strips may be easily wound over irregularly shaped joints, such as elbows, knees, and fingers. Although a roller bandage should be secured by adhesive tape, if tape is unavailable, the gauze may be torn or cut at the closing end into two strips which then are wrapped around the extremity and tied into a knot. Wrap and tie once again for a more secure bandage.

SPLINT AND SLING. When a bone has been broken, care should be taken not to move the limb unnecessarily until a doctor can set it. You may apply a splint to keep the limb immobile until professional help is available. A splint may be made from any sturdy, unbending material—wood, heavy cardboard, plastic strips—long enough to reach beyond the joint nearest the fracture.

Tie the splint with cloth at three points: at the fracture, above it, and below it. Be careful not to cut off the circulation.

For arm fractures, a sling made of a three-cornered piece of cloth helps limit movement after a splint has been put in place. (*See* SLING.)

TRIANGLE BANDAGE. Because it is so versatile, a triangle bandage is an essential item in any home first-aid kit. It may be used as a sling, as a tourniquet, or as a dressing. A good size for a triangle bandage is fifty-five inches along the base and thirty-six inches along the sides.

TOURNIQUET. Never use a tourniquet to stop bleeding unless the victim is hemorrhaging so severely that bleeding cannot be controlled by the application of a pressure bandage. If a large artery has been severed, or a limb amputated, a tourniquet may be the victim's only chance for life. But

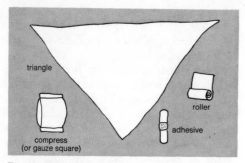

Four types of bandages.

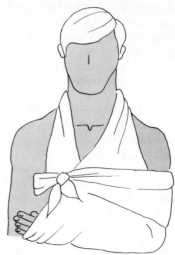

An arm sling may be made from a triangular bandage. Tie two ends of the triangle together behind the neck, draw the third end around, and tie or pin in the front.

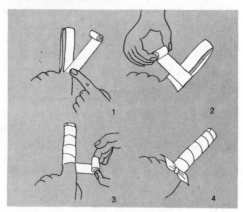

Steps in applying the finger bandage.

Spiral reverse forearm bandage. Start by making several turns to anchor the bandage, then make a spiral turn every time you make a wrap around the arm. With care you can make a flat, snug bandage. Overlap one-third or more of the width of the bandage.

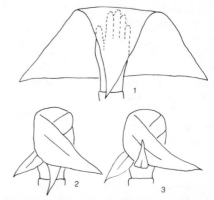

Triangular bandaging of the hand. Place hand on bandage, then fold down point of triangle. Bring ends around, fold up point of triangle, then complete by bringing ends around hand and tying with a square knot.

Steps in applying the figure-of-eight bandage to the ankle.

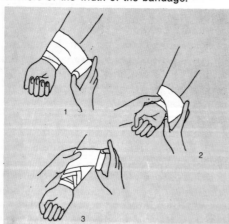

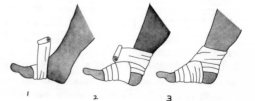

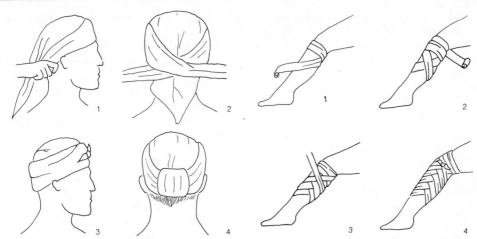

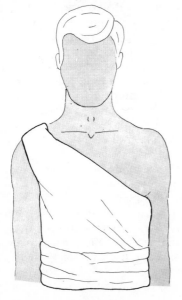

Triangular bandaging of the head. Place the triangular bandage so that one point hangs down over the back of the neck. Bring the other two ends around and tie at the forehead. Then fold up and tuck the point of the bandage around the other two tightened ends at the back of the head.

The figure-of-eight bandage is useful for bandaging the leg or the arm. First make several circular turns to anchor the bandage. Then criss-cross as you overlap the bandage slightly. Finish by tying with a square knot. The last illustration shows how the bandage may be brought over the bend of the knee.

Triangle bandage for the chest. Cover the chest with the bandage as shown at left. One point of the triangle is over the shoulder, and the other two are under the arm. Tie two ends around the back so that one strip remains longer than the other. Tie the long end to the point of the bandage hanging over the shoulder. For a back bandage, cover the back with the flat of the bandage, and tie in the front.

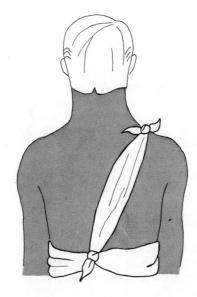

these are the only instances where the use of a tourniquet is justified. (*See* BLEEDING.)

The danger in applying a tourniquet is that it may injure the skin or tissues around the wound. Or it may entirely cut off the blood supply to the lower part of the affected extremity, inviting gangrene and perhaps eventually necessitating amputation.

A tourniquet should be made of flat material, such as stockings or a belt or a wide piece of cotton, rather than of rope or similar material that will cut into the skin. Wrap the flat material around the bleeding limb twice tightly and tie a half knot. The material should be placed two to four inches above the wound.

Place a short, thick stick or similar object on the half knot and tie a full knot. Twist the stick to tighten the tourniquet until blood stops flowing. Then tie the stick in place with the ends of the tourniquet or with another strip of material. The tourniquet should be secure yet loose enough for a finger to fit under.

The tourniquet should not be removed until the victim is under the care of a doctor or other medical personnel who know how to control hemorrhage and replace blood. (*See* TOURNIQUET.)

Banti's Syndrome. An enlargement of the spleen (congestive splenomegaly) associated with deficiency of red and white blood cells is also known as Banti's syndrome. (*See* SPLEEN.)

Barber's Itch. Years ago infections involving the beard were spread by contaminated shaving articles and towels in barber shops.

That is why such infections today are often called barber's itch. State laws which govern sanitation in barber shops have mostly controlled the original source of barber's itch. Nowadays the term usually refers to bacterial infections (sycosis barbae) of the beard.

Sometimes fungus infections of the beard (tinea barbae) are also called barber's itch. (*See* TINEA.)

In sycosis barbae, red, inflamed sores filled with pus form around hair follicles—the skin depressions from which hairs grow. This condition, which is more common among men who wear mustaches and beards, occurs most frequently on the upper lip, but the chin and neck region are often involved.

If neglected, sycosis barbae may get much worse and become chronic and difficult to cure. Early treatment almost always cures it, also preventing destruction of the hair roots and scarring. Although antibiotics are the preferred treatment, various other treatments are also used. Hot, wet compresses or dressings made by dipping soft cloths or gauze pads in solutions of boric acid can be applied to the skin and will help the inflammation.

Shaving can usually be continued while the disease is being treated, but a brushless shaving cream should be used (so the brush won't reinfect the beard) and the razor should be dipped in alcohol before each shave.

Barbiturate Poisoning. When taken under a doctor's supervision, barbiturates and other drugs are relatively safe, but because the therapeutic (helpful) range of a drug is very close to the toxic range, many persons experience an adverse reaction. Due to different bodily rates of absorption, metabolism, excretion, or susceptibility to the action of a drug, a barbiturate may cause an unexpected excessive sedation effect.

Toxic reactions to barbiturates are varied, depending upon the type of barbiturate taken. They may or may not be associated with the size of the dose or how long the drug is taken. Many deaths are due to the short-acting barbiturates, whereas few have been linked to the slow-acting ones such as phenobarbital. (*See* ADDICTION; BARBITURATES; DRUG ABUSE.)

Barbiturates. The "sleepers," or depressants, are a wide range of drugs which were first medically introduced in 1903 to induce sleep. Since that time, almost two thousand different barbiturates have been manufactured, each being assigned a name ending in the letters *al:* secobarbital, pentobarbital, amobarbital, phenobarbital, and so on.

Prescribed as tranquilizers and sedatives, they depress the nervous system so as to eliminate fear, anxiety, and excitement. The barbiturates are reported to be the number-one drug of addiction and of suicide (from overdoses).

Depressant drugs produce both physical and psychological dependence. If addiction occurs and the drug is then suddenly withdrawn, the effects of the withdrawal process from barbiturates can be more dangerous than those from narcotics. A period of restlessness, anxiety, fear, and tremor is followed by hours of nausea, vomiting, and abdominal pain. On the second and third day after withdrawal has begun, severe convulsions can occur. Barbiturate abusers usually recover from these, but some have recurring delirium, hallucinations, and exhaustion.

A person who takes barbiturates over a long period of time will have slurred speech, a staggering walk, and loss of coordination. He will be sluggish, emotionally unstable, depressed, and may lapse into a coma.

An overdose of a barbiturate—a common occurrence—may result in death. Children may die accidentally from barbiturates not kept out of their reach. Also fatal is the mixing of barbiturates and alcohol, which depresses the respiratory system. (*See* ADDICTION; DRUG ABUSE.)

Barium. This chemical is a metallic element which occurs in minerals in combination with other elements. Barium sulfate is a nonpoisonous, insoluble, white powder used as a pigment in paints, printing inks, and medicines. A "barium cocktail" is given a patient before an X ray because barium is opaque (does not permit passage of X rays) and therefore allows the physician to perceive the digestive tract. (*See* X RAY.)

Barium carbonate is a heavy, odorless, and tasteless compound which is toxic to rats in small doses, soluble in the hydrochloric acid of the stomach, and in large doses lethal to most animals and man.

Bartholin's Glands and Ducts. Located beside the female vagina are the small, paired Bartholin's glands. They secrete mucous materials that aid lubrication during sexual stimulation. They are believed to be similar to the Cowper's glands in the male. (*See* COWPER'S GLANDS.)

Each of the tiny Bartholin's glands empties through a duct running down along the side of the vagina and opening into a fold between the hymen and the labia minor. (*See* FEMALE ANATOMY.)

When one or both ducts or glands become infected, the condition is called Bartholinitis. Large quantities of pus are secreted so that the ducts, and sometimes even the glands, become red and swollen. Drainage becomes blocked, and the ducts can be felt along the side of the vagina. Sometimes so much pus collects that the entire labia are swollen. Periodic swelling on either side of the entrance to the vagina causes pain, especially during sexual relations. The infection may clear up, only to recur by itself or through reinfection. Each recurrent infection further enlarges the Bartholin's duct and causes local tenderness. It can occur in one duct at a time, causing swelling only on one side, or can involve both ducts. Occasionally it may even spread into the glands themselves.

Local heat packs and broad-spectrum antibiotics usually cure the infection. The cause may be the venereal disease of gonorrhea or other infection.

In extreme cases an abscess may develop

that must be opened surgically for drainage. The duct itself may need to be reopened and cleaned after the infection is cured. Physicians must also check the possibility that the passage may be blocked by an inclusion cyst, that is, a sac of fluid or semisolid material inside another sac or passage. This is especially possible after the vulvar tissue is torn or cut surgically during childbirth.

Blocking of the Bartholin's duct also may be caused by large sebaceous cysts, hydradenoma (tumor), or a physical defect tracing back to the woman's own birth. Cancer of the Bartholin's duct or gland is rare.

Basal Metabolism. Metabolism simply means the total of all chemical reactions occurring in the body. (*See* METABOLISM.) In order to compare one person's metabolism with normal values, it is measured while he is at rest. This resting level of metabolism is called the basal metabolism.

As a result of the chemical reactions in the body (the metabolism), heat is given off. The rate at which it is given off is the metabolic rate. Heat production and therefore metabolic rate can be measured directly in a device called a calorimeter, but this is awkward to do. Instead, the exact amount of oxygen used by the patient over a given period of time is measured by a device with an oxygen supply and mouthpiece called a metabolimeter. We know that the body produces 4.825 calories of heat for each liter of oxygen it uses. Therefore, if we measure the amount of oxygen a person uses, we can easily calculate the heat produced by his body.

The measurement of the basal metabolic rate (BMR) must be done while the patient is at absolute rest, but awake. He must not have eaten any food for twelve hours before the test, and must have had a full night of restful sleep. The person must lie perfectly quiet for thirty minutes before the basal metabolic rate is determined, and any form of excitement during the test must be eliminated. The temperature of the room must be kept constant, somewhere between 62° and 87° F.

Once the patient's BMR is determined it is compared with normal values. The test results are considered normal if they fall in the range from 10 percent below to 10 percent above the standard.

Various thyroid gland disorders that result in the production of large amounts of thyroid hormone, will increase the basal metabolic rate; so will tuberculosis of the lung and fever-producing disorders.

The BMR has not been used recently to diagnose thyroid disease since better tests have become available. (*See* THYROID TESTS.)

Basedow's Disease. An excessive functioning of the thyroid gland, characterized by an increased basal metabolism, is known as Basedow's disease, or, more popularly, as hyperthyroidism. (*See* HYPERTHYROIDISM.)

Basophil. Certain components of structure cells of blood are known as basophils. (*See* BLOOD CELLS; LEUKOCYTES.)

Baths. The technical definition of a bath might be something like this: "Immersion of the body or body parts into a fluid medium (usually water) for therapeutic reasons." The purpose of a bath may be to cleanse, to soothe, to stimulate, to warm, or to cool the body. A body part after injury may be immersed in a cold bath (water temperature about 50° F. or 10° C.) to reduce swelling. A continuous warm tub bath (water temperature about 95° F. or 35° C.) is often used to calm an agitated patient. A bed bath or sponge bath is given to a patient in his own bed. A bath given in a special tub which allows immersion of only the patient's lower back, hips, and thighs is called a sitz bath. Warm baths are often used in physical therapy to increase the blood supply to a certain body region and to relieve muscle soreness. (*See* PHYSICAL THERAPY.) Many skin diseases respond well to frequent soaking in water or some other liquid. (*See* SKIN.) Muscle stiffness and joint injuries are often treated in a hot bath of whirling or churning water called a whirlpool bath. (*See* WHIRLPOOL BATHS.)

Battered Child Syndrome.

In two recent consecutive years, there were 12,610 physically abused children scattered throughout the United States. (Many others, of course, were not reported.) Over one-fourth of them were under two years of age; almost half were over six years; nearly one-fifth were teenagers. All were victims of the battered child syndrome—a condition in which children are roughly handled by adults. This syndrome is now recognized as a significant cause of failure to grow, of disability, and sometimes even of death. (*See* GROWTH RETARDATION.)

Investigation of families in which children have been repeatedly injured or beaten show that many of the offending parents (or parent-substitutes) are of low intelligence; others are alcoholic, sexually promiscuous, unstable, immature, self-centered, or impulsive. They may have poor control of their aggressive feelings, or may psychologically reject the child. On the other hand, this syndrome is also found among people with stable financial and social backgrounds. Here, too, a defect in character structure accounts for the free expression of aggressive impulses.

In most states, private or hospital physicians are now required by law to report any instances of suspected willfully inflicted injury among their child patients. If it seems probable that a child will continue to be battered, steps should be taken to remove him from the home. Perhaps legal action will be necessary. (*See* MENTAL HEALTH.)

BCG.

Known in the medical world as Bacillus Calmette Guérin, BCG was developed in 1927 by Camille Guérin and Leon Calmette, bacteriologists. BCG is a prophylactic (preventive) antituberculosis vaccine. (*See* TUBERCULOSIS.)

Bedbugs.

The bedbug has become far less familiar than it was a few generations ago, at least in some parts of the world. It has not disappeared, but in those areas of the temperate zone where there is a higher standard of living and better sanitation, the bedbug is no longer likely to be a part of daily (or nightly) experience. It can still be found in an occasional motel, a few bad cheap hotels, and more than a few rooming houses, camp buildings, and poultry sheds.

Today the very idea of the bedbug may seem repellent—a red-brown insect that eats blood by thrusting out a segmented nose to stab down through the skin and suck. Its body is covered thickly with a stubble of bristly hairs; it sucks and engorges itself on blood for minutes at a time; emits a foul odor; and leaves behind a black tarry excrement.

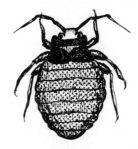

BEDBUG

The bedbug does not seem to be a carrier of disease, germs or parasites, either human or animal. (*See* INSECT BITES.) Neither is the bedbug necessarily the result of unsanitary conditions. Bedbugs are found in filth, but may also be found in clean surroundings. They require only some form of transportation—a suitcase, a package, secondhand furniture, or a basket of laundry. If there is no suitable conveyance, and they are hungry, bedbugs will travel long distances to get to their host sources of food.

The bedbug is related to many common insects, such as stinkbugs, plant lice, giant water bugs, leafhoppers, cicadas, and various kinds that feed on bats and on birds ranging from the swallow to condor. Varied though they are, all are alike in one way: they suck the vital juices from their plant or animal hosts. This is not stinging, as done by the wasp or bee, but puncturing with a sharp, sucking, noselike extension and drinking for minutes at a time. Although each of these bugs has its favorite victims, they are not choosy about tapping other species as well. Plant suckers will bite humans; bedbugs will go after animals; and bird bugs will attack man.

Bedbugs can betray their presence by their unpleasant smell, an odor from secretions of a scent gland. They are nocturnal feeders, but this does not mean they will feed only during the nighttime hours. Light itself, plus the perspiring attractiveness of the host, seem to be the decisive conditions. Bedbugs will come out of their hiding places and bite during the day if light is subdued.

Since they are small (about 2/10 in. long by 1/10 in. wide [5 by 2.5 mm.]) and so flat, large numbers of bedbugs can hide in the skimpiest space in the most unlikely locations. They congregate in large numbers, and masses of them can fit into cracks in plaster, along the joint between baseboard and wall; in the welts and tufts of mattresses; in the upholstery of chairs and in the joints of wooden bedsteads; in cracks around window frames; and behind wallpaper.

Bedbugs do not feed frequently. They can go months or even a year without food. But when they do feed they engorge themselves. A single feeding may take ten minutes. They then crawl back into their hiding places and spend perhaps several days digesting the blood. Over a period of time these mass congregating places become coated and thick with the black tarry excretion of the bugs, the digested remains of blood.

From hatching to maturity may take as little as a month or as much as four months. Going through five stages of increasing maturity, lasting a week or more each, the bedbug must eat at each stage to bring it to the next. This means at least five feedings in a lifetime. In each of the stages the bug molts, and at the last stage it grows rudimentary stub wings.

If temperature conditions allow, the female can produce at least three generations in a year. Bedbugs are sensitive to temperature and humidity, and the females are most productive at the fairly warm temperature of 70° F. (21° C.) or higher. Below 50° F. (10° C.) they lay no eggs.

The eggs are easy to see—pale yellow, large, laid at the rate of about three a day in groups of ten to fifty, until the female has deposited a broad mass of two hundred to five hundred. Hatching, again, varies with temperature. It may be as soon as four days or as long as three weeks, but most often is six to ten days.

As with other insects, not everyone reacts in the same way to the bites of bedbugs. Some persons feel hardly anything. Others have sore swellings, caused by local infection or an allergic reaction to the bedbug's saliva.

Once bedbugs have been located and their hiding places found, these pests can be eliminated without too much difficulty. Every possible nook, crack, and crevice in floors, walls, ceiling, and furniture should be suspect. Bedbugs will pack by the thousands behind loose wallpaper. This must be peeled away to get at them and their eggs. Metal furniture should not be exempted from the search; if it has cracks or hollow legs or hidden surfaces, it can harbor bugs.

Bedbugs are killed by at least two natural enemies, temperature and humidity, and a number of man-made conditions. If humidity is high they die at temperatures of

100° F. (38° C.) or more. When it is in the mid-50's or colder, the bugs stop crawling, feeding, and laying eggs. Local attacks on cracks, loose wallpaper, and furniture with household insect sprays is a good start in eradicating the pests. Successful general attacks on whole rooms or buildings include fumigating with sulfur candles and insecticides, and heating to temperatures well over 100° F. (38° C.) for several hours at a time. (*See* PESTICIDES.)

Next should come removal of the dead bugs, a thorough scrubbing, and then a regular schedule of cleaning and inspection to ensure that these visitors do not return.

Beds.   The average healthy person probably gives little thought to the bed on which he sleeps, but the bed is medically important in several ways. A soft, low-slung bed may seem adequate to many people, but poor support for the lower back during sleep can put undue stress on the lumbar spine and cause backache. (*See* BACKACHE; SPINE.) The best sleeping surface is a firm mattress, which offers support for the lower spine.

The hospitalized patient usually finds himself in a bed equipped with a special mechanism that allows its contour to be changed. Either by hand or electrical control the head or foot of the bed can be raised or lowered; the entire bed can be tilted and raised up and down. Not only does this variation in position add to the comfort of the patient, but certain disorders are treated by elevation of the feet or head.

Several specialized beds are sometimes used in the hospital. One which is designed to protect the postoperative patient and allow for his care is called an ether bed. A patient with broken bones may be placed in a fracture bed, which is fitted with traction equipment. A Fisher bed is used in the treatment of various disorders of the spine.

Patients who are forced to stay in bed for long periods of time may develop bedsores.

(*See* BEDSORES.) An air mattress placed beneath the sheets often helps prevent these. Also beneficial is a special rubber mattress filled with water, known as an Arnoth's bed.

Bedside Care.   The service rendered a bedridden patient by a nurse or nurse's aide is called bedside care. It includes bed baths, back rubs, changing bed sheets, supplying bedpans, and any other service which will make the patient more comfortable. The art of providing good bedside care is a vital part of the nurse's training. (*See* NURSING CARE.) Good bedside care can improve the patient's mood and ease the tedium and discomfort of his hospital stay.

Bedsores.   Decubitus ulcers, commonly known as pressure sores or bedsores, are a distressing complication for the bedridden patient. Hospital personnel and physicians spend a great deal of time and effort preventing and treating these painful and serious skin lesions.

The problem is due to a combination of factors. It is most likely to occur when a patient is very weak, paralyzed, or unconscious, and thus unable to change his position in bed from time to time. In normal sleep the healthy person will turn one way or another perhaps two to three dozen times during the night. If a hospital patient will not or cannot move his body sufficiently, the nurse must help him. In many hospitals it is the practice to turn the patient at least once an hour.

Continued pressure on the skin or fat tissue overlying bony prominences impairs the blood supply and nutrition of the tissues. The first signs of bedsores are erythema, or reddening of the skin. If the condition is not arrested, the skin darkens or takes on a bluish cast. Necrosis (tissue death) occurs, and the skin and tissue slough off. The ulcers may deepen even to the bone.

Maceration of the skin—softening by soaking—must be avoided. Bed sheets wet from perspiration or urine must be changed as soon and as often as possible. This is important if the bedsores are to be healed or kept from worsening. Wrinkles in the sheets irritate the condition, so careful bed-making is essential. Plastic sheeting instead of rubber under the cloth coverings is recommended when the mattress needs protection.

Special mattresses, sponge pads, inflated plastic pillows and rings, and other devices to relieve pressure are used in hospitals, and may be obtained in drug or hospital supply stores for home use. Rolled blankets or pillows are handy to place under the patient's knees to shift pressure, or for propping the patient on his side.

Bedsores are often complicated by infections, which may be treated with antibiotics. Special absorbent bandages are also used. Surgical removal of loose skin and tissue may be necessary. In some cases, the decubitus ulcer areas require skin grafts.

Careful attention to washing and drying the skin and the use of a dusting powder will help prevent or retard bedsores. The bed patient should be given a balanced diet, as poor nutrition will increase the danger of necrosis of tissues. (*See* NUTRITION.)

Bedwetting. The medical name for bedwetting is enuresis, which means unintentional or unconscious wetting during sleep by a person over the age of three. When the child or adult urinates involuntarily during waking hours also, the problem is known as incontinence. (*See* URINARY INCONTINENCE.)

In both cases, the cause of the problem can be either physical or emotional. Of the two enuresis is usually the milder problem and is easier to cure, since the patient still has control during conscious waking hours and loses it only when asleep.

PHYSICAL CAUSES. Among the physical causes of enuresis are various infections and inflammation of the urinary tract—surprisingly common among small children. Pinworms and irritation from strictures (narrowing) of the urethra (urine passage) or meatus (opening) are other causes. Irritation can set off the nerve reflex which initiates urination.

Ill or weakened persons may encounter this problem also. Among them are patients with systemic diseases such as tuberculosis, diabetes, hypothyroidism, epilepsy, spina bifida, or mental retardation.

In adults, drinking too much liquid, especially just before sleep time; the intake of too much diuretic-type beverage, such as coffee; or eating spicy foods which irritate the urinary system can also produce enuresis.

Extreme tiredness or exhaustion may cause a child to sleep so heavily he cannot awaken to normal urinary impulses. Sometimes his problem is simply due to a new schedule or new demands for which his urinary muscles are not yet adequately prepared, or which leave him exhausted. A good example is the child who is used to napping early and has just begun kindergarten. His new schedule means that his usual daily nap is postponed until after school—at about the same time he formerly awoke and went to the bathroom.

EMOTIONAL FACTORS. Another example is a child who is acutely afraid he will have a urinary accident, or one who in the past has reacted severely to punishment or embarrassment. As a result he has nightmares about the accident or about going to the bathroom—and during the dream urinates into the bed. Punishment and shaming will only increase and perpetuate such a problem. The only solution is to reassure the child and relieve his fears.

Nervous tension can affect the child's bladder muscles by causing periodic spasms and contractions which result in unplanned urination. An explosive overreaction of a parent or teacher to other situations or disciplinary problems can have such an effect, either temporary or of a chronic long-term nature.

Frequently a skilled and understanding counselor is needed to locate and explain the contributing habits and reactions of child, parents, teachers, and others such as playmates and neighbors. But parents themselves can do much to help prevent or correct less severe problems.

DISCIPLINE. Discipline is definitely necessary for every child, and the child wants such guidance. However, it should be administered in a consistent fashion with understanding and warm affection.

Both the discipline and the child suffer when the same infraction is punished one day and ignored the next, or punished in one child and ignored in another, unless the unpunished child is old enough and responsible enough to have been awarded such extra freedom.

Teachers, parents, and grandparents should try to reinforce a child's successes and reward his good behavior by compliments and special extra privileges.

PHYSICAL RETRAINING. If the cause of enuresis is physical, it should be medically treated and cured. If the cause is emotional, the contributing factors should be identified and positive steps taken to start correcting them.

However, in either case the child also should be physically retrained in his toilet habits. This will help restore coordination of the mental, neurological, and physical impulses involved. It will also help prevent future accidents and relieve the worries, fears, and pressures on the child while the other problems are being treated and cured.

Begin by figuring out the approximate times when bedwetting occurs. List the factors preceding bedtime which might also contribute. Give the child less liquid in the hour or two before going to bed, but make up for this with a glass of milk or juice on awakening, so that the proper body-fluid balance will be maintained and the urine will not become too concentrated.

For instance, if the enuresis usually occurs two hours after the child has gone to sleep, awaken him a little before that time and have him go to the bathroom as a preventive. Set a timer or alarm clock, if necessary, to help you remember. But never scold him if you get there too late, whether it is your fault or not. Train his reflexes during waking hours. Have him visit the bathroom immediately on feeling the first impulse, at least during the hours outside school.

Awaken him in the middle of the night at the risk of losing some of your own sleep for a short while. And don't be grumpy. The results will be well worth the effort!

As time passes, gradually lengthen the time before you rouse him for a bathroom visit, until he can get along until his nap or sleep ends naturally.

Bee Stings. Stings by bees, wasps, hornets, and yellowjackets usually cause only a painful local area of redness and swelling. If you are stung and any other symptoms appear, by all means call a physician promptly. You might have an allergy to the substance left under the skin by the insect.

Some people who have been stung by bees or similar insects have died within a half hour from violent allergic reactions. Watch out for such symptoms as dizziness, nausea, vomiting, stomach cramps, diarrhea, and breathing difficulties. Prompt medical attention is also essential for someone who has had multiple stings or has been stung in sensitive areas such as the eye or tongue, even if he shows no unusual reactions.

The sensitivity of a person allergic to these insects may not be noticed the first time he is stung, or may increase suddenly when he is stung again later. So don't be smug and careless just because you were bitten once and had mild or no ill effects.

Once a person has demonstrated that he is sensitive to stings, he should avoid areas where bees and other insects may be found.

Or he may be desensitized over a period of time by a series of injections of minute quantities of venom from bees, wasps, hornets, and yellowjackets. (*See* ALLERGY.)

Emergency kits are available which may be carried by persons who have bee allergies. These contain a tourniquet for stopping the passage of the venom through the body, a hypodermic syringe and needle for an epinephrine (adrenalin) injection, and oral preparations such as antihistamines. Consult your physician regarding the use of the kit.

First aid for simple bee stings of nonallergic persons includes removal of any portion of the insect's stinging apparatus which remains in the skin. Use tweezers if there are any available.

Relief for the pain of a sting may be obtained by applying ice, calamine lotion, baking soda, or a compress of very diluted ammonia water. Wash the sting wound and keep it covered with a bandage to prevent infection.

Behavior.   The way a person acts, performs, and reacts to various needs and in various situations constitutes his behavior.

The behavior of any individual shows recurring patterns. These patterns are partly determined by the brain and central nervous system, but largely by the feelings and experiences built into his personality during childhood.

Behavior is the result of the striving of a human being (or an animal) to fulfill his biological and social needs. Part of his behavior is determined by his needs for food, water, oxygen, elimination of waste products, warmth, and protection against attack. Other needs assure his social existence—sexual activity and mating, communication, and curiosity. A person's behavior is then directed toward the goal of fulfilling all these needs, to provide satisfaction and a state of well-being.

When his needs are not met because some frustration interferes, the individual must make adjustments and modify his behavior. If he can do this with fair success, then his behavior remains normal. But if he cannot find a way to surmount his difficulties, his behavior may become disordered.

Normal behavior varies according to cultural norms and to such factors as age, sex, status, role, and type of personality. What may be normal in one set of circumstances, may be completely abnormal in another. Normal also are variations in behavior patterns from time to time. An emotional event or physical illness can trigger a change. And the processes of growth and maturation will slowly change the behavior of a child.

The observable behavior of a child or an adult, while only part of his whole personality-picture, often reveals his underlying conflicts and tensions. If an individual of any age is unable to satisfy his needs and cannot resolve his conflicts, he may feel unable to cope with his world. At this point his attempts at adjustment appear to other people as disorganized behavior or mental illness.

Some examples of behavior signifying emotional trouble are constant belligerence; excessive moodiness; exaggerated worry; suspiciousness and mistrust; selfishness about almost everything; helplessness and dependency; poor emotional control, with outbursts out of proportion to the cause and at inappropriate times; a resort to daydreaming and fantasy in place of facing reality; and hypochondria. (*See* CHILD BEHAVIOR.)

Belching.   The common burp, or belch, comes from the swallowing of air or from gas in the stomach caused by the chemical reactions of food and digestive juices. (*See* FLATULENCE.)

Belladonna.   The meaning of this word in Italian is "beautiful lady," an allusion to the striking effect of the drug on the human eye: it dilates the pupil. The drug is derived from a plant called deadly nightshade in allusion to Atropos, one of the three Fates in Greek mythology. The plant is a perennial herb with attractive, small flowers, and shiny purple-black berries. The active substance, obtainable from the roots, leaves, and berries, is an alkaloid, atropine.

In excessive doses atropine is a deadly poison; characteristic symptoms are dryness of the mouth, inability to urinate, fever, a rash, and delirium. In precisely controlled doses it is one of the most important of drugs. It was formerly much used before administration of ether anesthesia to prevent the excessive flow of saliva that tended to choke the airways. Its derivatives and drugs with similar actions are important to the ophthalmologist for several reasons, especially its effect in keeping the pupil widely dilated to permit ophthalmoscopic examination of the interior of the eye. In general it acts as antidote to pilocarpine and related alkaloids.

Bell's Palsy.   A paralysis of one side of the face from an unknown cause is termed Bell's palsy. It may occur on either side, but seldom on both sides at the same time.

Sometimes the paralysis occurs after the patient has had a chill, or has exposed his face to a raw wintry wind. It is not known, however, whether the chilling is the real cause, or whether it has just brought to the surface some preexisting problem.

Some people get the condition repeatedly. The symptoms take a long time to disappear, at least several weeks and once in a while up to a few years.

The affected side of the mouth will sag and may need to be supported by a tape or some other sling applied by the physician. Upward massage of the face with the hands, electrical stimulation with a special device at the clinic or hospital, and dry heat from a lamp help to tone up the face muscles and maintain circulation during the period of paralysis.

Persons who have a tendency toward Bell's palsy should keep their faces covered when in a cold wind. Knitted caps which extend down over the cheeks are recommended.

The problem occurs most frequently during adulthood. Professional diagnosis is im-

U.S. Department of Agriculture

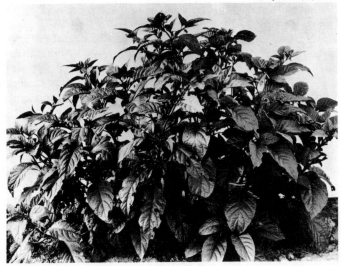

The belladonna plant, also known as deadly nightshade, is poisonous if eaten. It is nonetheless valuable as a base for several useful alkaloid drugs, such as atropine and scopolamine, sometimes used in the treatment of Parkinson's disease.

portant, for this relatively mild disorder may be confused with symptoms of a stroke. (*See* STROKES.)

Bends. At one time the bends, also called caisson disease or decompression sickness, were a problem confined to deep-sea divers and workers in compressed-air compartments of tunnels and caissons. Today, however, it may also strike careless followers of the sport of scuba (self-contained underwater breathing apparatus) diving.

The bends occur when a person has been under high atmospheric pressure for a prolonged period, usually a matter of hours, and is suddenly exposed to a lower pressure. Atmospheric pressure on the surface is rated as one atmosphere. For each thirty-three feet below the surface of water, the pressure is increased an additional atmosphere. When a man stays underwater at a depth of more than sixty-six feet for several hours, his body fluids and tissues conform to the pressure sufficiently so that he may have difficulty if he does not decompress himself slowly on rising to the surface.

When blood passes through the lung capillaries, it picks up nitrogen, along with oxygen, from the alveoli (minute air sacs). The amount of nitrogen picked up depends on the pressure of the air or atmosphere. As pressure increases, so does the amount of nitrogen picked up by the blood. (And so does the oxygen, but this presents no problem, as the extra oxygen diffuses rapidly and metabolizes into the system.)

The additional nitrogen in the blood is carried to the body tissues and gradually saturates them under continued high atmospheric pressure. If the atmospheric pressure is suddenly dropped, the nitrogen (unlike oxygen) forms bubbles, which can block small blood vessels and do other damage by their pressure. In bends, these bubbles affect portions of the central nervous system, especially parts of the spinal cord.

The usual first symptom of the bends is pain in the legs and sometimes the arms. The pattern of other symptoms will vary with the individual and with the degree and suddenness of the atmospheric change. The patient may have dizziness, disturbances of vision, paralysis, a rash, a choking sensation in the chest, headaches, and inability to speak (aphasia), and may lapse into a coma.

It is urgently necessary to rush the patient to the closest decompression chamber and to call a doctor. (The local health department, fire department, and U.S. Navy unit have information on the location of suitable chambers.) The patient is put under gradual compression until the symptoms disappear, then is slowly decompressed. Nitrogen can be released from the tissues and body fluids without bubbles if decompression is gradual.

Symptoms of decompression sickness may appear within a few minutes or not until as many as six hours have passed. Usually they will develop within an hour. Oxygen administration is a useful first-aid measure, as it helps remove the nitrogen.

Full recovery depends on whether there has been serious damage to the patient's spinal cord; if the damage is minor, it usually repairs itself.

Deep-sea and scuba diving are best limited to people in good physical condition; they will be most able to cope with decompression emergencies should they occur.

Bends have also affected pilots and passengers who have soared rapidly in airplanes to altitudes of some 25,000 feet or more above sea level without pressurized suits or cockpits. Commercial and most other high-altitude planes avoid the problem by pressurizing the cabins.

Benign. The term benign is used to describe a condition, such as that of a tumor, which is not malignant. Benign conditions are usually favorable for recovery. (*See* MALIGNANCY; MALIGNANT.)

Benzedrine. This is a trade name for amphetamine sulfate. (*See* AMPHETAMINE.)

Benzene. This is a distinct chemical substance, sometimes called benzol, which is obtained from coal tar. (It must not be confused with the "benzine" that is obtained as a mixture of hydrocarbons from petroleum. Benzine has been much used as a fuel and as a solvent for dry cleaning. It is flammable, but its effects on the body are much less dangerous than are those of benzene.)

Benzene is too dangerous to be used in the home. It is widely used in industry as a starting point for many coal-tar products, but chiefly as a solvent for latex in the manufacture of rubber products. Since the continued inhalation of air containing benzene vapor may lead to bone marrow destruction, with irreversible anemia, industrial plants go to great lengths to reduce the concentration of benzene vapor in the air of their factories.

When inhaled, benzene produces dizziness, stomach pains, difficulty in breathing, vomiting, coma, and potential death from respiratory failure. Since the respiratory problems are aggravated by vomiting, vomiting should not be induced as with other poisoning problems. The patient should be placed in fresh air, and artificial respiration given if necessary to resume breathing.

When ingested, benzene causes burning in the mouth and stomach, headache, nausea, and vomiting. Fresh air is also called for, and nothing should be administered to induce vomiting. If the patient is not breathing, use artificial respiration. (*See* ARTIFICIAL RESPIRATION; POISONING.)

Beriberi. A severe nutritional deficiency may result in a condition called beriberi. The major symptoms are caused by lack of thiamine, but often there is also a lack of ascorbic acid, riboflavin, niacin, and vitamin A. (*See* VITAMINS.)

The disease was once widespread in Oriental countries where most of the population lived on highly milled rice. Now it is less frequent there, because of social and economic improvements and consumption of a better diet with more foods containing thiamine. Beriberi rarely occurs in Europe and the United States, except in alcoholic patients who consume very small amounts of thiamine. (*See* THIAMINE.)

Beriberi may follow infection, or minor illness accompanied by fever, or hard physical labor, or pregnancy and lactation. The disease can usually be stopped at any stage in its course by improving the diet and especially by therapeutic doses of thiamine.

There are three main types of beriberi: *wet beriberi,* in which edema and heart failure occur; *chronic dry beriberi,* found only in older adults and often associated with prolonged consumption of alcohol; and *infantile beriberi.*

The patient with wet or dry beriberi may notice a loss of appetite, nausea, a feeling of malaise, and weakness of the legs. He may have a swelling of the legs or face, tingling and numbness in the legs, tenderness in his calves, and a burning sensation on the soles of his feet. The condition may persist for months or even years.

In wet beriberi, the patient becomes bloated with fluid, may have a rapid heartbeat, and complains of breathlessness. The veins on his neck may become enlarged and throb visibly. He may have high blood pressure and a diminished output of urine. The patient with severe wet beriberi may be in danger of a sudden increase in edema, along with acute failure of his circulation, increased difficulty in breathing, and even death.

The most outstanding feature of dry beriberi is a wasting and weakening of muscles with absence of edema. There may be a numbness and partial paralysis of the legs. Reactions and reflexes may be considerably slowed down. Thin, emaciated patients first use a stick or cane as an aid in walking, and finally become bedridden.

Infantile beriberi occurs in breast-fed infants, usually between the second and fifth months. While their mothers may have no signs of beriberi, their diet—and hence their milk—probably have a low thiamine content.

The infant with the chronic form of beriberi may be restless, cry a lot, pass less urine than normal, and show signs of puffiness. In severe cases, the infant may turn a bluish color and have trouble breathing. His cry may become thin, with a plaintive whine. He may have convulsions and coma, and death may occur within twenty-four to forty-eight hours.

The best preventive of beriberi is a well-balanced diet containing enough thiamine. Important sources of thiamine are pork, liver, yeast, whole cereals, and fresh green vegetables. Less adequate sources are nonenriched flour, rice, and processed cereals. Even human milk is a relatively poor source of thiamine.

Many foods lose thiamine during cooking and serving. Freezing, however, causes little or no loss in the thiamine content of foods.

Berylliosis. Persons employed in the manufacture of fluorescent lamps may inhale particles of the beryllium compounds used as phosphorus. The resulting lung problem is called berylliosis, one of a class of diseases known as pneumoconioses. (*See* PNEUMOCONIOSIS.)

Bicarbonate of Soda. Better known to chemists as sodium bicarbonate, this white, alkaline powder can be purchased as baking soda. Its uses vary, from a substitute for toothpaste to a bathing solution.

Acid burns are usually treated by flooding the injured area with a solution of four tablespoons of baking soda to one quart of tap water. Insect stings and bites also respond to this treatment.

Biceps. The muscle on the front side of the arm that bends the elbow is called the biceps. It starts above the shoulder and ends just below the elbow. Its name comes from the Latin words *bis,* meaning "two," and *caput,* meaning "head," because this muscle is shaped like the letter Y, with two heads at the top and only one tail at the bottom. Its full name is *biceps brachii* (biceps of the arm), to distinguish it from the *biceps femoris,* one of the muscles on the back of the leg that bend the knee. (*See* MUSCLES.)

Bidet. Most Americans are not familiar with the bathroom fixture called the bidet, although it is still found in bathrooms in South American and European houses. It may be described as a "sit-down bathtub," or a form of lavatory providing facilities for local or spot bathing, particularly of those regions of the body not easily washed when a person is fully dressed.

The bidet is a low-set basin or bowl equipped with hot and cold water, valves, a pop-up plug, and an integral douche or jet that directs a stream of water upward from the bottom of the bowl. The entire apparatus is designed to maintain a constant cleanliness in the user's genital and anal areas.

Many people believe that the bidet should be considered a hygienic necessity rather than a luxury. They point out that after a bowel movement it is better to cleanse the anus with soap and water than with even the softest toilet tissue. They add that if it is sensible to wash one's hands after going to the toilet, it is even more so to wash one's bottom.

In addition to cleansing and vaginal douching, this apparatus can be used in many other ways. It is excellent for sitz baths. (*See* SITZ BATHS.) The bidet is also useful as a foot bath, either for cleansing or for therapeutic purposes.

Bifocals. Eyeglasses that help one see at two different distances, and may be used for reading as well as for distant vision, are called bifocals.

The normal lens of the eye can adapt

itself to seeing at different distances. However, with age, particularly in people over forty, the eye loses some of this adaptability and requires bifocals to aid in seeing both far and near.

Sometimes trifocals are necessary to give an additional intermediate visual range. Bifocals or trifocals come in many variations and can be adapted to an individual's needs.

All glasses, single vision or multifocal, are available with glass or plastic lenses.

Bile. Gall, or bile, is a digestive juice manufactured in the liver. It is stored and concentrated in the gallbladder. (*See* GALL-BLADDER.)

Bilharziasis. Infestation with schistosomes, or blood flukes, causes a severe bladder inflammation called bilharziasis. This flatworm-caused disease is common in the Middle East but is rarely found in the United States. (*See* FLATWORMS; WORMS.)

The adult worms are up to one inch in length and spend various stages of their development in the lungs, liver, and urinary bladder. Eggs are laid in the lining of the bladder and passed into the urine, where

These are parasitic worms called liver flukes. They cause the disease bilharziasis, also called schistosomiasis.

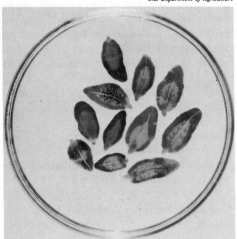

they hatch. Before being passed to another human, the eggs pass through another stage of development in a snail. Persons swimming, drinking, or bathing in the snail-infested water can then contract bilharziasis.

Once the disease is diagnosed, two medical steps are taken: A drug is prescribed to eradicate the parasite, and the damage to the internal organs is corrected by surgery.

Bilirubin. The orange or yellowish pigment in bile is bilirubin. It is produced by the liver. (*See* BILE; BILIRUBINEMIA; BLOOD; LIVER.)

Bilirubinemia. When the red-yellow pigment of bile, called bilirubin, becomes more concentrated in the blood than the relatively low levels considered normal, the condition is known as bilirubinemia. If the concentration becomes quite high, the condition is called hyperbilirubinemia.

Increased bilirubin concentration in the blood and lymph is one aspect of an abnormal hepatic condition, either jaundice or icterus (*hepatic* means related to the liver). (*See* JAUNDICE.) This excess of bilirubin in the blood gives the skin and whites of the eyes the yellow color typical of jaundice. Just as bilirubinemia is a symptom—of whatever causes the higher pigment concentration—so jaundice also is not a disease in itself but a symptom of some other disease.

The basic causes of jaundice may be liver disease (called hepatogenous jaundice), obstruction of the bile ducts (obstructive jaundice), or heavy production of bilirubin caused by large-scale destruction of red blood cells (hemolytic jaundice). Most often bilirubinemia results when there is an interference either with the production or elimination of bilirubin, which is a normal part of the bile, gallstones, blood, and urine. Its normal concentration in the circulating blood is about 0.5 milligrams for each 100 cubic centimeters of blood. This normal concentration is relatively light.

The way bilirubin is made tells something that is not always well understood about the way the body develops and lives. In the human body, life is based partly on death. To stay alive and well the body must not only develop and grow new cells; it must also destroy old cells. These old cells are destroyed mainly in various areas of tissue that, taken together, constitute what is called the reticuloendothelial system (R-E system) of the body. In these tissues, cells called phagocytes destroy invading cells (thus preventing infection) as well as old cells and excess matter no longer essential for life. Yet this destruction may not completely dispose of all the component material.

Bilirubin is a by-product or, to view the process in another way, a waste product of the destruction of erythrocytes or red blood corpuscles that have been circulating in the blood for 120 to 130 days. (*See* ERYTH-ROCYTES; HEMOGLOBIN.) As the red cells are destroyed, bilirubin is made by degrading the red coloring matter in the cells, hematin or heme, which is a combination of iron and a red-purple pigment, protoporphyrin, also found in chlorophyll. More specifically, bilirubin is produced in a way that makes it iron-free but rich in the coloring matter of the heme.

Most of this conversion probably takes place in the liver, spleen, and lymph nodes. As formed in the blood, the basic bilirubin compound is $C_{33}H_{36}O_4N_6$. From the blood, bilirubin is transferred in plasma and is processed through the liver which removes it from the blood, feeding it into the bile. Some of the bile is temporarily stored in the gallbladder; some is fed into the intestines. The golden color of bile is caused by this pigment, as is the pale yellowness of blood plasma. In various parts of the body, bilirubin is found in modified form—as soluble sodium bilirubinate in the bile and insoluble calcium salt in one type of gallstones.

In trying to determine whether the concentration of bilirubin in the blood is too high, medical scientists sometimes use what is called the icterus index. This is a measure of the yellow color of the serum as compared with the normal. A more accurate measure is obtained by chemical analysis of the serum for bilirubin.

A common cause of bilirubinemia is excessive destruction of red blood cells (hemolysis). This may occur as a congenital or as an acquired condition. One example is the erythroblastosis of infants due to Rh agglutins from the maternal blood.

Too little transfer of bilirubin to the liver may be caused by one of the novobiocin drugs or iopanoic acid, by heart surgery, or by congestive heart failure.

Bilirubin processing in the liver of the newborn and infants may be impaired by congenital defects. In premature babies the cause may be incomplete development of the hepatic system. Defects in liver enzymes cause the Crigler-Najjar syndrome of children. This is a condition in which a persistent and increasing jaundice develops in infants from the time of birth, because the liver does not develop the enzymes required to remove bilirubin from the blood. The brain is damaged by the excessive deposits of bilirubin. Most of these infants die before the age of fifteen months, but a few live several years.

Excessive bilirubin in the blood—jaundice—also can result from too little excretion of the pigment into the bile flow. This may result from liver injury caused by virus hepatitis or by medications such as the hormones estrogen and testosterone, and the drug chlorpromazine. Gallstones, cancer, and inflammation of the hepatic system are other causes.

Binet Test.   This popular test for measuring intelligence of school children is more commonly known as the Stanford-Binet test. (*See* STANFORD-BINET TEST.)

Bioclimatology.   The science that studies the interactions between atmospheric and biological processes over long periods of time is called bioclimatology. This science involves an experimental approach that seeks information on the kinds of environmental situations that produce specific reactions in living organisms.

Throughout the earth's history, there have been tremendous changes in climate, such as those created by advancing and retreating ice sheets. These have exerted a profound effect on the evolution, health, and life styles of all living things. (*See* BIOMETEOROLOGY; CLIMATE.)

Biodegradable. Waste materials in sewage, surface waters, and soils are biodegradable if bacteria commonly found there can attack them, break them down, and utilize them as food. Materials that are not biodegradable accumulate in the environment, possibly becoming a threat to health.

When metal, glass, or plastic containers for foodstuffs are discarded in or near bodies of water, they make perfect breeding places for mosquitoes and disease-carrying rodents.

In the early 1960's there were many complaints about foam on lakes and streams. This was caused by substances in detergents that were not decomposed readily by bacteria and therefore were transported with other wastes into the natural waterways. (*See* DETERGENTS; PHOSPHATES; WATER POLLUTION.)

Bioflavonoids. A group of substances, which include rutin, quercitin, and hesperidin, have become known as bioflavonoids. Prepared from the rinds of citrus fruits like oranges and lemons, they were believed at first to have special nutritive virtues. It was found later that these substances, when taken by mouth, were destroyed by the intestinal bacteria and had no significant pharmacological effects. In the words of the U.S. Food and Drug Administration, bioflavonoids are "ineffective for man in any condition."

Biological Warfare. The use of bacteria and viruses to produce disease or death in man or animals is biological warfare. (*See also* CHEMICAL WARFARE.) To be an effective weapon, a disease agent must have a high degree of infectiveness; a high degree of resistance to heat, sunlight, and drying; the ability to disperse rapidly; and the ability to cause mortality or crippling.

Some disease agents act directly upon animals, while others are zoonotic and may exist in the warfare area for years, spreading sickness and causing death. Thus these agents are a source of long-range economic loss.

Another aspect of biological warfare is the destruction of plants by the use of chemical hormones called "growth regulators." This method is often used by ground troops to prevent the enemy from gaining advantage through hiding places in foliage.

Biological agents can be diffused into a target area years before an initial outbreak of war. They will cause human sickness and eliminate a productive work force. Because of crop and animal sickness, the health of the target area becomes undermined and resistance to war is lowered.

Biometeorology. This new science, representing a mix of physicians and weather experts, involves the study of ways in which atmospheric conditions, climate, weather, and seasons are related to human health. Biometeorologists chart the courses of certain diseases under varying weather conditions. The following conclusions have been reached by some investigators.

Asthma attacks appear to increase with sudden cooling and low barometric pressure, but are infrequent during high pressure and fog. Most acute glaucoma occurs on very hot or very cold days. Urinary tract pain is common after an influx of cold, humid air. Peptic ulcer perforations occur mainly during drastic changes in air masses, and the incidence is highest in May and November. The toxicity of central nervous system stimulants, such as caffeine and amphetamine, rises as the temperature falls. Digitalis is dangerous in rising atmospheric temperature.

There have also been reports that traffic accidents rise during thunderstorms, not only because of road conditions but because of slowed driver-reaction time due to changes in the atmospheric electricity field.

Biopsy. A procedure which involves obtaining a portion of a living tissue from the body for microscopic examination is termed a biopsy. A biopsy is performed so that a specific diagnosis can be made. Many infections, tumors, and other disease entities look and feel so much alike that actual microscopic examination of the diseased tissue is required before the disorder can be identified and proper treatment started.

There are two basic types of biopsy procedures: the closed biopsy and the open biopsy. A closed biopsy can be performed without making a surgical incision and is usually done with needles or punches, using a local anesthetic (Novocain). Sternal biopsy, in which bone marrow is obtained from the sternum or breastbone, is a commonly performed closed biopsy.

Open biopsy entails a surgical procedure during which the diseased organ is directly visualized and part or all of it is obtained for examination. This procedure is a good deal more risky than a closed biopsy, but guarantees that a good specimen will be obtained.

There is in addition a third category—the surface biopsy, in which cells obtained from the surfaces of body organs are specially stained and examined under the microscope. George Papanicolaou, a Greek physician, developed this process and adapted it for use on the female cervix, upper respiratory tract, and the stomach. Today we primarily use it for detecting early cancer of the cervix and commonly refer to the procedure as a "Pap smear." (*See* CANCER; CANCER DETECTION; PAP SMEAR TEST.)

Biotin. A vitamin necessary for many of the complex reactions of metabolism that take place within the cells of the body is known as biotin. It is part of the B vitamin group and is found mostly in egg yolk. (*See* EGGS; VITAMINS.)

Biotin has been called a "micro-micronutrient" because very minute traces of it perform its metabolic task. It is very potent, and natural deficiencies are unknown. In addition to egg yolk, other excellent food sources are liver, kidney, tomatoes, and yeast. The human requirement for biotin has not been established because intestinal bacteria synthesize enough of the vitamin to supply the body's needs.

Birth Certificate. The legal registration of a person's birth is called a birth certificate. The birth of each child in this country is now recorded, and a certificate of it is important because it is legally the only proper evidence of a person's date and place of birth.

State birth records date back to the middle 1800's, although some states did not start such records until 1919. Many city and county records are older than state files.

Copies of birth certificates can be obtained by applying to the state or local government.

Birth Control. From earliest times women have tried to limit the size of their families or avoid becoming pregnant by practicing birth control. Birth control generally refers to the temporary prevention of pregnancy by various means rather than permanent prevention brought about by sterilization. Recently the practice of contraception has been referred to as family planning, a term that carries a more positive connotation and includes other factors as well.

Concern over population growth as well as public health and the environment has led to an increased interest in birth control. The health of the mother and her family is dependent in part on the spacing and limitation of the children she conceives.

A variety of birth control techniques are available, though not all are equally effective. So-called folk methods include *coitus interruptus* (withdrawal of the penis before ejaculation), prolonged lactation, and postcoital douching. The two latter methods are largely ineffective. It is known that nursing does inhibit ovulation, but the length of time this effect persists is highly variable. Ovulation can occur even without menstruation.

Selection of a birth control method should depend on the guidance of a physician as well as the preferences of the woman and her husband. (*See* BIRTH CONTROL, MECHANICAL MEANS; BIRTH CONTROL PILLS; RHYTHM SYSTEM.) The failure rate of any method depends largely on whether it is used properly and consistently. At present, birth control pills are the most effective, though not all women can tolerate them. No one method is suitable for everyone.

Work on male birth control pills and other techniques continues. Sterilization of either sex is of course 100 percent effective in preventing conception. Abstinence during the fertile period, the basis of the rhythm system, can also be effective.

Although birth control methods of one sort or another are being utilized with ever greater frequency, in some quarters birth control itself remains a controversial issue. Various religions, the Roman Catholic Church perhaps chief among them, have yet to pronounce unequivocally on the subject. (*See* BIRTH CONTROL, MECHANICAL MEANS; BIRTH CONTROL PILLS; IUD OR IUCD.)

Birth Control, Mechanical Means.
The use of special devices to prevent conception and/or implantation is considered a mechanical means of birth control. The devices include diaphragms, intrauterine devices, the condom, and jellies, foams, and other spermicidal preparations.

The intrauterine device, or IUD, has become one of the more frequently used methods of modern times. Once it has been inserted into the uterus it can be worn without further manipulation. According to some studies, 70 to 80 percent of its users

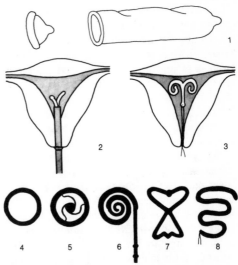

Among the oldest known contraceptive mechanical devices is the condom (1), a rubber sheath which is used to cover the male penis. It is shown rolled and unrolled.

Even older historically, but less commonly used until very recently, is the intrauterine contraceptive device. This is popularly referred to as the IUD, or IUCD.

Illustration 2 shows an IUD being inserted into the uterus with the aid of a tube through the cervix. 3 shows this IUD, called a Robinson Saf-T-Coil, in place in the uterus with strings extending through the cervix.

The remaining drawings illustrate some of the many other types of IUD's available for use: 4, Hall-Stone stainless steel ring; 5, Ota ring; 6, Margulies coil; 7, Birnberg bow; 8, Lippes loop.

will still retain the device at the end of one year. At the end of two years 60 to 70 percent will still be using it. (*See* IUD OR IUCD.)

Spotting, cramps, and occasional pelvic inflammation are the most common side effects of IUD use. Generally these symptoms tend to disappear after several months, though occasionally they are severe enough to warrant removal of the device.

The diaphragm was at one time considered the standard and most dependable method of birth control. When used properly and consistently, it had a failure rate of only two to three pregnancies per hundred women per year. (*See* DIAPHRAGM.)

The condom is a sheath worn over a man's erect penis during coitus to prevent sperm from entering the vagina. If the condom is of high quality and used regularly, pregnancy rates of as low as seven per hundred women per year have been reported. The condom was widely used before the introduction of birth control pills. It also helps curb the spread of venereal disease.

Jellies, creams, foams, and suppositories, all containing spermicidal chemicals, are inserted into the vagina and used for birth control. They are less effective than other methods, however, and some couples consider them offensive. Douching after coitus is not considered a particularly effective means of birth control. (*See* DOUCHING.)

A physician will advise a couple on their selection of birth control methods. No one technique is suitable for all persons. (*See* BIRTH CONTROL.)

Birth Control Pills. Oral contraceptives are commonly referred to as birth control pills. They are a popular and highly effective means of family planning. (*See* BIRTH CONTROL.) As an indication of their widespread distribution, they are often referred to as simply "the Pill," even though a number of types exist.

Oral contraceptives used today generally consist of synthetic or semisynthetic estrogen and progestin hormones. Used as directed, they suppress ovulation and prevent pregnancy. With the smaller doses sometimes prescribed, ovulation occurs, though pregnancy still seems to be prevented. This phenomenon is currently being studied, and scientific conclusions are as yet by no means clear.

Birth control pills are usually prescribed in either combined or sequential doses. With a combined dosage, the woman's pill contains both progestin and estrogen. She takes one each day from the fifth to the twenty-fourth or twenty-fifth day of her menstrual cycle. (*See* MENSTRUATION.) Using a sequential schedule, she would take pills containing only estrogen for fifteen or sixteen days, followed by five days of pills containing both estrogen and progestin. To help her maintain a daily routine, inert tablets are sometimes given for the remaining days of the cycle.

The combined dosage has been found to be somewhat more effective in preventing conception than the sequential. A pregnancy rate of 0.7 per hundred women per year is usually quoted for the combined dosage based on use effectiveness, as contrasted with 1.4 per hundred women per year for the sequential dosage. Nonetheless, oral contraceptives are significantly more effective than other methods now in use. (*See* BIRTH CONTROL, MECHANICAL MEANS.) Failure to take one or more pills during a cycle is the primary reason for impregnation.

Reactions to birth control pills are usually similar to those associated with early pregnancy: nausea, vomiting, breast engorgement, and some breakthrough bleeding. Headache, dizziness, and weight gain are also among the possible side effects. These reactions are usually related to the hormone estrogen and will decrease or disappear after a few months of using the Pill. They are usually not considered serious.

A relationship has been found between the use of oral contraceptives and an increase in blood-clotting disease. For this reason, women who have a tendency toward blood clotting or who have vascular disease are advised to use some other method of birth control.

It is difficult to determine how many of the so-called side effects of the Pill would occur even if the woman was not taking it. But because she is aware of the regular medication and is being supervised by a physician, she is more likely to report any unusual conditions.

The effect of prolonged use of estrogens on the body is still under investigation. Indirect evidence suggests that they might be carcinogenic (cancer promoting), though this has not been proved. Estrogens may produce a variety of changes in the cervix and breasts, the significance of which is also not known. The changes do, however, alter metabolism of sodium and water and various other body constituents. There is little evidence that such drug-induced changes constitute serious hazards to health.

Not all these symptoms appear in every woman who takes the Pill. Although no single method of contraception is best for all women, birth control pills have proved highly acceptable to an increasing number of them.

Birth Defects. Any abnormalities present in a child at birth can be considered birth defects. They may be the result of genetic disorders or of a faulty maternal environment (i.e., in the womb). An abnor-

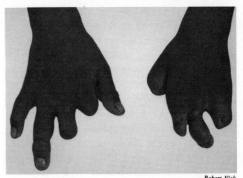

Robert Vick

"Mitten hands," produced by a congenital birth defect.

mality produced by a mechanical injury or some other difficulty during delivery, however, is considered a birth injury. (*See* BIRTH INJURIES.)

Some birth defects are apparent at delivery, while others do not appear until later in life. But since they do in actual fact begin in the womb, they are considered congenital (present from the beginning).

Congenital abnormalities appear in one of every forty births. They are considered responsible for 20 percent of all deaths within the first month after birth, as well as many miscarriages. The 80 percent of those infants who survive the first month generally live to adulthood. (*See* CONGENITAL DEFECTS.)

Fully half of all congenital problems involve the central nervous system. Among them is anencephaly, a condition in which the forebrain is deficient and the part of the skull which would cover it is missing. A child with this condition can not survive. Nor can the child with microencephaly, in which the skull and brain are disproportionately small.

A child may be born with hydrocephalus, an unusually large head due to fluid trapped within the skull. This condition is sometimes referred to as water on the brain. It results from an obstruction to the flow of cerebrospinal fluid and at times can be corrected surgically. (*See* HYDROCEPHALUS; WATER ON THE BRAIN.)

A congenital anomaly, such as this double big toe, is a defect that exists at birth. Other abnormalities may occur at the time of birth but may be due to problems of delivery of the infant.

Armed Forces Institute of Pathology

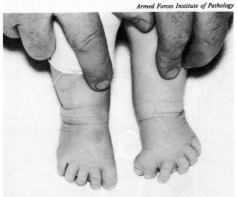

A defect in the closure of the vertebral canal is known as myelomeningocoele or meningocoele, depending on its location. Three of every thousand births exhibit this problem. Myelomeningocoele sometimes leads to weakness or paralysis of the legs and to incontinence.

Anencephaly and spina bifida (a hole in the spine) and similar conditions seem to be related to birth order, since they appear rarely in a firstborn child and more frequently in later children. The precise cause, however, is unknown.

Women are usually advised to avoid all drugs not prescribed by a doctor during their pregnancy. During the first three months, when organs and body parts are forming, the embryo is particularly vulnerable to changes in the mother's system. The safety of most drugs during pregnancy has not been established. The tragedy of hundreds of children born with defective limbs because their mothers had taken the drug thalidomide bears witness to this.

It is known that tetracycline, taken early in pregnancy while the embryo's tooth buds are forming, will produce yellowed teeth in the child. Even drugs given during labor can cause respiratory distress and other difficulties for an infant.

Genetic defects can cause such conditions in an infant as extra fingers and toes (polydactyly), dwarfism, and metabolic disorders. One of the more common metabolic problems is known as phenylketonuria, or PKU, involving a difficulty in assimilating the amino acid phenylalanine. This condition can be detected in an infant's blood very early, and his diet henceforth can be adjusted to avoid complications. But if it is left untreated, the child can become mentally retarded.

At least several hundred other hereditary metabolic defects have been identified, including common and uncommon, benign and serious diseases. Newly recognized metabolic disorders are constantly being reported.

Metabolic diseases can affect almost every class of biochemical substance and all the organs and tissues of the body. Cystic fibrosis is a metabolic disease characterized by repeated lung infections, although actually it involves dysfunction of the exocrine glands of the pancreas. No cure is known. Both Down's syndrome (mongolism) and cretinism bring mental retardation. (*See* CRETINISM; DOWN'S SYNDROME; MONGOLISM.) Maternal rubella (German measles) during early pregnancy can result in mental retardation, cataracts, heart abnormalities, deafness, or jaundice in the infant, depending on when the mother contracted the disease.

A baby's clubfoot—one that turns inward or outward to an unusual degree—is thought to be caused by mechanical malpositioning within the womb. It can be corrected by a brace, cast, or surgery. (*See* CLUBFOOT.) Skeletal problems, such as curvature of the spine and unstable hips that tend to rotate, can sometimes be corrected by splints.

One child in every six hundred births will have a cleft lip or cleft palate. The child's chances of having this defect increase to one in fifty if a parent had it, since it is inherited. Cosmetic surgery can often correct this condition which only occasionally is severe enough to interfere with eating. (*See* CLEFT PALATE.)

The cause of birthmarks is unknown. Some will disappear as the child grows older. Others may be removed by surgery, or covered with makeup. Common birthmarks include the so-called port wine stain and the strawberry nevus. (*See* BIRTHMARKS; PORT WINE STAIN.)

Congenital heart disease can include improper hookups of the arteries and veins, the absence of septa separating the chambers, or holes between the chambers. Heart murmurs, cyanosis, and sometimes even death can result. Many of these defects can be corrected by surgery if they are detected early enough.

Other physical defects detectable at birth include various hernias, fistulas (particularly the tracheo-esophageal fistula in the throat), and imperforate anus. Early diagnosis of these conditions permits successful surgery.

In view of the many types of birth defects, it is remarkable that so many children are born normal. Research into the causes and treatment of birth defects remains a great challenge, especially to such organizations as The National Foundation.

Birth Injuries. Any injuries sustained by the infant during labor and delivery are considered birth injuries. Such conditions can be the result of either physiological or mechanical difficulties. They are not considered congenital problems because those would have arisen earlier in development. (*See* CHILDBIRTH.)

As the baby's head passes through the birth canal, it can become bruised. Usually the head is molded to fit the canal, much like a piece of clay; the bruising occurs when it is pushed through too quickly.

Bleeding within the skull can produce brain damage and sometimes death. Forceps used during delivery to ease the child's head through the pelvis can also cause bleeding on the brain.

Sometimes squeezing and twisting the infant during birth, or pushing or pulling him too rapidly, leads to broken bones or to ruptured blood vessels or internal organs. Lack of oxygen can also be a problem if the mother has a long and difficult delivery.

But babies are quite resilient at birth and most of them escape injury. Moreover, birth injuries are becoming less common because of improved obstetric technique.

Birthmarks. Skin blemishes or discolorations that are determined before birth (congenital) are called birthmarks, or nevi. Nevi include pigmented lesions such as moles as well as skin abnormalities involving blood vessels, called hemangiomas (vascular birthmarks). Although some birthmarks do not develop until long after birth, the skin defect has been there since the time the skin was formed during prenatal life.

Nothing can be done to prevent birthmarks. Contrary to popular belief, they are not related to anything that may happen to the mother during pregnancy, nor are they related to anything that happens during birth.

Birthmarks may be small and insignificant or huge and disfiguring. Often they appear on areas of the body where they can be concealed; but when they appear on exposed areas, such as the face or arms, they present a significant cosmetic problem.

Birthmarks, especially some of the hemangiomas, may grow larger during the first few months after birth, increasing to many times their original size. Parents may understandably become frightened and think that immediate medical treatment is required. However, most of these birthmarks begin to diminish in size after a variable period and disappear by the time a child is seven or eight years of age.

On the other hand, some birthmarks

This birth injury was the result of an instrument wound to the infant's head, which occurred during delivery. *Armed Forces Institute of Pathology*

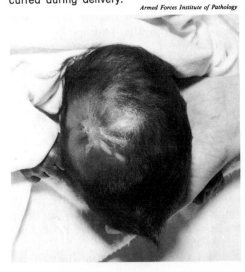

must be removed by medical treatment or surgery. Common treatments include cryosurgery (treatment with dry ice slush), electrodesiccation and electrocoagulation (destruction of tissue with an electrical current), X-ray and radium treatments, and the as yet experimental laser beam. All these treatments have merit, but they may also leave skin defects that are considered undesirable, such as scars.

Other birthmarks, like the so-called port wine stain, neither increase in size nor disappear. Unfortunately, there is no really effective medical treatment for such birthmarks. (*See* HEMANGIOMAS; MOLES; PORT WINE STAIN; STRAWBERRY MARKS.)

Bisexual. An individual who has both male and female organs is known as a bisexual or a hermaphrodite. (*See* HERMAPHRODITE; SEXUAL ABNORMALITIES.) This is a natural condition in some lower forms of animal life.

This term is also used to describe persons physically attracted to both sexes.

Bite. The proper contact of teeth is known as bite or occlusion. Teeth which come together properly, like well-working gears, can carry out their function effectively and with no harm to the bone in which they are embedded. The condition of teeth coming together improperly is called malocclusion. (*See* MALOCCLUSION.)

Black Death. An acute epidemic infection, usually transmitted to man by rodent fleas, is the Black Death, or bubonic plague, as it is medically known. (*See,* BUBONIC PLAGUE.)

Black Hairy Tongue. The tongue is covered with small projections of the mucous membrane that are called papillae. In some persons these papillae are irritated by smoking, poor mouth hygiene, or drugs taken by mouth, such as penicillin or chlortetracycline.

The result is elongation of the papillae.

There is also a darkening of the tongue, apparently from microorganisms. Sometimes the papillae grow so long they may be mistaken for hair. Treatment includes cleaning the tongue with a toothbrush, scraping, applying hydrogen peroxide solutions, and destruction of the tissue (cautery) by a chemical.

Blackhead. Too many youngsters in their teens have been scolded and sent to the bathroom to give themselves a good scrubbing because they have blackheads. Many people still persist in believing that these pimples with dark centers are caused by dirt clogging the pores.

The blackhead—in medical terms a *comedo* (plural *comedones*)—is thickened sebum, which in its normal state is the more liquid secretion from the sebaceous glands of the skin. In the comedo, the sebum is combined with other material. Some of it is dead keratinocytes, cells that form keratin, the chief substance of the outer layer of skin. The comedo may also contain minute hair fragments or parts shed from the walls of the sebaceous glands.

Light and air react chemically with the end of the comedo, producing the dark spot of the blackhead. Washing the face helps to loosen some of the skin cells that are constantly being shed, but hard scrubbing will not make blackheads go away. In fact it may irritate the already inflamed skin and cause complications.

The plugging of the follicles of the sebaceous gland and of the pilosebaceous units—hair follicles into which some sebaceous glands open—produces the pimples of acne. The reasons for the formation of comedones are not certain, but they are related to the hormonal balance of the system. It is well known that blackheads and acne are most common during adolescent years, when sex-related hormones are especially active.

For information on the treatment of blackheads, see ACNE.

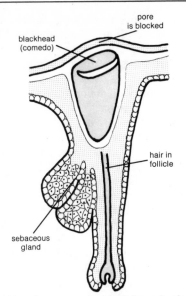

A blackhead, or comedo, is thickened sebum, the oily secretion of the sebaceous gland. The blackhead also may contain hair fragments, dead cells, and other skin debris.

Black Lung Disease. An occupational disease of miners who inhale coal dust is called black lung disease, or anthracosis. The dust particles inhaled contain carbon which causes coughing, shortness of breath, chest pains, and in many cases, premature death.

First noted in 1700 as an industrial disease, anthracosis usually develops after a ten-year period of working in the mines. Although most cases are diagnosed because of the above-mentioned symptoms, many are discovered when routine X rays are taken. The patient usually does not realize that anthracosis has begun until a cough sets in (without fever) or gradual shortness of breath develops.

No cure for anthracosis has been discovered and the only method for controlling it is to practice industrial hygiene.

Black Widow Spider Bite. Many think that a bite by the black widow spider, *Latrodectus mactans,* is fatal. This is not always true, but the bite is generally quite serious. The spider is widely found throughout the U.S. and may be identified by a red hourglass-shaped mark on the underside of the abdomen. About three-quarters of an inch across, the black widow is usually found around old wooden buildings and in dark places.

Once bitten, the victim experiences severe abdominal pain because of muscle spasms but no nausea or vomiting. Following the spasms, he may collapse and the pupils of his eyes may dilate. This is followed by swelling of the face, legs, and arms. Convulsions often occur.

The doctor treats a black widow spider bite by first making a crisscross cut over the bite. The poison is then sucked from the wound. Immediately after the bite occurs, a tourniquet may be applied just above the bite, but not so tightly that it cuts off the blood supply. (*See* TOURNIQUET.)

Some doctors feel that these measures do little good, because the amount of venom injected into the victim is small and is absorbed quickly by the tissues. Instead, they recommend that the wound be washed with hydrogen peroxide, alcohol, or an antiseptic because spiders are dirty and the wound could become infected.

In all cases, the victim should be taken to a hospital. An antivenin may be administered to stop further toxic symptoms. Where muscle spasms are severe, intravenous injections of calcium lactate or calcium gluconate can be given to lessen the pain.

Bladder. The bladder is a thick, balloon-like, muscular organ designed to receive and store urine until it is periodically discharged.

Located in the lower front of the pelvic abdominal cavity, the bladder is just behind the symphysis pubis and in front of the male rectum or the female vagina. Its functions are kept completely separate from those of the reproductive tract in women,

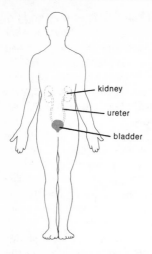

kidney

ureter

bladder

but in men the two systems share one common urethral outlet. (*See* URETHRA.)

Freely movable, the bladder is held secure by its placement between the perineum (muscular floor of the pelvic cavity) and the peritoneum, a strong membrane which lines the abdomen and surrounds most of the other abdominal organs. In infants, the bladder is shaped more like a cone and projects farther upward along the abdominal wall than in later years. Birth defects of the bladder are rare.

When the adult bladder fills, it rounds upward like a balloon, first oval and then round, pushing the peritoneum with it, possibly as high as the navel. The full bladder presses the peritoneum against the rectum in the male or against the vagina and uterus in the female.

When it empties, the top of the bladder falls flat. The peritoneum drops back down with it, almost parallel to the pelvic floor.

URINATION PROCESS. At the bottom of the bladder, circularly arranged muscle fibers form a sphincter ring around the opening to the urethra. Normally contracted to close the opening, these sphincter muscles only relax when the pressure of a full bladder sets up a reflex impulse.

The process of emptying the bladder is urination. Once urine pressure sets off this reflex, it continues until the bladder is emptied completely. However, a person can also start and stop this emptying action at will.

Involuntary or uncontrolled urination is called incontinence. This is normal in infants and varies greatly in young children. Some learn easily to control urination, even at night; others are slower, for various reasons. (*See* TOILET TRAINING.)

When an older child or adult loses normal control of urination either all or part of the time, this becomes an uncomfortable and embarrassing problem. There can be many causes which require medical attention to be located and treated. In stress incontinence, on the other hand, the patient has normal control except under conditions of extra internal pressure such as sneezing. (*See* STRESS INCONTINENCE; URINARY INCONTINENCE.)

CONTRACTION AND DISTENTION. The capacity of the bladder changes somewhat at different periods in a person's life, as well as varying greatly from one individual to another. However, the average adult bladder holds over three-fourths of a quart (about 700–800 ml.).

A bladder with progressively reduced capacity is called contracted, hypertonic, or spastic. This often results from spasms due to bladder injuries or lesions in the central nervous system which control the urination reflex. It also can occur temporarily from irritation or infection of the bladder, or during periods of emotional tension.

Urgent and frequent urination and bladder spasms, with pain that is often severe, are among the symptoms of this bladder trouble. Sometimes the bladder capacity becomes so low that it cannot hold any urine at all. Correction depends on locating and curing the cause, either psychological or physical. Meanwhile the discomfort can be eased with hot sitz baths (sitting in hot water over the hips), hot douches, heating pads, or diathermy (electrowave) treatments. Drugs may relieve the pain and spasms.

When the bladder does not empty properly, the condition is called retention. The problem becomes progressively worse as more urine flows in from the kidneys, gradually overfilling it. If this persists, the bladder becomes distended, and increasingly larger amounts of urine are required to produce the urination reflex. Eventually, involuntary voiding or overflow leakage (incontinence) will occur.

Treatment of this problem consists in emptying the bladder with a catheter (inserted drainage tube) until the muscles have contracted back to their original size. If the retention is due to obstructions, these must also be found and corrected.

Retention of urine is one of the primary causes of cystitis, or inflammation of the bladder with or without infection. It seems that the bladder's protective system depends partly on periodically ridding itself of the old urine and whatever bacteria or other contamination it contains. (*See* CYSTITIS.)

Another cause of urine retention in at least part of the bladder is malformations such as diverticula, little saclike pouches projecting outward from the organ walls. Often these have narrow necks restricting the flow of new and old urine, so that a diverticulum itself becomes inflamed and the trouble spreads to the rest of the bladder. The diverticula may need to be removed surgically.

INJURIES AND REPAIR. Repair of the bladder is somewhat like that of the teeth in dentistry, in that its tissues cannot be replaced by new growth. Instead, the surgeon must remove any diseased or damaged portions and close up the openings, salvaging as much remaining bladder function as possible.

The bladder is so elastic that it is unlikely to be injured, but it can be damaged by external blows and penetrating wounds or by internal foreign objects. However, seldom does anything get into the bladder from the outside except through the urethra as the result of self-exploration or of sadistic sexual practices. Under such conditions both inflammation (cystitis) and infection of bladder tissues generally follow within a few days. Blood and pus appear in the urine, and urination is burning, urgent, and frequent.

If a foreign body remains in the bladder for a few months, it will be encrusted with layers of hardened material from the urine and become a bladder stone (calculus). However, most calculi are formed in the kidney or bladder from minerals or organic materials such as blood clots. Additional damage, infection, and severe pain occur when these are forced into the narrow bladder neck or the urethra by urination. (*See* BLADDER STONES; KIDNEY STONES.)

Injury to the bladder may result from moderate blows to the external abdominal wall, causing blood in the urine as well as frequency and urgency of urination. But the injury usually heals rapidly.

BLADDER RUPTURE. Severe blows, penetrating wounds, or fragments of broken pelvic bone can cause rupture (tearing) of the bladder walls. Bladder wounds are common war injuries.

Less often will the bladder burst because of internal pressure. When this happens, it may be due to severe distention from urinary blockage or to weakening of the bladder wall by infection or some other disease.

If there is blood in the urine following an accident or injury, bladder rupture is probably the reason. Urination is painful and difficult, and shock may set in. (*See* SHOCK.)

When the bladder is ruptured, the urine escapes into the adjoining cavities and tissues. Most bladder ruptures open below the "roof" formed over the bladder by the peritoneal membrane, so that the urine fills the spaces between the bladder and rectum (and vagina in women) on the floor of the pelvic cavity.

If the bladder was full (distended) at the time of the injury or if the injury was serious, the peritoneum is likely to have been ruptured with the bladder. Then bladder pressure will force urine into the peritoneal cavity. Urine will collect in pockets lower than the top of the bladder. This is more of a problem with men, whose peritoneal membrane and cavity dip down between the bladder and rectum to fill the space occupied by the vagina and uterus in women.

When the peritoneum also is damaged, the problem is more serious, as peritonitis (inflammation of the peritoneal membrane) is likely to set in. (*See* PERITONITIS.) If the peritoneum is not involved, small bladder wounds will usually close up without surgery. However, drainage of urine by a catheter must be maintained for at least ten days, whether surgery is performed or not, to give the wounds time to heal.

When bladder wounds also involve injury to adjoining organs, the problem and its treatment are much like those of a fistula. In fact, if they fail to heal properly, a fistula can result.

A fistula is something like a rupture in that it forms a tubelike passage from the bladder to another organ or the external skin. Through this, urine can escape and other materials can enter the bladder. (*See* FISTULA.)

TUMORS AND CANCER. Bladder tumors grow in two forms—lacy, cauliflower-shaped protrusions into the bladder cavity or large, hard ulcerous lumps that spread rapidly outside the bladder. If the tumor is still small and involves only the superficial internal lining of the bladder, it can be removed along with the adjoining part of the bladder wall.

Usually, however, few symptoms are noticeable until the tumors are large or multiple. It may be necessary to remove the whole bladder and to divert urine into the large intestine or an external receptacle in an operation similar to a colostomy. (*See*

COLOSTOMY.) The tumors have a tendency to recur and spread through the bladder wall to adjoining tissues.

Bladder tumors are several times as common in men as in women, for reasons that are unknown.

Many bladder ulcers can be removed successfully if medical care is obtained promptly after the first symptoms are noticed. These are a frequent cause of cystitis.

Bladder Stones. Deposits of calcium salts may accumulate in the bladder in the form of calculi, or bladder stones. These stones may arise elsewhere (for example, in the kidney) but become trapped in the bladder.

Symptoms of bladder stones include various degrees of blood in the urine, bladder spasms, and difficulty in urination. They are often crushed by physicians with an instrument looking rather like a cross between scissors and pliers. Larger stones may require surgical removal.

Bladder stones are sometimes a complication of catheters in bedridden patients. Prevention is by means of regular irrigation. (*See* BLADDER; CATHETER.)

Blastocyst. During the first two weeks of pregnancy, the fertilized ovum (egg) is known as a blastocyst.

As soon as the ovum is fertilized, its cell begins to divide and duplicate into more cells, while it travels down the uterine tube to the uterus. At the end of the first week, it becomes embedded in a blister in the wall of the uterus and forms rootlike attachments which develop into the various organs and tissues needed for pregnancy. (*See* IMPLANTATION; PRENATAL DEVELOPMENT.)

Blastomycosis. A fungus causes the disease called blastomycosis. There are two types, North American and South American.

North American blastomycosis has been

found in parts of the central and eastern United States and Canada, less frequently in some tropical countries. The fungus of this North American variety, called *blastomyces dermatitidis,* usually attacks only the skin, but it may spread widely through the body organs and central nervous system. When the lungs are involved, the patient may spit up mucus and blood, have chills and fever, and lose weight. The bones of his chest and back may deteriorate. The disease is treated with the drug amphotericin B, and sometimes with surgery to remove lesions (tissue changed by the disease).

The South American type of the disease is caused by the fungus *Paracoccidioides brasiliensis,* which is also found in Mexico and the Central American countries. It starts with ulcers of the pharynx. These may enlarge and destroy the vocal cords and other parts of the throat and mouth. When the lymph nodes enlarge, the fungus may find its way into the stomach and intestines, with further destruction of tissue. Malnutrition and death often occur.

The South American blastomycosis is much more severe than most cases of the North American variety. It also is treated with amphotericin B, but relapses (recurrences of the disease) are frequent.

Bleeding.

An injury that breaks a blood vessel causes different kinds of blood loss, depending on the type of vessel.

When an artery is cut, bleeding is rapid and dangerous. Blood spurts out under pressure and must be stopped immediately by using a tourniquet or pressing on the arterial pressure points between the wound and the heart. (*See* CLOT; COAGULATION.)

Bleeding from a vein is less rapid, but if the vein is large it also must be stopped immediately. Even in twenty seconds enough blood can be lost to be dangerous.

Bleeding from a wound goes through several successive stages.

First, immediately after the wound, the blood runs freely. This has the effect of

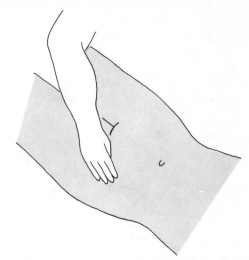

Pressure on the femoral artery, just below the waistline, may be used to stop the flow of blood from a leg or foot injury.

flooding away dirt and germs and bringing a large number of anti-infectious blood elements to the wound.

Second, the ends of the broken vessels begin to crimp shut rather quickly, stopping the blood flow. Then within about two to six minutes a clot forms. (*See* CLOT; COAGULATION.)

Third, in anywhere from thirty minutes to two or more hours, the wound begins to redden and swell painfully again, as more blood enters the injured vessels. There is no bleeding because the vessels have been closed securely by smooth-muscle contraction and clotting. As this happens the capillary walls become more permeable. Plasma and infection-fighting white cells move through these walls into the intercellular spaces and begin repairing the wound.

Bleeding can also be an abnormal condition not connected with wounds. The causes may be various, including a shortage of the blood protein substances needed for clotting (prothrombin and other factors) and a shortage of blood platelets, also essential in clotting. More rarely, abnormal bleeding is caused by a shortage of clot-forming fibrinogen in the plasma and by an

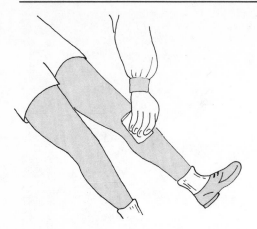

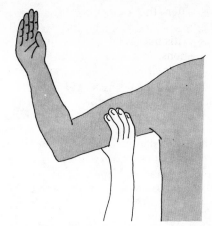

Direct pressure on a wound is often sufficient to stop the flow of blood until you can get the patient to a physician.

Finger pressure on the brachial artery may be used to stop bleeding from the arm or hand.

inherited hemorrhagic disease, the best known being hemophilia.

In physical examinations bleeding is tested to see how long it takes for the patient's blood to stop flowing out of a break in the skin and form a clot. The simplest of these "bleeding-time" tests is a test of coagulation. A finger or ear lobe is pricked and length of time before the bleeding stops is recorded. For the finger it should be two–three minutes; for the ear, four–five minutes.

In another test for clotting time, blood is taken into a test tube and allowed to stand, without agitation. In about six minutes it should be coagulated.

Bleeding Time. The length of time required for bleeding to stop after a puncture wound of the ear lobe or ball of the finger is known as bleeding time. Drops of blood are wiped away from the puncture every thirty seconds. Normally the bleeding stops within one to six minutes, as the blood vessels constrict. (*See* BLEEDING; CLOT.)

Blennorrhea. A discharge from mucous surfaces, such as gonorrheal discharges from the urethra or vagina, is called

blennorrhea. (*See* GONORRHEA; URETHRA; VAGINA.)

Blepharitis. When the *Staphylococcus aureus* germ infects the edges of the eyelids, the result may be a condition known as blepharitis. This also is called granulated eyelids, because drainage from the infection produces sticky or dry granules or scales on the eyelids.

The eyelashes may fall out, the eyelids may become sensitive and itchy, or there may be a burning sensation. Ulcerated sores may develop.

Usually the staphylococcus infection is complicated by seborrheic blepharitis, which is characterized by seborrhea, an excessive secretion of sebum, the oily substance of the sebaceous glands. Seborrhea of the eyebrows and scalp is often present, because of the spread of the infecting microorganisms. (*See* SEBACEOUS GLANDS; SEBUM.)

The granules and greasy secretions on the eyelids should be removed with a damp piece of cotton. Sulfa or antibiotic eye ointments are used. It is important to keep the scalp, brows, and eyes clean, or the infecting organisms may remain to reinfect the eyelids after the ointments are discontinued.

Blepharitis may be associated with other eye infections. When it is combined with conjunctivitis, it is known as blepharoconjunctivitis. (*See* CONJUNCTIVITIS; EYE; STY.)

Sometimes the basic problem lies in a skin disorder which also involves other parts of the body, and a consultation with a dermatologist (skin specialist) is required. Blepharitis with dermatitis (skin disease) is called blepharodermatitis, and may be related to eczema, psoriasis, pemphigus, or an allergic reaction. The possibility of an allergic irritation by eye makeup or some other cosmetic preparation should also be considered.

Blindness. There are few accurate figures on the number of blind people in the world. In the United States, estimates place the total number at close to one million.

This figure may strike you as tragic, but the real tragedy is that more than 50 percent of these cases could have been prevented. This is the opinion of the National Society for the Prevention of Blindness, which has been active for over half a century.

Agencies for the blind have worked long to erase the notion that the sightless individual is a pitiful creature who must beg with a tin cup or seek charity in other humiliating ways. What the blind really want is to be accepted as individuals not very different from the rest of us, and be helped to become as independent as possible.

FACING BLINDNESS. Despite great advances in the protection of the eyes as well as new medical and surgical techniques, many people today are losing their eyesight. The greatest number are over the age of sixty-five and are suffering from systemic disorders, such as diabetes and circulatory disease, which contribute to eye problems.

If you were facing inevitable blindness,

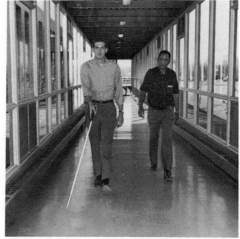

VA Hospital, Hines, Illinois

The first decision a blind man or woman must make is to continue with life—but according to a different pattern than the one previously followed. Here a young man practices with a cane.

what could you do? Here are some suggestions:

Make the best use of what eyesight you have. Talk this over with your eye doctor.

Learn how to be as independent as you can, but accept assistance when you need it. Either extreme—wanting everything done for you or refusing all aid—will be an unsatisfactory and unhappy adjustment.

Get in touch with agencies for the blind that can help you learn how to live with your handicap. Your local health department, medical society, or public library will enable you to locate these agencies.

Learn how to use the many aids for the blind, such as braille books, a standard or braille typewriter, "talking books" (recorded material), a guide dog, and so on. (*See* BRAILLE.)

If you are of working age, get a job. Agencies for the blind will help you do this.

Get a hobby, if you don't have one already. You could, for example, learn to play a musical instrument, compose music, sing in a choir, write poetry or short stories, or knit. Many blind persons, however, have more active hobbies. Some swim, play golf, bowl, ride a bicycle (one built for two), or give lectures.

Keep up your education. Day or night classes not only can be fun but can lead to a career. There are many blind professionals, such as lawyers, teachers, psychologists, even judges and doctors.

If you face blindness, one of the most important things to do is to associate with positive, happy people. Avoid friendships with persons who continually look on the dark side of life and offer you only pity.

And don't let yourself stagnate. Listening to radio or television most of the time is not enough. This is too passive. You must keep both your mind and your body active.

AIDS TO THE BLIND. Braille is printed with raised dots on paper, which you read by passing your fingers over the dots. A variation of this consists of braille letters on a tape which moves rapidly beneath the reader's fingers.

Hundreds of special household aids that can be operated by touch or sound rather than sight have been developed for the blind—for example, measuring devices with embossed numbers and letters. Among other products so adapted are electric cooking devices, thermometers, tape measures, bathroom scales, needle threaders, hem gauges, clocks, watches, timers, and braille tape markers. Many industrial measuring devices, such as calipers, micrometers, compasses, protractors, T-squares, and slide rules are also available for the blind. For their recreation there are specially designed playing cards, chess sets, Scrabble sets, bingo boards and numbers, dominoes, crossword puzzles, and many other games.

In the developmental stage are many electronic devices to aid the blind. One consists of a light and dark sensing device which is connected to a radio in the form of a helmet. The radio waves are transmit-

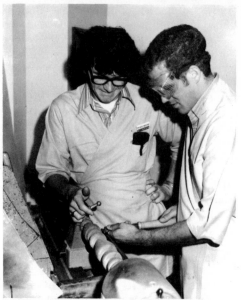

VA Hospital, Hines, Illinois

Learning a new skill is a critical task for a blind person. It provides the man or woman with a sense of worth as well as a possible means of livlihood. Here wood-turning has been chosen for study.

ted to receptors implanted under the skin of the skull for stimulating parts of the brain. The result is that the blind user can visualize the general shape of objects before him.

Another black and white sensing device works like a television camera by stimulating a panel placed against the blind person's back. The panel is covered with dots which vibrate against the skin, giving general image patterns.

CAUSES OF BLINDNESS. Among the major causes of blindness are cataracts, glaucoma, amblyopia, diabetes, and trachoma. Separate articles under these titles give details on these problems. Other eye problems which may cause blindness are summarized in the articles EYE; EYE INJURIES; EYESIGHT.

A summary of measures to save eyesight is included in the article EYE CARE.

Blind Spot. The spot on the retina not affected by light is known as the blind spot. This is the place where the optic nerve leaves the retina. (*See* EYE; OPTIC NERVE; RETINA.)

Blister Beetle. Widely distributed all through the United States are about two hundred species of insects which cause blisters when just barely touched. They contain a very large amount of an irritating substance called cantharidin. (*See* APHRODISIAC; CANTHARIDES.)

If one of these insects walks across a person's skin and is not harmed or touched, it will probably not cause damage. If, however, it is brushed or touched, a clear amber fluid will flow from many parts of the insect's body.

In about ten minutes the affected skin area will start to tingle. Several hours later, blisters appear; their number and size are determined by the amount of fluid left on the skin. (*See* BLISTERS; CANTHARIDES.)

Blisters. The fluid-filled sac which forms on the skin after irritation or disease is called a blister. So-called water blisters, with clear fluid, are frequently caused by rubbing, chafing, or a tight pinch. Blisters may also fill with blood from injured small blood vessels. Or they may be formed from the fluid by-products of insect bites, surface infections, skin disorders, or systemic disease.

In general, leave blisters alone. The fluid will be absorbed and transported away naturally as the lesion clears. If your blisters are widespread and you do not know the cause, check with your physician.

If you have a large clear-liquid blister caused by rubbing or chafing—one that will probably be broken because it is located on the foot, heel, or another vulnerable spot—then you may puncture the blister. Pierce it in two places with a needle and gently force out the fluid with a piece of gauze. Be

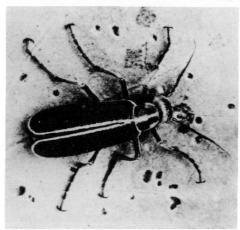

U.S. Department of Agriculture

The margined blister beetle and the skin injury which it causes. Dark spots result from the secretion of cantharidin from the insect's wings.

sure to sterilize the needle first by holding it in an open flame. Then cover the collapsed blister with a clean gauze dressing to protect it from infection.

Small blisters, with little chance of breaking, should be washed carefully with soap and water and covered with a bandage to keep them intact.

If the blister already has been torn open, exposing the raw underskin, wash the area with warm water and mild soap, and dress it as you would a small wound. Infection is the major risk in open blisters.

Do *not* puncture blisters due to burns. (*See* BURNS.) Small blisters which often accompany skin disease are called vesicles, and the process of blister formation is termed vesication. A vesicant is a drug or some other substance which causes blisters.

Bulla is the medical term for a blister larger than five millimeters in diameter.

Bloating. When the tissues beneath the skin become puffy from abnormal fluid accumulation, the condition is called bloating. The more correct term, however, is edema. (*See* EDEMA.) Congestive heart failure and low levels of protein in the blood are common causes. (*See* HEART.)

The term bloating is also used to describe the full, distended feeling in the abdomen which comes from overeating. (*See* INDIGESTION.)

Blood. The main function of blood is transportation. Blood picks up oxygen, one of the body's most necessary substances, from the lungs and returns waste carbon dioxide. It also takes up nourishment from the intestines when foodstuffs have been adapted to body needs, and carries them to tissues throughout the human system.

After the nutrients have been used by tissue cells and processed through various organs, such as the skin, intestines, and kidneys, the residues are taken up by the bloodstream to be passed out (excreted) from the body.

Hormones, which control vital functions, are taken in by the blood from various points and discharged at others, following instructions from elaborate sensing systems located along blood vessels and within the brain, glands, and organs. (*See* HORMONES.)

The blood also aids in maintaining a chemical and fluid volume balance in the tissues, helps keep the body temperature at normal levels, transports infection-fighting substances to sites where they are needed, and forms clots to block loss of blood after injury.

Unfortunately for man, his blood is also a handy transportation system for bacteria, viruses, and lifeless chemicals that cause and spread disease.

The means by which blood is pumped through the body is described in the articles BLOOD CIRCULATION and HEART.

COMPOSITION OF BLOOD. Almost half of the blood volume consists of red and white cells (many more red than white). The rest is a fluid called plasma, which surrounds the cells. The cells are also termed corpuscles. A simple laboratory test, using a tube of blood whirled around in a centrifuge, separates the red blood corpuscles from the plasma and determines the percentage of these cells in relation to the whole blood. Both the ratio of red blood cells to whole blood volume and the instrument used to obtain it are called a hematocrit.

The average hematocrit for an adult male is about 47 and for women about 42. This may vary upward or downward as much as 10 or 15 percent and still be within the normal range. Corpuscles are described in the article BLOOD CELLS.

Cholesterol is an important somewhat fatty substance found in the blood and tissues. Its many functions include aiding information of bile salts, important to the digestion of fats; helping to produce essential hormones; and preventing excessive water evaporation from the skin.

The unfavorable aspects of cholesterol are probably more familiar to modern man than its vital functions. An excess amount of cholesterol is sometimes found in the blood, a condition known as hypercholesteremia, which has been blamed for the formation of atherosclerotic deposits on the walls of blood vessels, restricting blood circulation. (*See* ATHEROSCLEROSIS; CHOLESTEROL.)

The blood plasma also contains a large variety of minerals, chemicals called electrolytes, nutrients, nitrogen-containing compounds, and antibodies, important in the fight against disease. All these are carried in a liquid state, for plasma is about 90 percent water.

BLEEDING AND CLOTTING. When clots form within the bloodstream, they may cause serious problems. The blood contains two substances to prevent internal clotting: antithromboplastin (or antithrombin for short) and an antiprothrombin substance called heparin.

In addition there are a number of substances that produce clotting of blood when it is needed. These include prothrombin, fibrinogen, and calcium ions. There are at least ten other substances involved in the process by which prothrombin is converted to thrombin, which changes soluble fibrinogen into the insoluble strands of fibrin.

This pattern of clotting can be upset by many factors. Clotting occurs faster, for example, when a coarse substance is placed on the bleeding wound. This is why gauze bandages help stop bleeding. A hot towel is sometimes applied to a wound to raise the temperature to at least 115° F. (about 46° C.) and speed up the chemical action that causes clotting.

Why, then, are ice packs also used to stop bleeding? Although cold may interfere with the clotting of blood, it has another characteristic that often outweighs this disadvantage. Cold causes blood vessels to contract, rapidly reducing blood flow.

Deficiencies of blood substances such as fibrinogen, calcium salts, cells called thrombocytes, and vitamin K also hinder clotting. The introduction of other chemicals into the blood, either by a natural or an abnormal reaction of the body or by hypodermic injections, can also vary the speed of clotting. Anticoagulants such as heparin are valuable in the treatment or prevention of diseases in which there is abnormal clotting, with blockage of blood passages.

BLOOD DISEASES. Blood testing is common during routine or special physical examinations. The chemical nature of blood is changed not only in specific blood diseases but in nearly every other kind of disease that is systemic (spread throughout the body) rather than confined to a small area.

Changes in a person's diet, the drinking of alcoholic and other beverages, drugs taken by mouth or injection, smoking or inhalation of other gases into the lungs, and emotional responses also may cause alterations—often rapid and dramatic—in the character and composition of the blood.

A common blood condition is anemia, in which there is a shortage of either ery-throcytes or hemoglobin or both. Hemoglobin is a large molecule that contains iron, vital to proper health. (*See* ANEMIA.) In leukopenia there is a deficiency in the number of white cells. Polycythemia is a condition characterized by too many ery-throcytes. (*See* BLOOD CELLS.)

Leukemia is a fatal condition, sometimes termed cancer of the blood, in which there is an abnormal increase in the number of leukocytes. (*See* LEUKEMIA.)

Thrombocytopenia is an abnormal decrease in platelets, also called thrombocytes, which are essential to the clotting of blood. Another disorder in which the blood does not clot properly is hemophilia, which occurs in males although it is passed on from one generation of males to another by females who show no signs of the disease. (*See* HEMOPHILIA.)

Various abnormalities of the blood are termed dyscrasias and are frequently caused by the effects of medication. During therapy with certain drugs, periodic blood sampling must be made to detect unfavorable reactions.

Cancer of the bone has a severely deteriorating effect on the blood, because bone marrow is the site of formation of ery-throcytes.

In addition to disorders of blood chemistry, there are blood problems that result from improper circulation. This may be due to defects in the blood vessels, blockage of veins and arteries by clots, or a wide variety of heart malfunctions. (*See* BLOOD CELLS; BLOOD CIRCULATION; BLOOD DISEASES; HEART.)

Blood Bank. If all human blood were exactly the same, and if we could predict the need for it in transfusions according to a predetermined schedule, there would be no point in storing or banking it. However, all human blood is not the same.

Facilities called blood banks collect whole blood from donors; test it; identify it according to type; process it in various ways; store it in several forms; and either transfuse it or supply blood, or portions of the blood such as plasma, to other facilities for transfusions. (*See* TRANSFUSIONS.)

The blood bank, like a financial bank, takes "deposits" of blood when it can get them. It then makes this blood available in several "denominations," or kinds of blood material, according to need—whether to a single patient in surgery or to the many victims of a major disaster.

The most important blood bank denomination, whole blood, is stored for as long as three weeks, cooled to a normal refrigerator temperature of about 42–44° F. (6–7° C.). Plasma may be stored for months in fluid form or almost indefinitely when frozen or freeze-dried.

Whole blood is preserved by the addition of small amounts of several citrate or oxalate compounds to prevent coagulation, plus sugar (glucose) to nourish the erythrocytes (red corpuscles). Dried plasma is reconstituted for transfusion by adding sterile water. The various other fractions of blood, blood substitutes, and blood expanders are concentrated and preserved in a variety of ways before transfusion into the recipient's bloodstream.

The development of blood banks is fairly recent, having come about mostly during and since the 1940's. Actually the techniques that made the first blood banks possible were known some decades earlier, but there had been no pressing demand for blood banks until a major need suddenly loomed up in the 1940's. That need was World War II.

The technical innovations that made blood banking possible were (1) the recognition of blood types at the beginning of this century and (2) the first successful storage of whole blood about fifteen years later, during World War I.

The Austrian-born pathologist Karl Landsteiner discovered that the red blood cells carry a protein substance on their stroma (surface) that is a type of antigen

(substance that stimulates production of an antibody) called an agglutinogen. (*See* ANTIBODY; ANTIGEN.) From this discovery, Landsteiner and his associates in 1901–1902 went on to develop what came to be known as the International Classification of Blood Types. This classification is simpler than the clumsy numerical classifications used previously. It includes the four well-known blood types, A, B, AB, and O, and is based on the sensitivity reaction of antigens or agglutinogens A and B in one person's blood to the antibodies or agglutinins alpha and beta in another person's blood. Combinations of agglutinogen A, for example, and agglutinin alpha cause agglutination or clumping of red cells, and this in turn causes serious problems in the circulatory system and kidneys. (*See* BLOOD TYPES.)

Once doctors understood how bloods can be incompatible, they were able to safely match the blood of donor and recipient.

Safe storage of blood became possible when researchers found the right chemical additives and temperatures to preserve it. The use of sodium citrate as an anticoagulant was first perfected in 1915 by Richard Lewisohn. During this same World War I period, Oswald Robertson, a U.S. citizen, successfully demonstrated to the British Army that whole blood could be safely stored for later use in transfusing the wounded.

Transfusions, as such, did not begin with these twentieth-century developments. They were originally tried experimentally as far back as the seventeenth-century and included the use of some nonhuman blood. However, because this animal blood caused some deaths—apparently not in all cases—the practice of transfusing was condemned in the written laws of some European nations and not tried again to any great degree until the nineteenth century.

Before the establishment of blood banks, a physician would test a patient's relatives and friends until he found the right blood

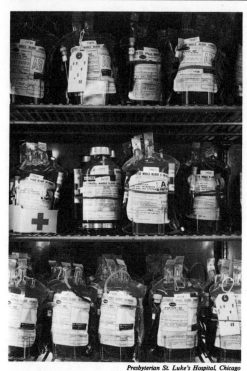

Presbyterian St. Luke's Hospital, Chicago

Fresh whole human blood in a refrigerator at
a blood bank.

type, performed a cross-match test for
compatibility (mixing small amounts of donor's and recipient's blood), and transfused
the donor's blood directly to the patient.

By the 1930's, the techniques for preserving the freshness and preventing the coagulation of blood had progressed to the point
where blood banking became feasible. In
1937 Dr. Bernard Fantus established at
Cook County Hospital, Chicago, the first
blood bank in the United States.

The 1940's were a period of many developments in the science and technology of
blood banking. Many new specialized blood
types were discovered. Cross-matching of
blood was further expanded and refined.
The result was that the collection, testing,
storage, and transfusing of blood became
such a specialty that the practicing physician began to have less responsibility for the

technical side of transfusing blood. More
and more this responsibility was put in the
hands of the professionals and technicians
who worked full time in the blood bank.

Progress in blood banking was so great
that just twenty-five years after the first
U.S. bank was established at Cook County
Hospital there were 5,537 banks in the 50
states and in U.S. possessions.

Today the blood bank performs even
more complex kinds of testing than in the
past to safeguard its users. The present-day
blood bank may be anyone of several kinds
of facilities and may offer a wide variety of
services.

Tests are now performed not only for the
red-cell-clumping problem but also for
other kinds of potentially dangerous
incompatibility. Testing now includes
elaborate blood typing and cross-matching
for all major blood types and additional
types, such as the Rh factor, as well as the
use of Coombs serum (and other methods)
to test both for specific sensitization to the
Rh factor and other conditions and for the
degree of sensitization.

Such testing may be performed for legal
purposes in questions of the paternity of a
child. But the tests can establish fatherhood
only by exclusion—that is, show that because of the blood type inherited by the
child the person tested cannot be its father.

Blood banks are of several types, including hospital transfusion services; community transfusion clinics; Red Cross transfusion centers; blood collection services
operated by hospitals; and hospital-
operated facilities that primarily store
blood.

More goes on in these centers than just
the taking and giving of straight blood.
They may take blood directly from donors;
process blood and blood compounds; give
blood transfusions; store blood; and test
blood and plasma. And whole blood is by
no means the only material they offer. Today's blood bank *can* transfuse whole
blood, but it also can offer such specialties

as dried and irradiated blood plasma; pooled plasma (from several donors); platelet-rich plasma; anti-hemophiliac plasma; platelet concentrates (to control bleeding); "packed" or concentrated red blood corpuscles (to treat anemia); fibrinogen (to improve clotting ability); albumin (to enlarge total blood volume in treating shock); and gamma globulin (to prevent or lessen the effects of measles).

One recent development is a deep concern about the possibility that blood contaminated with infectious organisms is being received from certain commercial blood-collection facilities. In particular there is concern about blood services that receive blood from donors who provide it purely for the fee received, as in the transient and Skid Row areas of large cities. Infectious hepatitis, among other diseases, is thought to be spread from some such agencies and donors.

As a result there is a growing movement to develop volunteer community sources for the needed blood; to impose stricter rules of hygiene and testing; and to discontinue the use of questionable blood sources.

Blood Cells.

Corpuscles, or blood cells, compose about half the volume of blood; the rest is a fluid called plasma. Most of these cells are red. They are also called erythrocytes. An amazingly large number of them, from 20 to 25 trillion, circulate through the body. There is only one white blood cell, or leukocyte, for every 600 or 700 red blood cells.

The cells pick up, transport, and discharge various vital materials as they move through the bloodstream, as well as fight disease. Blood cells are examined under the microscope and by means of various tests to determine their condition and "count"— the number of each type of cell in a given volume of blood. The results help in the diagnosis not only of diseases of the blood, but of other diseases that affect the bloodstream.

RED CELLS. The most important role of red blood cells is the transporting of a red pigment known as hemoglobin. Several million molecules of hemoglobin are contained in one human red cell. It is hemoglobin that picks up oxygen during the journey of blood through the lungs and takes this vital gas to body tissues.

Only the red cells can carry hemoglobin in the blood. When a red cell disintegrates, as it does after about four months, the hemoglobin seeps out into tissues or organs, where it is broken up into simpler chemical components.

Some of it is transformed into chemicals that form the basis of the bile pigment, bilirubin, in liver secretions. If there are too few red cells in the blood or if there is too little hemoglobin within the cells, anemia results. (*See* ANEMIA.)

A medical problem that may be considered the opposite of anemia is polycythemia, an abnormal increase in the number of red cells. One cause is prolonged residence at high altitudes. (*See* POLYCYTHEMIA.)

WHITE CELLS. The white cells of the blood are called leukocytes. There are several varieties of fully developed leukocytes, generally classed as lymphocytes, monocytes, and granulocytes. These are further divided into a number of subclassifications.

Lymphocytes take their name from lymph, because most of them are produced in the lymph glands. A monocyte is typified by a single (mono) nucleus, or center portion. A granulocyte appears granular (grainy) under the microscope.

The blood also contains platelets (thrombocytes), which are not complete cells, but fragments of white cells called megakaryocytes. In addition there are cells in various stages of development. Their names end with -blast, from the Greek *blastos,* meaning bud or shoot.

The lymphocytes are produced not only in the lymph nodes but also in the spleen, thymus, and other lymphoid (lymphlike) organs. Monocytes may be formed by the same organs, but most of them are produced in the marrow of bones.

The granulocytes, also called polymorphoneuclear cells, are produced in bone marrow. Three classes of granulocytes are neutrophils, eosinophils, and basophils. Basophils are important because they carry histamine, a substance related to allergic reactions. (*See* HISTAMINE.)

FUNCTIONS OF LEUKOCYTES. Each type of leukocyte has a specialized function, although the prime role of all of them is combating infection.

Lymphocytes may change their forms when they are called into action to fight infection. Some become monocytes, and function as phagocytes or macrophages—cells that surround and consume bacteria and cell debris by a process called phagocytosis. The phagocytes also contain chemical substances that have bactericidal (bacteria-killing) properties.

Granulocytes also act as phagocytes. Eosinophils increase rapidly during the course of diseases caused by parasites, such as trichinosis, apparently for the purpose of nullifying the poisonous effects of the disease.

Basophils, in addition to transporting histamine, release heparin into the bloodstream. This substance helps prevent blood from clotting and aids removal of fat from the bloodstream.

Neutrophils, functioning as phagocytes, are among the first cells to function during infection. When many are found in the blood, the condition is known as neutrophilia. This occurs during the body's fight against bacterial infection, cancer, hemorrhage, poisoning, and other critical problems. Large numbers of neutrophils also circulate normally during heavy exercise, apparently because they are carried from storage areas in the capillaries by the increased flow of blood.

White cells can move out through the blood vessel pores and tissue spaces, although these openings may be smaller than the normal diameter of the cells. This is accomplished by diapedesis, a process in which the cells are squeezed through the openings in much the same way as a water-filled balloon may be forced through a narrow hole. The cells enter injured tissue in this fashion to help rebuild new tissue after injury.

Blood platelets, or thrombocytes, adhere to each other during bleeding and help stop blood loss. They also change form when exposed to air, and aid clotting. (*See* BLEEDING.)

In leukemia (cancer of the bloodstream) there is a large production of white cells, many of which are unable to function normally. The leukemic cells also invade the bone marrow and other parts of the body. (*See* LEUKEMIA.)

Bacteria of many varieties are ordinarily present in various passages of the body, but usually are kept within harmless limits by the action of white blood cells. If insufficient white cells are produced, however, the bacteria multiply without restraint and severe infection can result.

Agranulocytosis is a disease in which this occurs. The bone marrow stops production of neutrophils and monocytes and the bacteria gain headway. Often the cause is traced to drugs that have a side effect of suppressing white cell production. Overexposure to radiation, as by X rays or a nuclear explosion, can have similar results.

The treatment of agranulocytosis must be twofold. First, the cause of the bone marrow deficiency must be eliminated. Second, antibiotics or other medication must be given to kill off the runaway bacteria. If the bone marrow is damaged beyond recovery, the disease will be fatal.

Blood Circulation. In order to perform its many functions, blood must continually circulate through the body. It takes two main pathways as it circulates through the body. One, the pulmonary, carries blood to

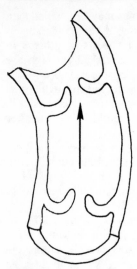

Cutaway sketch shows how valves operate in the veins. When there is a blood flow in the direction of the arrow, the valves open as shown. If the pressure is reduced or stops, the flaps of the valves close, to stop backward blood flow.

the lungs to release waste carbon dioxide and return loaded with oxygen. The second pathway, the systemic, delivers oxygen to tissues throughout the body, where it picks up carbon dioxide and other wastes and transports nutrients, hormones, enzymes, and other chemicals to sites where they are needed.

THE ARTERIES. The blood vessels that carry blood from the heart are called the arteries. The aorta, or great artery, is about one inch in diameter at its exit from the heart. As the blood continues its trip to every corner of the body, the arteries carrying it become smaller and more numerous, with many branches. Close to the end of its outward trip, it passes through narrow branches called arterioles, then into arterial capillaries. These are even smaller vessels that diffuse blood nourishment into the tissues and pick up waste material.

THE VENOUS SYSTEM. Joining the network of arterial capillaries are the venous capillaries, which start the blood on its way back to the heart. The blood next flows into the small veins called venules, then into fewer veins of ever widening diameter, until it reaches the heart.

At every gland through which there is circulation, the blood makes a delivery of some substance and picks up others. One important stop is the marrow of bones, where new red blood cells are made.

VESSEL STRUCTURE. Both arteries and veins are flexible tubes that can constrict (narrow) and dilate (expand) according to the needs of the body. This is accomplished by the tightening and relaxing of involuntary muscle fibers that make up the vessel walls, as well as by pressure from voluntary muscles surrounding the vessels.

Such muscles play an important part in forcing blood back to the heart. This function is called a venous pump. The tightening of leg muscles by walking or some other exercise squeezes the veins, forcing the blood to flow upward. It cannot normally flow downward, as the veins are equipped with one-way valves.

In varicose veins, these valves do not work properly, and the venous pump cannot send enough blood upward. The veins then dilate, the walls deteriorate from the strain, tissues are poorly nourished, and fluid collects in the limbs. (*See* VARICOSE VEINS.) Inflammation of the veins is called phlebitis. (*See* PHLEBITIS.)

The walls of arteries are subject to a number of disorders. They may harden and deteriorate, or the passages may be narrowed by spasms or cholesterol deposits. (*See* ARTERIOSCLEROSIS; ATHEROSCLEROSIS; CHOLESTEROL.)

Sometimes the sheath or covering of the nerves, arteries, and veins in legs or arms becomes inflamed. This condition is called Buerger's disease, or thromboangiitis obliterans, and results in pain from intermittent claudication. (*See* BUERGER'S DISEASE; CLAUDICATION.) Vasoconstriction (narrowing of vessels) commonly occurs during cool weather; this condition may be extreme in individuals with Raynaud's disease. (*See* RAYNAUD'S DISEASE.) Very cold temperatures, however, cause the opposite reaction in normal individuals—the vessels dilate to permit an increase in the amount of blood circulating through the extremities in order to keep them from freezing. This extra blood is what makes noses and ears red in winter.

Blocking of blood flow through arteries or veins (ischemia) can cause tissues to die from lack of oxygen. If this continues, gangrene may set in, and amputation may be required to save the patient's life. (*See* GANGRENE; ISCHEMIA.)

BLOOD PRESSURE. In order for blood to keep moving properly, it must be kept under pressure. This pressure is provided by the action of the heart, although many other factors can alter it in favorable or unfavorable ways. The pressure is greater when the heart is in the period of contraction, or systole, than when in diastole, the phase of relaxation and expansion. Blood pressure usually is measured on the brachial artery of the upper arm with an instrument called a sphygmomanometer. This device indicates the pressure required to raise a column of mercury in a tube marked off in millimeters (mm.). Thus if a given blood pressure raises the mercury to the 100 mm. mark, the reading is 100 mm. of pressure.

The average adult has a systolic pressure of about 100 to 120 mm. and a diastolic pressure of 65 to 88 mm. There are individual differences in normal levels, and also variances in response to normal activity. Exercise, stress, and excitement, for example, will raise the pressure. Your doctor will try to take your blood pressure at a time when you are calm and rested. On your medical record, your blood pressure will be noted in abbreviated form, with the systolic reading first, such as 160/104. If your regular reading was at these figures, by the way, you would have hypertension, or high blood pressure. Regular low read-

This diagram shows the circulation of blood in the body. Starting at middle left and following the arrows, the old blood is pumped from the right ventricle of the heart out through the pulmonary artery to the lungs at top, where fresh oxygen replaces the stale carbon dioxide.

This freshened blood returns from the lungs through the pulmonary veins into the left atrium of the heart.

The blood and its fresh oxygen are pumped out through the left ventricle into the aorta and distributed via smaller arteries and capillaries to all parts of the body and its organs.

The used blood is gathered back into small capillaries and veins and through the vena cavae into the right atrium of the heart, to begin anew the cycle through the lungs.

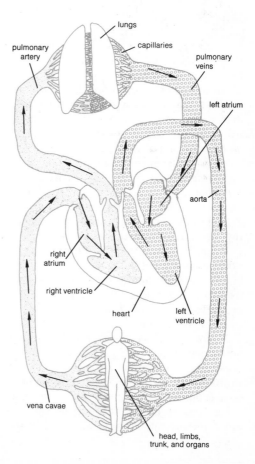

lungs

capillaries

pulmonary artery

pulmonary veins

left atrium

aorta

right atrium

right ventricle

heart

left ventricle

vena cavae

head, limbs, trunk, and organs

ings mean low blood pressure, or hypotension. (*See* HYPERTENSION; HYPOTENSION.)

Loss of blood, like the opening of a valve on a pressure tank, results in a drop in blood pressure, and the body reacts at once to compensate for the loss. Blood is forced into the arteries from parts of the body that hold substantial supplies of it. One of these reservoirs is the venous system, which holds about half of the body's volume of blood. Others are the spleen, liver, heart, and lungs. Also, fluids from the tissues are forced back into the blood vessels, thus restoring blood volume but lowering the concentration of red blood cells.

When the body loses much blood, the reservoirs may raise the pressure close to normal, but the person will then go into shock from insufficient blood to handle tissue needs. (*See* SHOCK.)

Blood pressure can be raised by the constriction of blood vessels, which is in fact how the reservoirs compensate for pressure drop. In response to an opposite problem, pressure that is too high, the vessels may dilate, making more room for blood. Such responses are called autoregulation (automatic controlling) of blood pressure.

Messages from the brain and other parts of the nervous system play a part in autoregulation, as do hormonal and other chemical substances that flow from glands during body crises and stimulate constriction or dilatation of the blood vessels.

During exercise, the body produces some of these substances, such as carbon dioxide and lactic acid, in greater quantities than usual. The arteries dilate, bringing increased quantities of oxygen-carrying blood to working muscles.

Nitroglycerin is an important rapid-acting vasodilator drug that lowers blood pressure during attacks of angina, a heart problem. Excess salt retained in the kidneys is a cause of high arterial pressure, and other body organs react in special ways to affect vessel tonus (normal state) and blood pressure.

AGE AND BLOOD PRESSURE. Younger people have lower blood pressures. The systolic pressure is only around 40 mm. at the time of birth, and doubles during the first year of life. At age twelve it usually is slightly above 100 mm. Old people usually develop some degree of arteriosclerosis, and the resulting inelasticity of the aorta and large arteries acts to raise systolic pressure quite high, sometimes over 200 mm. Women tend to have lower blood pressure than men until after the menopause (change of life), when it goes higher.

Some persons are born with defects that keep their blood pressure abnormally high. Alterations in pressure upward or downward are important signs to the physician, since they often accompany systemic disorders and infections. (*See* BLOOD; HEART.)

A separate circulation system, which joins the blood system in many places, is that of the lymphatic vessels, ducts, and nodes. (*See* LYMPH.)

Blood Diseases. Most blood diseases are diseases of another organ or several organs, and they affect the body generally. Blood is the body's lifeline. Whatever affects it, affects all of the interrelated experience we call "good health."

While some diseases do affect the blood itself—its cells, plasma, or the clotting processes—to call these purely diseases of the blood is like saying that the common cold is a disease of the nose and chickenpox a disease of the skin. At the same time, some blood-related conditions can be explained more fully if discussed under their own headings. These include ailments of the heart and blood vessels, and the kidneys, liver, spleen, bone marrow, and reticuloendothelial system. (*See* VASCULAR PROBLEMS.) Some of these are referred to in this article, but only when they directly relate to a specific disease involving the blood.

Blood diseases are numerous. They have many causes ranging from synthesis of proteins to ingestion of arsenic. Some originate as problems of nutrition or of metabolism. Others involve infection, cancer, chemistry, shock, burns, wounds, pregnancy, underdone pork, overdoses of medications, and ancestry going back to Greece, Portugal, or West Africa.

The four broad classes of blood diseases are conditions affecting (1) the red cells, (2) the white cells, (3) the platelets and other clotting and hemorrhagic factors, and (4) the plasma proteins. (*See* BLOOD CELLS; BLOOD PLASMA; CLOT; COAGULATION; WHITE BLOOD CELLS.)

RED-CELL DISEASES. Red-cell diseases are called anemias and polycythemias. Anemia is the production of too few red cells or too little hemoglobin, the oxygen-carrying red matter in the red cells. (*See* ERYTHROCYTES; HEMOGLOBIN; RED BLOOD CELLS.) Adult males normally have average red-cell counts of 5 to 5.4 million per cubic millimeter; women average 4.5 to 4.8 million. Blood that continues counting 4 million or less for some time is considered anemic.

Anemia is probably the most significant of the blood diseases simply because there are more forms of anemia than any other kind of blood disorder. Anemia can be a simple, benign condition detected in a young woman after she is first married and is thinking ahead to child-bearing; or it can be a deadly condition to the Rh positive infant, suffering from the disease called erythroblastosis fetalis. (*See* ANEMIA.)

Polycythemia is the production of red cells beyond the 5 to 5.5 million count. This may be temporary, caused by normal conditions such as hard exercise. Or it may be persistent, caused by too little oxygen, as in the case of some persons who live at high altitudes and respond poorly to a rarified atmosphere.

Anemias usually are symptoms rather than diseases in themselves. And, like some other blood diseases, they often involve not just the red cells but all parts of the blood—

the white cells, platelets, and plasma too. To the physician they are a sign that something is amiss not only in the bloodstream but elsewhere in the body. There may be a digestive problem, an improperly functioning organ, an unseen loss of blood, a flaw in red-cell production, or poisoning.

Anemias can be classified in various ways—by their cause, their effect, whether or not they are hereditary. One simple classification includes three groups: Red-cell process anemias, red-cell material anemias, and red-cell loss anemias.

Red-cell process anemias include abnormalities in the production of erythrocytes (red cells) in the bone marrow, the heart of red-cell production. Among these are conditions in which the bone marrow is destroyed (myelophthisic anemia) or red cells are destroyed (splenic anemia). Also, poisons and X-ray or gamma radiation may interrupt red-cell production by the marrow (aplastic anemia). Treatment may include discovery and elimination of the causative poison or radiation. Removal of the spleen helps in the splenic and aplastic types. Aplastic anemia often is quickly fatal.

Red-cell material anemias develop when the bone marrow cannot make red cells or makes them poorly because of lack of proper materials. This can be caused, for example, by a number of pregnancies within a relatively short time. The mother simply cannot produce enough red cells within the time span to keep up with her own and the fetuses' needs. Other causes may be intestinal ailments, stomach problems, or simply lack of proper nutrition. In fact there may be many causes (and one person can have several different types of anemia at the same time) or there may be a single cause such as the lack of the *intrinsic factor* that causes pernicious anemia. (*See* PERNICIOUS ANEMIA.) Beriberi, pellagra, and sprue are anemias directly related to poor nutrition and digestive abnormalities, as are two less familiar conditions, tropical macrocytic anemia and severe pregnancy anemia. Another diet-related type is chronic iron-deficiency anemia, which can affect infants too. It has a variety of causes including infection, poor diet, heavy menstruation, and diarrhea.

Treatment for these conditions includes potent vitamins, especially B-complex; greatly improved nutrition; and transfusions. (*See* NUTRITION; VITAMIN DEFICIENCIES; VITAMINS.)

Red-cell loss anemias include both chronic and acute anemias in which there is destruction of red cells or hemoglobin caused by injury, poisoning, or infection (acquired anemias); anemias in which this destruction is an inherited trait; and those in which there is an actual outflowing of blood from the body, red cells included.

In the acquired anemias, the body reacts to various conditions or materials by destroying its own red cells. These conditions and materials may be serious mutilating injuries or burns. They may be toxic substances such as arsenic, lead, toluene, benzol, or animal and vegetable poisons. The causes may be the products or effects of bacteria and immune bodies in the blood. Diseases of the white blood cells may trigger such anemias.

Inherited anemic diseases may be serious, leading to death, or they may be relatively minor. They are hemolytic or red-cell-destructive anemias. Thalassemia is one such disease. The minor form usually is a mild disease. Thalassemia major most often leads to death. (*See* THALASSEMIA.) Another such relationship exists in the sickle cell conditions. Sickle cell *trait* is not serious. It results when one parent contributes genes for fragile, crescent-shaped red cells. Sickle cell anemia is generally fatal at an early age. It develops when both parents contribute genes for the trait.

Another of these hemolytic anemias is familial hemolytic jaundice, in which the spleen affects the production of small, weak red cells.

Actual blood loss is the cause of the hemorrhagic anemias. The causes are varied, including all kinds of nonhealing wounds and ruptures in the vessels, such as hemorrhoids or chronic nose bleeds. Other causes are stomach ulcers and gastrointestinal cancers, and extreme bleeding during menstruation.

Rh disease, or erythroblastosis, is one of the hemorrhagic anemias. This disease, which takes the form of serious anemia and jaundice, can develop in the baby born of an Rh negative mother and Rh positive father. When this happens the newborn's blood must be slowly drained and simultaneously replaced with healthy blood. (*See* RH FACTOR.)

Treating the blood-loss anemias includes careful examination of stools and urine for blood, and the use of transfusions. Surgical removal of the spleen or tumors may help in some cases. Helpful medications include cortisone, ACTH, vitamin B_{12} and folic acid, and iron and liver extract.

The most serious of the red-cell excess diseases is polycythemia vera, or true polycythemia, in which the total number of red cells may double to 10 million or more per cubic mm. Hemoglobin increases greatly. Since the overall result is a great expansion in the total volume of blood, the number of the other two kinds of blood cells, the white cells and platelets, may increase two or three times. The blood also thickens, causing it to pump slowly, to cause more pressure, and to clot at critical points in the body, heart, brain, and legs and other extremities.

Treatment consists of reducing the volume of blood by bloodletting (*see* PHLEBOTOMY) and trying to reduce hemoglobin production by greatly reducing the intake of iron.

WHITE-CELL DISEASES. Like the red-cell diseases, the white-cell diseases of the blood include those in which there are too many white cells, not enough cells, and seriously damaged cells. Normal counts of white cells are 5,000 to 10,000 per cubic mm. This count varies with normal changes in the activity of a healthy person. Exercise, pregnancy, and menstruation all increase white-cell count for a while. Infections also greatly promote white-cell production, increasing the count by as much as four times. If white-cell disorders reduce the count too much, the body's protection against infection is decreased.

Various types of infections cause great increases in specific types of white cells. Pyogenic infections (pus-producing), the type caused by the cocci bacteria (streptococcus, staphylococcus, etc.), stimulate great increases in granulocyte production. Viral infections such as whooping cough prompt lymphocytosis, that is, great increases in lymphocyte production. Malaria and typhoid fever, among others, produce monocytosis, a rise in monocyte-making. And certain allergic reactions and parasitic invasions (trichinosis, hookworm) cause eosinophilia, an increase in circulating eosinophils.

Extreme reduction in white cells is a condition known as *leukopenia*. White-cell count falls to less than 5,000 cells per cubic mm. Causes include sensitivity reactions to drugs or other chemicals; infections such as typhoid and measles; enlarged spleen; and bone marrow disease. One of the most serious forms of leukopenia is agranulocytosis. (*See* AGRANULOCYTOSIS.) In this condition, usually set off by a sensitivity reaction to a drug such as the sulfonamides or an antibiotic, great numbers of the disease-fighting neutrophil cells are destroyed. The body becomes extremely vulnerable to infection.

The *leukemias,* on the contrary, involve great increases in white-cell production. So great are these increases that they literally crowd other vital cells out of the bloodstream and the organs. There is an acute form of leukemia, a chronic form, and variations that are intermediate. (*See* LEUKEMIA.)

Acute leukemia is almost always a disease of children. It begins suddenly and proceeds quickly. The blood-forming organs are damaged. Red cells and platelets are greatly diminished and may almost disappear. There is hemorrhaging in the skin and mucous membranes; infections develop throughout the body. The acute form can bring death in as short a time as a few weeks, but life may be sustained for six months or even more. Much hope for the eventual control and possible cure of acute leukemia is prompted by the work of a number of leukemia researchers who have been investigating the theory that acute leukemia is caused by a virus. Drugs are used to prolong life in acute leukemia and have been greatly improved in the past ten or fifteen years.

Chronic leukemia more often affects patients in their middle years. It begins quite gradually, in most cases, and may run its course to death in as little as one year or as much as four years or longer. In addition, there are less serious forms, such as chronic lymphatic leukemia, in which the disease may go on for ten years or more. Both X rays and tissue-killing drugs are used to attack and control this disease.

Other white-cell diseases include:

● Hodgkin's disease, a chronic lymphatic disease which until recently has been considered invariably fatal. New treatment may now bring a delay in its course. Starting as a painless lump in the neck, it leads to inflamed enlargement of the kidneys, liver, and lymph system. Before the most recent development in the treatment of Hodgkin's disease, life expectancy was one to twenty years.

● White-cell cancers, sarcomas that spread rapidly through the bloodstream and have their greatest effects on the bones and lungs.

● Bone-marrow cancers. Cells in this blood-forming tissue grow uncontrollably. Multiple myeloma is one of these. It is fatal but life may be prolonged for periods of a few months to a few years.

PLATELET AND CLOTTING DISEASES. Th· platelet-hemorrhagic diseases and conditions include all those disorders of the blood involving abnormal bleeding or clotting and the processes connected with these.

Problems involved in clotting failure may be *prothrombin deficiency* or certain plasma abnormalities in which fibrinogen is reduced. Causes may be liver disease, a lack of vitamin K, or an excess of artificial or natural anticoagulants in the bloodstream. Another cause of clotting failure is the disease thrombocytopenia, in which the damaging effects of poisons or radiation reduce the platelet count to 100,000 per cubic mm. or less. This is a progressive condition in which all the platelets eventually disappear and there is fatal internal bleeding.

Excessive clotting may be caused by atherosclerotic changes in the circulatory system; by too scant a supply of anti-clotting factors in the blood (heparin, antiprothrombin); high fat levels in the blood; or a variety of other metabolic or even emotional causes.

Other hemorrhagic diseases include the purpura conditions, in which the blood vessels break or leak blood beneath the surface of the skin, causing large blue, blue-black, or purple spots beneath the skin surface. These purpuras may be minor, as in the so-called "Devil's pinches" that are the blemishes of women who complain of bruising easily. Or they may be signs of more serious ailments, such as the vitamin-C-deficiency disease scurvy, and infectious diseases in which there is fever and internal rupturing of vessels.

The true bleeding diseases are those in which blood continues oozing or spilling from wounds without clotting. Generally these are called hemophilia, but this is not one disease but many. They are inherited, usually through the female side of the family, though in rare cases males also pass these disorders from generation to generation. A number of popular names have been given to hemophilia, including "Christmas disease," for the last name of a boy in whom a condition similar to hemophilia was found, and "royal disease" because of its incidence in the royal families of Spain, Imperial Russia, and Great Britain. Hemophilia is caused by the inability of the body to form a substance called clotting factor VIII or anti-hemophiliac globulin. Christmas disease, or hemophilia B, is due to deficiency of factor IX.

LOSS OF PROTEINS. Diseases affecting the plasma proteins cause a serious loss of the protein substances in the blood that are necessary for the processes that resist infection and preventing blood loss. The most serious form of this condition is the disease agammaglobulinemia. This is a great decrease or a total absence of gamma globulin, the blood plasma substance that transports the protein molecules called antibodies. A great decrease of this substance therefore cripples the body's defenses against infection. The cause may be malnutrition or a defect in protein synthesis in the body.

Several other conditions also result in losses of protein from the blood. Certain kidney malfunctions may cause too much secretion of proteins with the urine. And production of proteins may be hampered by liver disease or damage from cancer, abscesses, or other causes.

Blood Plasma. Although blood appears to be a uniform red fluid, it actually is a rather complex mixture of various kinds of cells suspended in a liquid. The cells are red and white corpuscles and platelets. The liquid is plasma. (*See* BLOOD.) Plasma-like liquid also is part of the lymph and intramuscular fluid.

Blood plasma is about 54–55 percent of the total volume of blood; the cells make up the remaining 45 percent. Like the whole blood of which it is a part, the plasma portion also is a complex mixture. A little of everything seems to be there, and this "everything" can be understood most easily if the plasma is viewed first in general and then in detail—like gradually sharpening the focus on a microscope.

Seen as a whole, plasma is a slightly alkaline liquid, rather like egg white but pale yellow or (in some cases) straw-colored. It is often clear unless the person has been eating fats; then it may be milky. Going to the next degree of focus, plasma contains many substances that are absorbed directly into it and carried along: digested materials like the fat globules that cloud it; bodily secretions of various kinds; enzymes (such as thrombin, which reacts with fibrinogen to clot the blood); antibodies; hormones; and waste products. And so plasma, seen in greater detail, is not just a liquid; it contains all three kinds of matter—solids, liquids, and gases.

EVERYTHING HAS A PURPOSE. About 90–92 percent of plasma is water; about 9 percent is solids. The gases, combined or associated with other substances, are oxygen, carbon dioxide, and nitrogen. The dissolved solids in the plasma can be classified as either organic or inorganic. The organic compounds are proteins (fibrinogen, albumin, and globulins) and non-proteins (sugar, creatine, urea, uric acid, and others). The inorganic compounds are especially the chlorides, bicarbonates, and phosphates of sodium, potassium, and calcium.

In addition to this overall function of the proteins, the individual protein substances have specific jobs. Serum albumin is the most plentiful and plays the biggest part in maintaining the osmotic equilibrium. The alpha globulins carry lipids and steroids. Lipids are fatty-waxy substances. Along with carbohydrates and proteins they are the basic stuff of animal tissue. Steroids are fat-soluble compounds and include a number of materials found naturally in the body, including many hormones. Beta globulin carries lipids, iron, and copper. Gamma globulin carries the blood's disease-fighting antibodies. (*See* GAMMA GLOBULIN.) Fibrinogen makes possible the clotting of blood. (*See* CLOT.)

PLASMA FOR TRANSFUSIONS. If blood is prevented from clotting by adding heparin, sodium citrate, or potassium oxalate, the red and white cells slowly settle, leaving

above them the clear plasma. The plasma now can be made to clot by various means, and when the clot shrinks, as it does on standing, it leaves a clear fluid called serum. Since the clot represents the fibrinogen that had been in the plasma and is now changed to fibrin, serum is essentially plasma minus fibrinogen. Serum is therefore easier to work with than is plasma, for it no longer presents a clotting problem.

When blood plasma is extracted from whole blood and transfused to a patient, it is usually adequate to meet all his needs for blood. Plasma used in transfusions contains all the ingredients in the complex blood mixture *except* the cells. Hence for most purposes the only difference between transfusing whole blood and plasma is that plasma may leave the patient a bit anemic. One exception, though, is when a patient has had massive hemorrhages, with extreme loss of blood. In such a case of hemorrhagic shock some whole blood must be given to replace the blood's hemoglobin, because this is the vehicle by which blood supplies oxygen to the body and removes waste products.

Beginning in the middle and late 1930's, blood plasma has been used increasingly to supply the needs of those requiring transfusions. It has two great advantages over whole blood: First, because plasma can be frozen or dried, it can be stored for several months before use—compared with a maximum of three weeks for whole blood. Second, because it contains no red cells, there usually is no danger of the mismatching, a problem that can cause serious trouble. It is the red cells that clump together—that is, agglutinate—when the wrong blood types are mixed. The collection and use of plasma is even further simplified, compared with whole blood use, because plasma from different donors can be mixed—possibly even to the advantage of the recipient. For example, plasma coming from donors of A type and B type blood would contain A and B substance, and this would neutralize the anti-A and anti-B agglutinins in the mixed plasma. The mixture, then, would be much less likely to cause mismatching problems than would plasma from a single source.

Plasma is available in various forms, prepared with a variety of chemicals to keep it from clotting. (Without any additives it is called *true blood plasma*.) Some of these anti-clotting additives are sodium citrate, ammonium oxalate, and other neutral salts. Anti-hemophiliac human plasma is plasma that is used to stop hemorrhaging in a bleeder (hemophiliac), at least temporarily; it must be prepared quickly to maintain the plasma's anti-hemophiliac qualities.

Blood Poisoning. Known medically as septicemia, poisoning of the blood is caused by toxins or microorganisms in the bloodstream. The infection is accompanied by chills, fever, sweating, and prostration. (*See* PYEMIA; SEPTICEMIA.)

Blood Pressure. If the human body were to be described in an engineering prospectus placed on the desk of almost any corporation executive, the inventor certainly would be dismissed as a maniac or at least an impractical genius, unfitted for corporate life. Consider the circulatory system, for example: a pump the size of a large fist or eggplant intended to impel a complex liquid at prescribed pressures through a system of tubing long enough to reach four times around the Earth. (*See* BLOOD CIRCULATION.) Yet this is what the system does, and with only a few exceptions does quite well despite the extremely variable demands made on it to pump faster and slower, increase and decrease pressure.

As used in medicine, the term "blood pressure" does not refer to pressure just anywhere in the circulatory system but specifically to pressure in the arteries. And, more specifically, it refers to pressure where it is easiest to measure, the large artery in the left forearm.

Like many hydraulic systems, the human circulatory system carries two kinds of

pressure. These correspond to the two kinds of heart pumping action. First, there is steady, or maintenance, or static, pressure, which is produced by the diastolic action as the aortic and pulmonary valves close at the end of pumping contraction and the heart fills with blood before the next outward push. Second, there is kinetic or

Average Normal Blood Pressures

Age	Systolic Pressure	Diastolic Pressure
10 years	103	70
15 years	113	75
20 years	120	80
25 years	122	81
30 years	123	82
35 years	124	83
40 years	126	84
45 years	128	85
50 years	130	86
55 years	132	87
60 years	135	89

Systolic pressure is the force with which blood is pumped by the heart during the period of the heart's contraction; *diastolic pressure* is the force with which blood is pumped by the heart during dilatation or relaxation.

U.S. Vitamin and Pharmaceutical Corporation

pumping pressure as the heart contracts to push blood out through the vessels. Diastolic pressure maintains the bloodstream in a steady, pressurized condition, ready for any varied needs. Systolic pressure delivers blood quickly through the system as needed in various parts of the body for greater and lesser activity. These pressures are like the two kinds of pressures in city water supply system, one to keep the water in the pipes, even at the top of a high building, and the second to give an extra push to make water gush out of a faucet when the handle is turned.

Unlike any other hydraulic system, the human circulatory system is subject to almost no reasonable or predictable rules of operation. Both internal and external conditions affect the blood pressure. Some of these change slowly, others quickly, some often, some infrequently, some predictably, others with no warning at all.

Internally, blood pressure is affected by:

• Contractive pumping action of the heart as the left ventricle forces the blood out.

• The volume of blood thrust into the aorta by the heart.

• The resistance of the arteries to the volume of blood delivered to them—this resistance depending on their flexibility, elasticity, and muscular response. (*See* AR-TERIOLES; ATHEROSCLEROSIS.)

• The condition of the blood, including its thickness or viscosity.

• The health of other organs and tissue, principally the heart, arteries, kidneys, and ductless glands such as the adrenal gland.

WHAT IS NORMAL? External conditions influencing the blood pressure are everything that happens during a lifetime or a day. Pressure varies with age, sex, the state of the emotions, the hour of the day, the number of good habits (good diet, plenty of rest) and bad habits (smoking, drinking). And some of the conditions that might seem to raise blood pressure, such as an infectious disease with fever, do not raise it. In fact, pressure may drop during an infection.

What is normal blood pressure? What is too high, too low?

These questions cannot be answered any more accurately than questions like: What shoe size is normal? What is too large, too small?

Blood pressure that is normal for one person may be higher or lower than another person's pressure. And the same person may vary in blood pressure from day to day or even hour to hour. This is the reason, for example, that some people show blood pressures in life insurance or military medical examinations that the examiners find questionable. The applicant or inductee may not really have, for example, high blood pressure; nervous tension caused by anticipation and the exam experience itself may drive the pressure up.

READING THE PRESSURE. Blood pressure is measured by an instrument called a manometer, used in detecting and measuring pressures in liquids and gases. The specific type of manometer used is a sphygmomanometer. It consists of a small squeeze-bulb air pump, an inflatable cuff, and a columnar scale (thermometerlike) which measures pressure in the cuff and arm. The column is filled with mercury; the scale is in millimeter increments.

To take blood pressure the physician or nurse buttons the cuff around the left arm and pumps up the cuff with the hand pump until the pressure in the cuff is high enough to cut off circulation in the artery feeding blood to the arm and hand. Then the examiner opens the valve in the bulb slightly, leaking air pressure and watching the mercury column as it sinks slowly. Meanwhile he is listening with his stethoscope for the "sounds of Krotkoff" over the brachial artery at the elbow. These sounds begin as sharp clicks when the pressure falls just low enough to let a spurt of blood pass through the artery with each heartbeat; the examiner records this as the systolic pressure. As the mercury continues to fall, the sounds become softer or duller, still keeping time with the heartbeat. At the moment they become inaudible the examiner again notes the height of the mercury column and records it as the diastolic pressure.

Blood pressure measurements are given in figures that represent the force needed to raise a column of mercury (*Hg*) to a certain height measured in millimeters. A figure for systolic pressure might be given as 130 mm.Hg.

Instead of exact target figures, there are *ranges* of normal pressure, high and low, but even these ranges are stated somewhat differently among various medical scientists. The normal range for systolic pressure in adult men is put at 100 to 150 mm.Hg, though some authorities say the high figure should be 140. The diastolic range is 60 to 88 mm.Hg. Normal average systolic pressures for adult males are considered to be about 120 to 130 mm.Hg. What happens to the so-called normal pressures during the course of actual living shows the true nature of blood pressure in the human body.

Every person's pressure, for example, goes through a diurnal (daily) variation. The busy man whose pressure may be 100/60 mm.Hg as he lies in bed before the alarm rings, may have a reading of 150/90 mm.Hg when he walks in the front door before dinner.

Women normally have somewhat lower blood pressure than men, but hormonal influences may make their pressure vary tremendously. After menopause, for instance, some women may have systolic pressure reaching to 250 mm.Hg and diastolic pressure of 120 mm.Hg.

Infants typically have lower blood pressure, often measuring about 80 mm.Hg systolic and 50 to 60 mm.Hg diastolic. As they grow older the pressure gradually increases.

Since there is so much variation in blood pressure in the same person and among individuals, there is no precise, clear-cut way to say when pressure readings should be called abnormal. The clue, though, is keeping a record of how much and for how long a person's blood pressure readings vary or deviate from what has been recorded as that person's normal pressure. This deviation, then, can be interpreted, seeing whether it is "too high" or "too low."

Some physicians feel that if a patient's pressure continues to read as much as 15 mm.Hg systolic and 8 mm.Hg diastolic higher than his normal figure, then he has high blood pressure, or hypertension. Or if a man's pressure drops below 110 mm.Hg systolic or a woman's below 100 mm.Hg systolic, this is often considered low blood pressure, or hypotension. (*See* HYPERTENSION; HYPOTENSION.)

These are not absolute high or low limits, however. Medical scientists do not yet know how to establish such absolute limits, and in fact there is much that is not yet understood about blood pressure, especially hypertension.

One problem that is well recognized is the limitation of detecting and measuring blood pressure. One of the greatest needs in learning more about blood pressure and treating abnormal pressures is a means for taking blood pressure readings continuously, around the clock. One means, developed so far, for greatly improving the accuracy or fidelity of extremely rapid pressure changes is an electronic instrument that replaces the mercury column with high-speed recorders and transducers. These are sensitive units that convert the mechanical action of blood pressure to electric impulses, driving the pens across the graph of the recorder.

VARIETIES OF HYPERTENSION. High blood pressure may be of several kinds and is classified in two main ways: how extreme it is, and what is causing it. When serious, high blood pressure causes various disabling and fatal conditions, including cerebral hemorrhage, heart failure, coronary disease, and kidney damage.

Benign hypertension may be of widely varying degrees of severity. One victim may live with it for life, never knowing he has it. Another may suffer constantly. Another may die of it. It may be controlled permanently or go beyond control and cause heart failure. Frequently it is found in the same family.

Malignant hypertension, which is not common, may not be a distinct malady but only a much more severe form of hypertension than benign. Once it develops—and it is more a disease of young people than older —it may cause death in months or in only a year or so unless it is discovered early and immediately treated.

Hypertension classified by cause includes

both *primary* and *secondary* high blood pressure. The primary type is known by several other names, including hypertensive cardiovascular disease, essential hypertension, and hypertensive heart disease. It is a disease in itself and quite difficult to control or cure. Both benign and malignant hypertension can be of the primary type.

Secondary conditions are a symptom, an effect of disease elsewhere in the body, particularly the kidneys. Cancer of the adrenal glands can be a cause.

Symptoms of high blood pressure vary with the seriousness of degree of the condition. They include hemorrhages of the skin, nosebleeds, hemorrhages in the conjunctiva of the eye with some visual disturbances, and, in more advanced cases, severe headaches. Examination may show that the heart is enlarged, or that the left ventricle has been damaged. There may be cerebral hemorrhage.

In hypertension, the blood pressure reading that is most significant is the diastolic. The reason is that this lower reading, taken when the heart is pausing, shows most clearly how much harder the next pumping action must be to reach the high of the systolic reading. It is this increase of heart effort and pressure on the arteries that slowly strains the heart, speeds the development of arteriosclerosis, and ruptures vulnerable arteries such as those in the brain.

Treatment for hypertension consists of diet control; sometimes surgery to cut autonomic nervous controls to the arterioles; and the uses of medication such as rauwolfia serpentina, hydralazine, tranquilizers, and diuretics. (*See* DIETS; DIURETICS; TRANQUILIZERS.)

LOW PRESSURE, LONG LIFE. Unlike high blood pressure, low blood pressure can be good for one's health. The clue to watch for in hypotension is whether it always is low and whether there may be some other disease that could be lowering it.

Hypotension can be a symptom of tuberculosis, cancer, rheumatism, and conditions lowering the secretions of the adrenal glands (Addison's disease), thyroid, and pituitary glands. Or it can result from malnutrition and extreme weight loss. Sometimes it accompanies changes in heart action and blood content or volume. Such conditions are slow heart beat, anemia, and bleeding. (*See* ANEMIA; BLEEDING; BRADYCARDIA.)

Such drugs as tranquilizers and other hypertensive drugs also can decrease blood pressure too much.

The most serious of the hypotension symptoms is fainting. This may have other causes than low blood pressure, but if it continues, abnormally low pressure should be suspected. Other symptoms are dizziness, constipation, and fatigue that becomes most serious in the mid-afternoon. (*See* FAINTING; FATIGUE; REST.)

If hypotension is caused by another, more serious condition, and is having serious effects such as repeated fainting or bad depression, it can be treated with a number of pressure-raising drugs such as mephenterminesulfate. But if no other disease or abnormality is involved, low blood pressure should be considered a blessing. The "victim" will lead a healthier, longer life.

Blood Transfusion. The procedure by which whole blood or certain elements of blood are introduced directly into the bloodstream is known as a blood transfusion. (*See* TRANSFUSIONS.)

Blood Types. When the term *blood type* is used, it may suggest that we all have a certain kind of blood that is absolutely different from the blood of some people and absolutely identical with the blood of others —almost as if it came out of large blood bank bottles labeled "Type A" or "B" or "O" and so on. But this is not what "blood type" means. (*See* BLOOD.)

Human blood is not uniform. It is a highly fluid gumbo of enzymes, hormones, sugar, proteins, salts, red cells, white cells, water, gas, minerals, and more; it varies in many ways and may even be as individualistic as fingerprints or voice sound. But blood typing is concerned with only one aspect: compatibility in transfusions. Probably the only "absolute" about blood is that if certain of these red corpuscle and plasma proteins are mixed with certain others, as in a transfusion, they will cause the red cells to go into an antibody reaction. They agglutinate—that is, clump together—and also rupture or hemolyze. What this means is that some of the protein cells in the recipient's blood are actually *immune* to some of the proteins in the donor's blood. They cannot combine normally, but instead go into this reaction that destroys the red cells and stops some normal bodily functions. This can cause death. (*See* TRANSFUSIONS.)

THE MOST IMPORTANT SYSTEM. It is because this one characteristic of blood—the blood-type protein content of red cells and plasma—is a matter of life and death that it is used as the basis for classifying blood into different groups or types. Once a person's blood type is known, doctors and nurses can avoid *giving* him blood that is the wrong type or letting him *donate* blood to another patient who has the wrong type to mix with his blood.

There are a number of blood classifications, but the most important, because it is the most widely used, is the International or Landsteiner Classification of Blood Types, also referred to as the A-B-O System. It was developed in 1901–1902 by Karl Landsteiner and his associates. Landsteiner, a pathologist, was born in Austria but did his research in the United States. For his pioneering work in developing the blood classification, he was awarded the Nobel Prize. (*See* BLOOD BANK.)

The Landsteiner Classification groups all human blood into four types. The basis of this typing is the presence or absence of two protein substances in the red cells and two in the plasma, and the interactions or lack of interactions of these proteins.

There are numerous proteins in the blood, but these are proteins that most commonly cause dangerous sensitivity or immunity reactions. The blood reacts violently to them. They are bad chemistry.

PROTEINS THAT ACT LIKE ANTIBODIES. The proteins in the erythrocytes, or red cells, act like antigens when they come into contact with certain other proteins. That is, they stimulate the formation of antibodies. These red cell proteins are called *agglutinogens*.

The proteins in the serum or plasma act like antibodies, moving in on foreign invaders to protect the body's health. Among other things, antibodies cause bacteria and cells to clump or agglutinate so that they will be destroyed. In this case it is the red cell proteins that are attacked and destroyed. These protective plasma proteins are called *agglutinins*.

For each specific red cell protein substance there is a specific plasma protein that agglutinates it.

To make identification simple, in the Landsteiner system the protein substances in the red cells and plasma are given letter designations. In the red cells these substances are called A agglutinogen and B agglutinogen. In the plasma they are called either alpha (α) or anti-A agglutinin and beta (β) or anti-B agglutinin. Alpha substance agglutinates or clumps red cell substance A. Beta clumps B. Blood with a certain red cell substance in it—for example, A—naturally cannot also contain the very plasma substance that would agglutinate substance A. It would have to contain either beta agglutinin or no agglutinin.

THE FOUR TYPES. The presence or absence of these substances makes the four types of blood. Blood red cells can contain A substance only, or B only, or both, or neither. Blood plasma can contain alpha, or beta, or both, or neither. Each blood type is a specific combination or lack of red cell substance(s) and plasma substance(s), as follows:

In type A, red cells have agglutinogen A; plasma has agglutinin beta.

In type B, red cells have agglutinogen B; plasma has agglutinin alpha.

In type AB, red cells have agglutinogens A and B; plasma has no agglutinins.

In type O, red cells have no agglutinogens, but plasma has agglutinins alpha and beta.

In addition, A type blood is further broken down into two subtypes. These subtypes are based on how strong the clumping reaction is. In most persons this is a strong reaction and they are type A_1. In a few, the reaction is much weaker, and they are called A_2. Yet even blood researchers do not completely agree about these subgroups. For one thing, if a so-called A_1 blood clumps more weakly and an A_2 blood clumps more strongly, the two are hard to tell apart. Some medical scientists believe that the difference is not just a matter of the titer (quantity) of anti-A. They say the difference is not quantitative but *qualitative* —that the stronger reaction is caused by a difference in this subgroup of A. If strong enough this reaction can even make some presumably A type blood incompatible with other A blood.

Blood type is inherited according to Mendel's laws of heredity. If a person inherits traits for both A and B substances he will have type AB blood; or if both parents contribute A or B or O traits, he will have those types. But if one parent contributes a B trait and the other an O, he will be classified as having type B blood because the genes for type O do not stimulate the formation of any red cell substances.

BEING SAFE AND BEING PRACTICAL. Health care personnel are careful to ensure the safety of transfusions in a number of ways. They learn the type of blood of both donor and recipient by a method called blood typing. They mix a sample of the person's red cells with two samples of plasma agglutinins, made from human, animal, or plant sources. By watching the red cells under a microscope to see what makes them clump or has no effect, they know which of the four types the blood is.

Also, they can cross-match the blood of a would-be donor and recipient to learn exactly what will happen if these particular bloods are mixed. (*See* TRANSFUSIONS.)

Compatibility of the actual combination of donor and recipient blood is the final answer because sometimes variations on the apparently standard rules of blood compatibility are not only permissible but necessary for the health of the recipient. He might not be given the blood he needs because of worry about the plasma agglutinins it contains, even though the donor's agglutinins are not the first concern in transfusions. Or he might be given blood thought to be safe—the universal type O— but really dangerous to him because of the high level of agglutinins it contains.

WHO CAN GIVE AND RECEIVE. The general rules of transfusing the four types of blood are:

The type A donor can give blood to type A or type AB recipients but not to type B or O. The type A recipient can take blood from type A or type O.

The type B donor can give blood to type B or Type AB but not to type A or O. The type B recipient can take blood from type B or O.

The type AB donor can give blood only to other type AB recipients, but the AB recipient can take blood from all donors. He is a "universal recipient."

The type O donor can give blood to anyone, and is called a "universal donor." But type O recipients can take blood only from type O donors.

These rules can be bent somewhat when it is necessary to save a life. If there is a shortage of certain types of blood, first consideration should be given to the type of red cells in the donor's blood and the type of agglutinins in the recipient's plasma. The donor's plasma is not so important, simply because there isn't enough of it—just a pint or a half-pint, and it is quickly dispersed through the recipient's whole circulatory system. But if the donor's red cells are wrong, the recipient's entire plasma supply reacts against it.

There are a few other exceptions to the general rules for mixing blood. Type O blood, for example, varies in the amount of alpha and beta agglutinins it contains, so it is not always used universally. Type O blood with the highest agglutinins is not given to type A, B, and AB recipients, but only to other type O's. Also, blood for transfusions can be altered to make it more compatible by adding A and B agglutinogens to use up or exhaust the clumping reaction of the agglutinins in it.

THE REAL DANGER—AFTER CLUMPING. What happens when the wrong type of blood is given to a recipient is not just a matter of the red cells clumping together. It is what happens after the clumping that may cause death.

When red cells are agglutinated they move in clumps along with the flow of circulation until they reach the smallest capillaries. There they block the vessels; but within minutes, or a few hours at most, the effects of jamming together, plus attacks by antibodies, are breaking up the red cells. This dumps their hemoglobin into the plasma. Then the real problem of the transfusion reaction begins. This free hemoglobin collects in the smallest passages of the kidneys, completely clogging them so that the kidneys may stop operating entirely. This can cause death in less than two weeks.

A transfusion reaction, however, does not inevitably cause death. Fast action can combat these effects. The patient must be given large quantities of fluids, alkaline compounds, and diuretics to flush the kidneys and break up the hemoglobin jams in the tubules. If the patient can be kept alive for the two-week period, the natural disintegration of the hemoglobin should then open up the kidneys again.

OTHER BLOOD-TYPE PROTEINS. There are other blood-type protein substances or factors in the blood, but because they do not

cause the problem of antibody reactions, with dangerous clumping and rupturing of red cells, they are of no importance in blood typing and the safety of transfusions. Some of them, though, are important for other reasons. All persons have one or both of two other blood-type substances, M and N—either type M or N or MN. Adding their main blood-type designation makes the complete designation AM or AN or BMN, etc.

Information about this additional type is used in legal cases when knowing a person's blood type can help prove his identity. In paternity cases (trying to prove who is the father of a child), knowing the child's A-B-O blood type is no help. This information alone cannot prove that any man is or is not the father. If his blood should be typed as A_1 or A_2 this would be more precise, but testing for M and N substances would be still more precise. It would show, for example, that a child with AN blood could not be the offspring of a man with BM blood or even AM blood. Or if a man were type AN, and a woman with AN blood had a baby with type AMN blood, the man could be excluded, on scientific grounds, as the baby's father.

NAMED FOR A MONKEY. One other protein substance, a red cell substance, is important because it can cause serious agglutination problems, but in a different way than the A-B, alpha-beta substances. This is the Rh factor. It was named for the rhesus monkey used in the research that led to its discovery in 1940 by Karl Landsteiner and Dr. A. S. Weiner, an immunologist.

A large majority of all people have this protein in their red corpuscles. They are called "Rh positive," and when their blood is typed this designation is added to their A-B-O type so that their complete blood type label is A-positive, B-positive, etc. The difference in the action of the Rh factor compared to the A-B, alpha-beta substances can be seen in the effect on those who do not have the Rh factor, the "Rh negative" persons (typed as A-negative, B-negative, etc.).

If the relationships were the same as for the A-B, alpha-beta substances, the Rh negative person would have Rh antibodies. This is the relationship in the case of the type A person who lacks B substance and so has the B antibodies called beta agglutinins. But for the Rh factor the relationship is not the same.

The Rh negative person normally has no Rh antibodies. But—and this is the problem—he can get them. He gets them by being given blood in a transfusion from an Rh positive donor. Then the recipient forms Rh antibodies in about twelve days. If he is given a second, a third, or more transfusions from an Rh positive donor, the antibodies will agglutinate the blood. This usually does not happen when Rh negative blood is transfused to an Rh positive recipient.

Such reactions can cause difficult transfusion problems, but the greatest danger caused by the Rh factor is to the life of newborn infants. The danger arises when an Rh positive man and an Rh negative woman conceive a second, third, or later child.

More than half the babies coming from this combination are Rh positive, but this in itself is no problem either to mother or child. Each is self-contained with a separate blood supply feeding through, but not mixing in, the placenta between them. The whole red cells of the fetus cannot get through the placenta capillary walls and enter the mother's bloodstream, causing an antibody reaction. Mother and child are a little like neighbors in adjoining hotel rooms, sharing but not meeting in the common bath between them. Solid walls and doors, like the capillary walls, separate them. But just as noise from a late poker game can penetrate the partition, or water from bad plumbing can leak out of the bathroom, some part of the red cells, such as the Rh protein substance, can abnormally diffuse through the capillaries. It can go from the Rh positive fetus to the negative mother.

Even when this "leakage" happens it usually has no bad effect. But in about 5 percent of the cases the mother's blood does react to the invasion of the Rh substance by forming agglutinins—that is, antibodies for Rh substance. These antibodies can diffuse back just as the positive substance leaked through. In the blood of the fetus they can combine with the Rh protein in the red cells and cause such serious agglutination of the red cells in the fetus as to produce a severe anemia.

The fetus either miscarries, is born dead, or has a jaundice and anemia that lead to death. This condition, called *erythroblastosis fetalis,* is treated by completely replacing the baby's damaged blood with fresh, healthy blood.

Usually there is no danger to the first Rh positive child born of an Rh negative mother. But if there are Rh positive babies in later pregnancies, they may be damaged by the Rh positive antibodies still remaining in her bloodstream at the time of these pregnancies. Fortunately there now are ways of diagnosing this danger before birth so that this Rh fatal condition can be prevented before it develops.

MOST INDIANS ARE TYPE O. One of the most interesting things about the different blood factors is their variation among racial groups. Caucasians, for example, have a higher percentage of type A than other groups: blacks, a higher percentage of B; and American Indians, a higher percentage of type O. Other blood types vary, too.

Racial differences are also found in the Rh factor. Eighty-five percent of Caucasians are Rh positive, as are 95 percent of blacks and approximately 100 percent of American Indians and Orientals.

Besides the A-B-O, Rh, and MN blood-type systems there are about a dozen others, some named for the families in whose members certain blood substances were found.

Among these other systems and factors are the Lutheran, Lewis, Duffy, Kell, Kidd, H, P, and Xg systems.

Blood Vessels. Blood and other fluids related to blood are transported through the body in tubes called blood vessels. The total length of all this tubing has been estimated at 60,000 to 100,000 miles. Yet the round-trip time for any single drop of blood to travel from the heart, through the body, and back to heart is only about one to two minutes, since this complete circuit is only about one mile. No single drop of blood travels through all the many branching vessels. (*See* BLOOD CIRCULATION.)

Just as any transport layout, such as a highway system, includes various classes or types of routes, the circulatory system consists of several sizes and kinds of tubes.

Like the multi-lane superhighways or expressways that take the great crush of high-speed rush-hour traffic outbound from the center of the city, the *arteries,* largest of the vessels, take blood at its greatest pressure and velocity from the heart out to the rest of the body. From the main arteries, blood flows into the smallest arteries, the *arterioles,* like main streets, and then into the smallest of all vessels, the *capillaries,* rather like neighborhood streets, lanes, and paths.

At their other ends, these capillaries lead back into the *venules,* like larger thoroughfares, and then into the *veins,* which branch into larger and larger vessels, carrying a heavier and heavier volume of blood as they lead back into the heart.

Not one but two circulatory circuits carry blood in the body. They are the lifeline, the transport and supply system that most directly serves the number-one need of the animal organism—metabolism. Everything that the body is or can become takes place in the chemistry that goes on in the protoplasm of the cells—burning energy, producing wastes, fighting invaders, giving way to destruction, making new protoplasm. Each cell "breathes" (burns

oxygen and food substances) and "exhales" (eliminates carbon dioxide and water). When this doesn't happen in any part of the body for even a short time, as in serious infection or freezing or certain other injuries, that part dies and must be amputated.

The two separate circulatory circuits meet these needs precisely, each in a different way. One circuit, much larger, is the *systemic,* or *greater,* circuit. It carries food and wastes between the heart and the body. The smaller *pulmonary,* or *lesser,* circuit runs the round trip between the heart and lungs, doing nothing but getting oxygen and leaving wastes.

Both circuits have three subsystems: the arterial, capillary, and venous systems. Yet the two circuits are not the equals or counterparts of each other. The systemic circuit is complex; the pulmonary is simple. The systemic is several almost independent sections, each consisting of arteries and arterioles feeding into branching capillaries in all the organs, and then back into the veins. The pulmonary circuit serves just one organ, the lungs, running a single loop from the heart to the lungs and back.

One of these semiautonomous sections, the liver and the vessels connecting it, is sometimes referred to as a third circulatory system, the portal system or circuit. It includes the portal vein, bringing nutrient-rich blood from the intestines to the liver; the sinusoids (somewhat larger than capillaries), branching from the portal veins through all parts of the liver; and the hepatic vein, carrying blood from the liver back to the main venous system.

If blood merely ran through the blood vessels like water through plumbing, the structure and operation of the vessels would be simple. The only thing needed would be some tubing with possibly a few valves here and there. But the body is alive, moving, growing. For example, the same vessels that supply blood to a woman in the deepest stages of sleep must be able to surge extra blood to her thighs and calves when she is

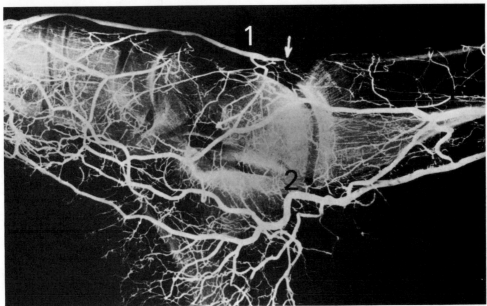

The blood vessels of this foot and ankle were injected with a dye so they could be seen in an X ray. The arrow shows abnormal closing of a vessel, but a large collateral (branch or secondary) network at 1 takes over the blood circulation. The foot is to the left, and the ankle joint is at 2.

running the hurdles and to her trunk and legs when she is giving birth. (*See* ARTERI-OLES.) The blood vessels do this, helping the powerful heart to propel the blood; rushing, channeling, and metering blood wherever it is needed most; easing it out to the farthest reaches of every organ, every muscle, the last horizon of skin.

Each type of blood vessel is unique in the job it does and the way it is put together. Arteries and veins in the two circuits, systemic and pulmonary, have reverse functions. Systemic arteries carry oxygen-laden blood from the heart out to the body. The high oxygen content makes this blood bright red. Blood returns from the tissues to the heart through the veins, dark red to red-blue now because it contains much less oxygen but a heavy proportion of carbon dioxide. Seen through the skin, the blood in shallow veins close to the surface has a dark blue or even greenish appearance.

Arteries are any large vessels taking blood *away from* the heart to other parts of the body. The largest of the blood vessels, they are heavier and stronger than the other vessels and help to propel the blood. Separate systems of arteries and other vessels supply each of the organs or organ groups.

Largest of the arteries is the aorta, about one inch in diameter. (*See* AORTA.) Blood pumping into the systemic circuit comes out of the heart (left ventricle) directly into the aorta, which branches into the coronary arteries, supplying the heart, and four other major arteries. These four are the two carotid and two subclavian arteries supplying the head and other upper parts of the body.

Below the diaphragm, blood is supplied by several more main arteries to major organs and groups of organs. Branches of the celiac artery supply the stomach, liver, pancreas, and spleen. The renal artery goes to the kidneys; the mesenteric artery, to the intestines; the iliac arteries supply the lower trunk and legs.

Arteries help propel the blood by a combination of elastic and muscular action interacting in their walls. The inner layer is endothelial cells—smooth, long cells only 1/10,000 of an inch thick. This is the kind of material that lines much of the body; its smoothness lets the blood slip along with little resistance. The middle layer is smooth muscle and elastic connective tissue, and the third, outer layer is loose connective tissue that includes its own blood vessels—to supply food to the artery walls.

It is this interacting elastic and muscular action that is felt as "pulse" in the arteries at the wrist or neck. As the mighty heart —so strong it might be referred to in the cartoons as "Supermuscle"—pumps out 1/4 cup of blood with each contraction (called systole), the elastic tissue gives way, expanding, but then returns resiliently to its original size during relaxation (diastole). This action protects the walls against the powerful pumping thrust, but it does more too. It spares the heart from pumping effort by evening or cushioning the force between the high pressure of the heart's contraction and the falling pressure of relaxation.

Near the heart, muscular tissue is a smaller proportion of the artery wall middle layer, but the proportion increases farther from the heart, as the arteries branch into smaller and smaller vessels. Here muscular action is more needed than elastic because at these outer points it becomes more important to regulate the flow rate and distribution of blood to get it quickly where it is needed most.

Arterioles are the second type of vessel that outward-bound blood from the heart passes through. As the arteries continue to branch into smaller and smaller vessels farther from the heart, they feed into this second type, referred to as the outer ends of the arteries, or the smallest of the arteries, or simply the connection to the capillaries.

The arterioles are so small they are barely visible, but once the heart has pumped the blood and the arteries have surged it outward, it is the arteriole action that puts large volumes where it is needed most.

Arterioles are the most important of the blood vessels for regulating blood pressure. These small vessels have literally muscle-bound walls. When nervous signals reach this smooth muscle, the walls cinch down on the vessels or relax, shutting off blood to the capillaries or turning it on. This faucet-like action is a response to autonomic nervous impulses that unconsciously sense and coordinate body needs, such as sending more blood to the intestines after a meal.

Capillaries receive blood from the arterioles by way of intermediate vessel sections that are ringed with sphincter muscles opening or closing each capillary mouth to blood flow. The capillaries are the terminus of the circulatory system, the end of the line, the point to which the blood is brought to perform its given task—sustaining life.

Among the blood vessels the capillaries are doubly unique. First they are microscopic in size, so small they cannot be seen with the naked eye. Their length is about 0.01 inch (250 microns), and their diameter, about 0.0003 inches (7.4 microns), is just enough to let one red cell through at a time. Second, they are integral parts of the organs they feed, not separate and distinct tubes connecting various parts of the body.

The walls of the capillaries are just one layer of endothelial cells, the same tissue as the artery lining. At just 1/10,000 inch (2.5 microns) thick, these walls are permeable to the movement of nutriments outward and the entry of wastes inward.

Venules receive the waste-laden blood from the capillaries at the far end of the capillaries—the end away from the heart. These are minute veins, the smallest in the venous system. They join together, forming larger and larger vessels, and finally link with the veins. The blood they carry contains the products of metabolism, including much CO_2 (carbon dioxide).

Veins take this darkest of the blood back to the heart for pumping to the lungs and purification. In several ways the veins are like the arteries. They are large and carry considerable volume of blood. In fact, their inside diameter is larger than that of the arteries, but this is because of a major difference between these two kinds of large vessels. The vein walls are thinner because they carry no thicknesses of elastic and muscle tissue to help control and move blood under pumping pressure. There is very little pressure here. The walls are thin and can collapse.

Blood does not return to the heart under pumping pressure from that organ. Instead a combination of valve action, muscular motion, and other motion in the body moves it along. Veins running between large muscles and the skeleton are pressed as the muscles flex to move the body. Blood in the veins is forced along the tubes, but in the tubes there are valves that open in the direction toward the heart and close against any backflow away from the heart. By this squeezing-damming process the blood is moved back, at a rather leisurely rate, to the two main veins carrying blood to the heart.

The *inferior vena cava* collects blood through four somewhat smaller veins from the lower part of the body. The *superior vena cava* collects blood from the upper part. Both drain into the right atrium of the heart.

From this upper right chamber of the heart, blood moves down into the lower chamber, the right ventricle, and is pumped up through the pulmonary artery to the lungs. This arterial blood, unlike that in the systemic system, is the dark blood, loaded with wastes. In the lungs it feeds into the maze of pulmonary capillaries. Lacing through the alveoli (air sacs) of the lungs, these vessels lose wastes and pick up oxygen by diffusion and osmosis through their permeable walls. Then the blood, now bright red because of its fresh oxygen, flows back through the pulmonary vein to the left atrium, for pumping by the left ventricle out to the systemic circuit. The circulatory cycle is complete.

Lymph is carried through the body by an auxiliary system of vessels. It is derived from the blood plasma and is the same type of watery liquid. At the outer reaches of the capillary network, some of the plasma moves through capillary thin walls and into the tissue spaces where it is then called *interstitial fluid.* (*See* PLASMA.)

This fluid moves through the tissues. Some of it goes directly back into the veins by osmosis. Some continues through the tissue spaces until it reaches lymphatic capillaries, where it is collected and then fed back through an ever larger network of lymph vessels until it reaches the thoracic duct. From this duct it goes to the superior vena cava, rejoining the main bloodstream once more.

Blue Baby. The infant who is blue, or, "cyanotic," at birth is often called a "blue baby." The word *cyanosis,* which is often used to describe this condition, is derived from the Greek word *kyanos,* meaning blue.

The bluish color of cyanosis in the infant is the result of an increased amount of reduced hemoglobin (i.e., the oxygen-carrying substance of the red blood cells) in the capillaries. For this reason, cyanosis is most easily seen where the capillary loops are numerous, as in the tips of the fingers and toes, earlobes, the tip of the nose, and inner membranes of the mouth. In poor peripheral circulation in the newborn infant, the color can range from the bright pink of generalized vasodilation to the progressive peripheral blueness of poor circulatory flow. Circumoral cyanosis (i.e., blueness about the lips) is not uncommon and, of itself, is seldom of importance. Also, from time to time, the infant may have a dusky color during the first few months of life, which can be due to the vasomotor instability of that age period.

Cyanosis is not uncommon in the newborn period. A wide variety of conditions can be responsible for its appearance. Sometimes the age (minutes, hours, or days after birth) at which cyanosis appears, and its distribution, may provide a clue as to its origin. The prognosis and treatment for each condition are different, so that it becomes necessary for a physician to make an early and accurate diagnosis.

Cyanosis of pulmonary origin is probably the most frequent reason for "blueness" in the newborn. Often there is an initial obstruction of the airway, and cyanosis appears soon after birth.

The respiratory distress syndrome can appear in infants of normal gestation but is more usually found in prematures. In this condition, an intense cyanosis can develop, which also requires immediate treatment. The cyanosis reaches a climax within twenty-four to forty-eight hours.

A number of other conditions in the newborn period also can produce cyanosis, such as pneumonia, diaphragmatic hernia, tracheo-esophageal fistula, cerebral damage, cardiac problems, lung disease, and so on. Expert care and prompt diagnosis are necessary for all conditions in which cyanosis is a component. (*See* CYANOSIS.)

Body Odor. People generally assume that perspiration, or sweat, is the sole cause of body odor, but this is not true. Perspiration itself is probably odorless. Some odor develops from the action of bacteria on secretions of the skin's glands. These bacteria are present on everyone's skin and are most active in warm, moist surroundings. Because of this, body odors are likely to arise in the parts of the body from which perspiration cannot evaporate immediately, such as the underarms, genitals, and feet.

Body odor is also related to the source and type of sweat secreted. Sweat is composed of the free-flowing liquid of the eccrine sweat glands plus a milky secretion of

the apocrine glands. (*See* APOCRINE GLANDS.) Eccrine glands are widely distributed over the body surface, with some concentration on the forehead, palms, and soles. Heat or nervous tension stimulates them to produce large amounts of sweat. As this evaporates, the body is cooled. Sweating brought about by heat alone does not usually cause an odor problem.

In addition to the sweat produced by the eccrine and apocrine glands, however, there are other secretions that contribute to the characteristic odors, not always unpleasant, of the normal body. Examples are the sebum secreted by the sebaceous glands of the hair follicles of the scalp and the water-repellent secretion of the tarsal (meibomian) glands of the eyelids.

Body odor seems to occur more often in times of emotional stress when apocrine sweat, as well as eccrine sweat, is secreted. The apocrine glands are restricted mainly to the underarms, the nipples, and the anogenital regions. Growth of the apocrines, which are closely associated with hair follicles, is stimulated by the same hormones that cause hair growth in the underarm and genital areas. This is why body odor is rarely a problem in children and old people.

Personal cleanliness is the primary means of controlling both bacterial growth on the skin as well as body odor. In addition, most women, but few men, remove underarm hair by shaving. Underarm hair collects both bacteria and perspiration, so better protection is provided if the area is shaved.

Because garments can also collect odors, clean clothing is just as important as clean skin. Underwear should be changed daily. Outer garments should be regularly washed or dry-cleaned. Women's clothing may be protected by dress shields, but these must be laundered after each wearing. Clothes which have acquired persistent odors, or appear to be associated with odor problems, should be discarded.

Deodorants and antiperspirants provide

additional protection from body odor but do not replace the need for cleanliness. (*See* DEODORANTS AND ANTIPERSPIRANTS.)

Sometimes other factors can play a role in producing an unpleasant odor. These include certain metabolic and infectious diseases, certain drugs, and foods, like garlic or onions.

If a body odor appears to be unusual and is not controllable through cleanliness and the use of deodorants a doctor should be consulted.

Boils. A large infection of a hair follicle with staphylococci is called a furuncle, or boil. When boils are multiple or recurrent the condition is called furunculosis.

The staphylococci enter the openings (follicles) from which the hair extends or find entry into other pores of the skin. The staphylococci, like other bacteria, multiply rapidly. A pocket, containing pus and particles of destroyed tissue, forms in the follicle and causes swelling and pain.

Certain conditions favor the development of boils. Pressure and rubbing, as under a collar, make the neck a frequent site; the belt line and the buttocks are also susceptible. Moisture, as from sweating, speeds multiplication of the bacteria.

Blocking of pores or follicles, a frequent problem on the nose, also provides a fertile bed for the staphylococci. Garage mechanics and other people who work with grease and oil have tendencies toward boils because of the damming up of follicles.

Other illnesses may weaken the body's resistance and can make it prone to boils. Thus we have an obvious means of avoiding the problem: Try to keep yourself in good health and your skin clean, so that follicles will be kept open and bacteria will have little chance to multiply.

People with boils are frequently in such great discomfort that they cannot resist squeezing and picking them. Such measures are hazardous. They injure tissues and further the spread of bacteria, causing other boils to appear.

By all means, do not fuss with boils on the upper lip or below the nose. The staphylococci may spread by following the veins into certain blood-sinuses about the brain—a severe complication that can be fatal.

Moist heat (hot packs) will help the boil come to a head and open, so that the pus may drain. But discontinue this measure as soon as the boil opens, for the moisture could increase bacterial activity.

Cover the draining boil with a soft, loose, sterile dressing. Keep the skin clean and wash your hands thoroughly after touching the boil or dressings. Medication to combat the bacteria may be prescribed.

Sometimes it will be necessary for the boil to be cut open for drainage. This is not a home remedy, however, and should be performed by a physician.

One simple way to reduce the pain of a boil is to avoid moving the part of the body where the eruption is located. The swelling of a boil is tightly confined, and movement of skin and tissues is irritating.

When a patient suffers from repeated episodes of boils, specialists may try to introduce another type of staphylococcus—one that does not produce boils—to combat the type that is producing the trouble. X-ray therapy also may help.

Most boils continue for a few days or weeks, but sometimes they may occur in crops off and on for years. Some develop into carbuncles, which are similar to boils except that they are larger and have more than one core of infection. Carbuncles and widespread boils may be accompanied by sickness throughout the body. (*See* CARBUNCLES; STAPHYLOCOCCUS.)

Bone Bank. When doing bone grafts or bone transplants, surgeons prefer to use bone from elsewhere in a person's body. However, when suitable bone is not available from the patient himself, it can be obtained from a bone bank. A bone bank is a collection of stored bone which comes from cadavers, from amputated limbs, or from other operations. It is preserved in antiseptic solutions or by freezing or freeze-drying. (*See* SURGERY.)

Bones. Certain connective tissues of the body are hard and rigid. These are called osseous tissues, and they are organized into structures called bones.

The bones have many functions. Along with muscle, they help you to remain rigid in various positions or to move, using the lever principle you learned about in school. They also protect various parts of the body: the brain, the heart, the lungs. The larger bones of man are hollow, and the cavity is filled with marrow.

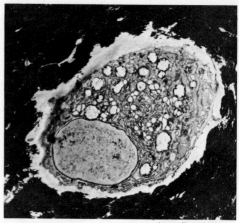

Argonne National Laboratory

Electron micrograph of a bone cell.

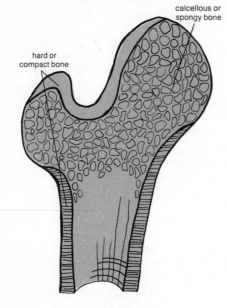

BONE TISSUE

One of the most vital functions of the bones is to assist the body in hematopoiesis, or the development of blood and blood cells. Before a child is born, the marrow of the bones in the embryo contributes to making both red and white blood cells. After birth, bones concentrate largely on the formation of red cells called erythrocytes. (*See* BLOOD.) If there is an abnor-

mal production of these cells in the bone marrow, a blood deficiency condition called anemia will result. (*See* ANEMIA.)

The composition of bones will vary in accordance with their size, shape, and use. The typical long bone, such as that of the arm or leg, consists of a relatively narrow shaft called the diaphysis. The diaphysis widens near the ends into the metaphysis, the part of the bone where most of the growing occurs during childhood. At the end of a long bone is an enlarged, rounded part called the epiphysis. This is covered with articular (joint) cartilage, which moves back and forth in the joint socket between bones. (*See* CARTILAGE.)

In the shaft of the bone is the marrow (medullary) cavity. The marrow lies in a framework of spongy (cancellous) bone. The marrow itself may be red or yellow. The red marrow is located in the wider ends of the long bones and contributes to the development of red blood cells. The yellow marrow is in the narrower part of the bone and contains many fat cells. Both the red and yellow marrow also contain several other types of cells, among them myelocytes, which are believed to have a role in producing certain white blood cells.

The outer layer of most bones is pro-

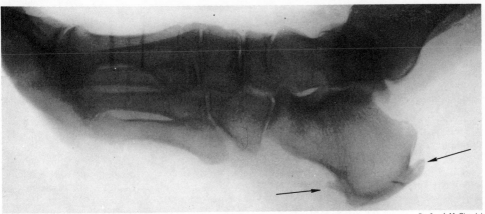

A bone spur is a projecting piece of abnormal bone. It is particularly
painful on the foot. At right in the X ray is a calcaneal (foot bone) spur.
The spur at left is called plantar, referring to the sole of the foot.

tected by the periosteum, a fibrous layer
that is attached to muscles and tendons.
The inside of canals and other openings in
the bones are lined with a membrane called
the endosteum.

There are also large air-filled cavities in
some bones, like those of the nose. These
cavities are called sinuses or antrums. A
small perforation in a bone for passage of
a nerve or blood vessel is termed a foramen.

Both blood vessels and nerves are found
in most bones. Most of the nerves regulate
the narrowing (vasoconstriction) or expansion (vasodilatation) of blood vessels to
meet circulatory needs of the blood system,
but some register pain. Often pain from disease or injury in a bone spreads or appears
to be located elsewhere in the body. When
this happens, the pain is said to be "referred."

Although the bones are hard and firm,
they are far from lifeless, and may change
in many ways after they have reached
maturity. They are almost continuously active, making blood cells and storing or ex-
changing calcium, phosphate substances,
and other body chemicals.

A shortage of blood supply to a bone,
lack of proper nutrition, imbalances of hormones in the system, infections, and other
factors may alter bone structure. Nutritional deficiencies do the most damage to
the bone during development. One of the
familiar diseases of poor nutrition among
children is rickets, in which the body does
not absorb enough calcium and phosphorus
to allow proper growth and development of
bones. This is most often due to deficiency
of vitamin D. Severe rickets may produce
deformity of bone, including bowlegs and
a narrowing of the pelvic outlet in women.

In adults, particularly women past the
menopause, abnormal rarefaction of bone
may occur, called osteoporosis. The cause
is controversial, but one factor in women
appears to be a diminished secretion of estrogens. (*See* OSTEOPOROSIS.)

If there is an abnormal secretion of
somatotropin (or STH) from the pituitary
glands, acromegaly may result. This is a
condition in which the bones keep growing
after adulthood has been reached. It is one
cause of giantism. (*See* ACROMEGALY.)

The bones also have the ability to grow
in order to compensate for physical injury.
When part of a limb must be amputated,
the strength and thickness of the bones adjoining the amputation are likely to in-

Major Bones of the Body and Their Location

Astragalus (*talus*). Immediately below the tibia and fibula, in the ankle, connecting with the heel bone.

Atlas. First vertebra below the skull.

Axis. Second vertebra in neck.

Calcaneus (*os calcis*). Heel bone.

Calvarium. Bones forming the top of the skull.

Capitate. The largest bone of the wrist, located near the center of the wrist joint.

Carpus. The eight small bones of the wrist: greater multangular, lesser multangular, lunate, capitate, hamate, navicular, triquetrum, and pisiform.

Clavicle. The collarbone.

Coccyx. The tailbone; vertebrae at the base of the spine.

Concha. A small, shell-shaped bone along the outer side of nasal cavity.

Costal bones. The ribs, 12 on each side, coming from the spinal column.

Coxae. The hipbone, composed of three fused bones: the ilium, ischium, and pubis.

Cranium. The skull, consisting of the occipital bone, 2 parietal bones, 2 temporal bones, 2 frontal bones, and the sphenoid and ethmoid bones.

Cuboid. A small bone in the foot.

Ethmoid. A small bone in front of the base of the skull.

Facial bones. Ten small bones which form the bony structure of the face: nasal, zygoma, maxilla, vomer, palatine, lacrimal, nasal concha, ethmoid, sphenoid, and mandible.

Femur. Thighbone, between hip and knee.

Fibula. Outer bone of the leg, from knee to ankle.

Foot bones. Seven tarsal bones (calcaneus, talus, cuboid, navicular, and three cuneiforms), 5 metatarsal bones, and the bones of the 5 toes.

Frontal bones. Bones of the forehead.

Humerus. Arm bone, from shoulder to elbow.

Hyoid. A thin U-shaped bone under the chin and above the larynx.

Ilium. The part of hipbone in which the femur fits.

Incus. One of 3 small bones of middle ear, adjacent to eardrum; called the anvil.

Inferior turbinate. Same as the concha.

Ischium. Part of the hipbone.

Lacrimal bone. A small bone of the front of the skull.

Malar. Cheekbone; zygoma.

Malleus. One of 3 small bones of the middle ear; called the hammer.

Mandible. The jawbone.

Maxilla. The upper jawbone.

crease. Bone may even form in soft tissues of the body as scarring occurs. When bones have been broken, they will knit themselves together efficiently if the parts are placed in the proper relationship. (*See* FRACTURES.)

Neoplasms (new growths) may also occur in the bones. (*See* CANCER; TUMORS.)

There are 206 bones in the human body, each with its own name. Not included in this count are numerous tiny bones that are not part of the regular bone system, but are embedded in the tendons over the bones of the knee, hand, and foot, and in parts of the skull.

Booster Shot. When an extra shot of immunizing substance is given in a booster dose or shot, it maintains or renews the effect of the original injection. (*See* IMMUNIZATION.)

Boric Acid. This is an inexpensive chemical readily prepared from borax and obtainable in the form of either crystals or powder. It is a very weak acid but useful in treating burns from lye and similar materials because it instantly neutralizes alkalies. It is used in powder form as an antiseptic on body surfaces; dissolved in water it is used to treat superficial infections of the eye. Boric acid is useful in foot baths, and skin diseases are sometimes treated with poultices of boric acid and starch. (*See* POULTICE.) Partly because it has no distinc-

Metacarpal bones. The 5 bones of the hand that the finger bones are attached to.

Metatarsal bones. The 5 bones of the foot that the toe bones are attached to.

Nasal bones. The bones of the nose.

Navicular bones. Small bones of the hand and foot.

Occipital. The back and part of the base of the skull.

Palatine. A bone that makes up part of the hard palate, nose, and orbit.

Parietal. A bone that makes up part of the side and top of the skull.

Patella. The kneecap.

Pelvis. Consists of the hipbones, sacrum, and coccyx.

Phalanges. Bones of the fingers and toes.

Pubis. The bone in front of the pelvis.

Radius. The long bone on the outer side of the forearm; extends from the elbow to the wrist.

Ribs. Costal bones.

Sacrum. Five fused vertebrae in the lower back.

Scapula. Shoulder blade (wingbone), which connects with the clavicle and the humerus.

Sesamoid. Small bones in tendons or places where muscles or tendons rub against larger bones, usually in the hands or feet.

Skull. The cranium.

Sphenoid. A bone making up the front portion of the base of the skull as well as parts of the orbit and nose.

Stapes. One of 3 small bones of middle ear; called the stirrup.

Sternum. The breastbone.

Talus. See astragalus.

Tarsal. See foot bones.

Temporal. The bone forming the front portion of the side of the skull and part of the base.

Tibia. The large inner bone of the leg between knee and ankle.

Turbinals. Three bones located on the outer side of the nasal cavity.

Tympanic bones. Three small bones of middle ear: the incus, malleus, and stapes.

Ulna. The long bone on the inner side of the forearm, between elbow and wrist.

Vertebrae. The spinal column, made up of 33 vertebrae: 7 in the neck, 12 in the chest (thoracic), 5 in the lower back (lumbar), and 9 that compose the sacrum and the coccyx.

Vomer. The back segment of the nasal septum that separates the two sides of the nose.

Wrist. See carpal bones.

Zygoma. The cheekbone; malar bone.

---

tive taste or color, it is sometimes taken internally by mistake and is fatal. It is also absorbed from skin surfaces in sufficient amounts to cause poisoning if large areas of skin are exposed to it for any length of time.

Botulism. The most dangerous form of food poisoning is botulism. The poison produced by the bacterium *Clostridium botulinum* is so deadly that as little as one part in ten million is enough to kill a mouse. The rod-shaped germs are found in soils everywhere. They are anaerobic (able to live without oxygen), and their spores (seeds) are so tough that they resist the action of the digestive juices and survive prolonged boiling. The poison itself, however, is destroyed by six minutes of boiling.

Since 1900 there have been between 500 and 600 outbreaks of botulism in the U.S. Many have been due to eating improperly processed and unheated home-canned vegetables, such as green beans, corn, and asparagus. Smoked fish and preserved meats as well as commercially canned soups have also been proved responsible. In general, all nonacid foods canned at home without the use of a pressure cooker are unsafe to eat without being boiled for at least six minutes, and commercial products cannot always be trusted. This is especially true if the cans are damaged or bulge at the ends. Infected food will show definite signs of spoilage, and it should be destroyed without being tasted. Even the smallest taste can be too much. Reheating foods may not improve their flavor, but it does make them safer.

The toxin of botulism may cause digestive upset, but the real damage is to the nervous system. Double vision, difficulty in swallowing, and ultimately paralysis of the breathing mechanism mark the course of the disease. Symptoms may develop quickly or over a period of several days. An antitoxin is available and, if used in time, can be lifesaving. However, it is not a cure for any nerve damage that may already have occurred. The only sure remedy is prevention—extreme care in food processing, commercially and in the home.

Compared with a number of less deadly forms of food poisoning, botulism is a rare disease. Commercial canning is done in huge pressure cookers. Relatively few housewives can vegetables at home, and many of them also use pressure cookers. However, *Clostridium botulinum* is so widely distributed in nature that the danger of poisoning can never be ignored. If processing temperatures are not high enough to kill the germs, and if the food so processed is eaten cold, the results can be fatal. (*See* FIRST AID; POISONING.)

Bovine Tuberculosis. Almost all mammals, including man, are susceptible to a zoonotic disease called bovine tuberculosis. (*See* ZOONOSES.) This is a widespread, chronic, bacterial disease closely related to that causing human tuberculosis. While man may contract bovine tuberculosis, cattle are largely insusceptible to human tuberculosis.

The bovine infection may be transmitted to man by drinking infected milk and milk products. Pasteurization is an effective safeguard. The disease may be controlled by quarantines and application of the tuberculin test to cows. The threat of human infection is very low, but repeated testing in all herds is necessary as long as the disease exists. (*See* TUBERCULOSIS.)

Bowels. The relationship between intestinal disturbance and emotional disturbance has been known for a very long time. Such biblical expressions as "bowels of compassion" may seem quaint, but the observation they represent has been confirmed by modern researchers. (*See* INTESTINES.)

People's bowels are literally moved by emotional stress. Excitement, anxiety, or anger can induce diarrhea in perfectly normal people. Others, equally normal, tighten up and become constipated. These reactions are not likely to be harmful, need no treatment, and are accepted by most individuals as simply "the way I am." When the excitement is over, or the new job becomes routine, they go back to their usual bowel habits.

For some people, however, the emotional stress and the bowel disturbances seem to be permanent. The complex of symptoms sometimes referred to as the "irritable bowel syndrome" includes generalized abdominal discomfort, gassiness (flatulence), diarrhea (sometimes alternating with constipation), and above all an overwhelming concern with the functioning of the digestive tract. It has been said that these people have "bowels on the brain." When asked how they are, they are likely to respond with a complete organ recital.

As a rule, nobody has to urge them to consult a doctor, and a diagnosis of irritable bowel syndrome should mean that really dangerous conditions, such as cancer and ulcerative colitis, have been ruled out. (*See* CANCER; COLITIS.) Psychiatric treatment, a nonirritating diet, and a compelling interest that takes the patient's mind off himself may be helpful. Cathartics and enemas only make matters worse. Medical faddists and out-and-out quacks will never lack for followers, or income, as long as there are people with irritable bowels. (*See* CONSTIPATION.)

Bowen's Disease. There are several skin disorders which indicate present or impending internal malignancy. (*See* MALIGNANCY.) One of these is a round, scaly, reddened skin lesion which may resemble psoriasis or eczema. (*See* ECZEMA; PSORIASIS.) Beneath this surface lesion, in the epidermal skin layer, is found carcinoma of the squamous cells—Bowen's disease. A high percentage of patients with this disorder will develop an internal carcinoma of some type even years after the onset of Bowen's disease. (*See* CARCINOMA.)

Bowleg. If a person's knees are far apart when his ankles are close together, he is said to have bowlegs, or *genu varum*. Most of the bowing actually occurs in the lower half of the leg, below the knee. The classic example of bowlegs is the cowboy who spends all day in the saddle.

Many children show some degree of bowlegs up to about the age of three. Often the bowing of their legs is not as severe as it appears: the turning-in of the whole leg, plus the presence of baby fat, make the legs look more bowed than they really are. Postural (or idiopathic) bowlegs do not usually need treatment, because the child will outgrow the condition. But bowlegs caused by rickets or some other disease may require surgical correction.

Brachial Plexus. The meshwork of nerves coming from the fifth through eighth cervical and the first thoracic nerve roots and going to the arm is known as the brachial plexus. (*See* SPINE.) It extends from the neck to the axilla (armpit). By various combinations of nerve root fibers, it forms all the nerves of the arm, both sensory and motor. The largest of these nerves are the radial, median, and ulnar. The radial nerve is motor to the triceps and all the extensor muscles of the forearm. The median and ulnar nerves are motor to the flexor muscles of the forearm. (*See* ARM.)

Injury to the brachial plexus produces a flaccid type of paralysis in the whole arm. (*See* PARALYSIS.) The arm hangs limply at the side with the palm of the hand turned toward the back. There is loss of feeling as well as loss of muscle power. Brachial plexus injuries can be caused by pressure— for example, from the straps of a knapsack or a baby back-pack. Leaning on the top of a crutch can also produce enough pressure to injure the brachial plexus, although the pressure is usually limited to the radial nerve.

Brachial plexus injury may accompany injury to the spinal cord. For instance an auto accident which forces the head to turn to the left and pulls the right arm backward can cause both spinal cord injury and right brachial plexus injury. (*See* SPINAL INJURIES.)

Brachial plexus injuries occasionally occur during delivery as the obstetrician is obliged to turn the baby and deliver the arm. They can also be caused by picking a person up by the arm when his muscle strength is not sufficient to prevent stretching of the plexus, as when he is asleep.

Brachycephaly. When a person has an abnormally short head, the condition is known as brachycephaly. (*See* ANATOMY; HEAD.)

Brachydactylia. When a person's fingers and toes are unusually short, the condition is called brachydactylia. (*See* FINGERS; TOES.)

Bradycardia. A slow heartbeat rate is called bradycardia. Usually it means a rate less than about sixty per minute. This may or may not be an important sign, depending on what other disease symptoms are present.

In older persons, a very slow rate may be associated with mental confusion or fainting. Administration of some drugs is effective in stimulating the heart to beat faster. (*See* ARRHYTHMIA.)

Braille. The system of writing or printing for the blind in which letters and characters are represented by raised dots or points that can be recognized by touch is known as braille. It was perfected in 1837 by Louis Braille, a French teacher of the blind who at the age of three was blinded as the result of an accident. He became one of the world's most famous pioneers in teaching the blind to read and to perform useful occupations.

The braille system, which has been modified slightly since its origin, is now almost universal. Special books, newspapers, and periodicals are available in braille.

A second system of printing for blind readers is known as Moon's type. This consists of raised lines and curves, and is available to the very small percentage of persons who are unable, for one reason or another, to learn braille. Books printed in Moon's type are costly, bulky, and rather scarce.

Braille literature is available in most public libraries.

Brain. The human brain is the largest and most complex portion of the nervous system. Lying within the skull, it also is the best protected. With the spinal cord, it is called the central nervous system.

The largest portion of the brain consists of the right and left cerebral hemispheres. They handle some of the more advanced processes of the nervous system.

Various parts of this area, the cerebrum, have been charted, so that when certain parts of the brain are damaged, we know that there will be corresponding changes in certain areas of the body. This fact is of great help in the diagnosis of nervous system disorders.

The cerebrum has separate portions devoted to three general functions. The sensory portions receive and interpret sensations of touch, pain, heat, pressure, seeing, hearing, and so on. Motor portions control muscles and movement. Association areas handle higher mental processes, such as reasoning, analysis, and memory.

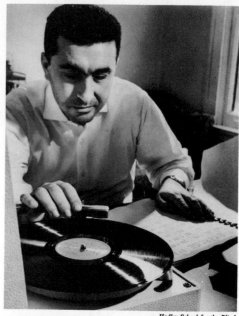

Hadley School for the Blind

Braille writing consists of raised dots on special paper. Here a romance-language instructor in a school for the blind reads an exercise in braille with his fingertips as he hears the same words played on a phonograph record.

The cerebrum is located in the entire upper portion of the skull. Below it, and toward the back part of the skull, is the cerebellum, which controls many activities of the body below the level of consciousness. It automatically handles reflexes of posture and balance, coordinates muscles, and maintains muscle tone. Most of the cerebellum is composed of white matter, although some near the surface is gray, like the advanced cells of the cerebrum.

Damage to the cerebellum, or inherited defects in it, make it difficult for a person to move parts of his body properly. If there is a malfunction of a portion of the cerebellum, only the parts of the body on the same side as the malfunction are affected.

In front of the cerebellum is an area called the midbrain, which functions, in part, to connect various divisions of the brain. Here also is the brain stem, which includes the pons, a connecting body of nerve fibers; the medulla oblongata (spinal bulb), a control and relay center for certain functions of blood circulation and breathing; and specialized nerve information relay centers called nuclei.

The spinal cord—the main trunk line of nervous system messages to and from the lower portions of the body—blends into the brain stem.

Above the midbrain is the thalamus, a very important center for processing and interpreting various sensations of the body. It is closely coordinated with the sensory parts of the cerebrum. The thalamus is believed to play a role in your general feelings—whether you feel elated or depressed.

Adjacent to the thalamus is the hypothalamus, which appears to have at least part of the brain's tasks of maintaining fluid balance in the body, sensing hunger, regulating body temperature, and signaling the need for sleep or wakefulness.

The hypothalamus secretes a hormone and other substances which aid in regulating water in the system and converting food and blood substances to energy (metabolism).

Obesity has been known to result from improper functioning of the hypothalamus. When a person sweats or when emotion makes his heart beat faster, it is the hypo-

thalamus that sends out instructions for these physical reactions through the nervous system.

Surrounding the brain structures and extending down to enclose the spinal cord are the meninges. These are membranes in three layers, the outer of which is called the *dura mater,* the middle the *arachnoid,* and the inner the *pia mater.*

The meninges form spaces for the cerebrospinal fluid. This liquid helps to cushion the brain and spinal cord against injury and to keep nerve tissue moist and lubricated.

The fluid changes in content with various diseases. As it is continuous from the brain down through the spinal cord, samples of the fluid are conveniently taken by what is called a lumbar (lower back) puncture. A needle is inserted between the lumbar vertebrae.

Infectious meningitis (inflammation of the meninges) may be diagnosed by examining the cerebrospinal fluid for microorganisms. (*See* MENINGITIS.) The germs causing syphilis may be similarly identified in the fluid of persons with this disease. Fluid pressure and content also are clues to the problems of brain hemorrhage or tumors.

The cerebrospinal fluid may increase abnormally because of disease or an inborn defect. When this occurs, the pressure may enlarge a child's head in a condition known as hydrocephalus. (*See* HYDROCEPHALUS.) One means of treatment is to tap the fluid and reduce the pressure. A newer method has been studied which would permit the extra fluid to be drained through a plastic tube to the child's stomach.

BRAIN-RELATED DISORDERS. Diseases of the brain often involve the spinal cord and other parts of the nervous system. Encephalitis is an example. It may be caused by a wide variety of viruses, and may be a part of other specific diseases, such as rabies or poliomyelitis. Combined with meningitis, it is called meningoencephalitis. (*See* ENCEPHALITIS; MENINGITIS; POLIOMYELITIS; RABIES; VIRUSES.)

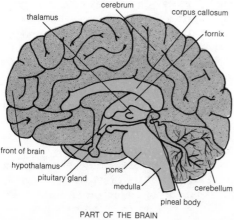

PART OF THE BRAIN
(SIDE VIEW)

Brain damage, sometimes occurring before or during birth, may cause varied mechanical difficulties with the muscles. The muscles may initially be in good condition, but without proper control by the nervous system they may quickly lose proper tone, strength, and coordination. In cerebral palsy, children have such mechanical problems of movement and coordination. Only a small percentage also have associated mental retardation. (*See* CEREBRAL PALSY.)

In epilepsy, the individual has problems of the brain which produce shaking or other abnormal body movements from time to time, with normal periods in the intervals between. The attacks may be due to a number of things, such as an infection, an injury, or a brain tumor, but often may occur without any known cause. (*See* CONVULSIONS; EPILEPSY.)

In parkinsonism, there are brain defects which result in tremors of the muscles, rigidity, slowness of movement, and weakness. (*See* PARKINSON'S DISEASE.)

METHODS OF DIAGNOSIS. The nerve messages through the complex pathways of the brain give off very weak electrical impulses, called brain waves. The rapid fluctuations of electrical potential may be detected by electroencephalography (EEG). This is a system in which electrodes (electric wire endings) are placed on the patient's skull and are sensed by a device called an electroencephalograph. The result is a series of wavy lines on paper (an electroencephalogram) which shows the fluctuations of the brain waves. Comparison of the recorded brain waves with those of normal individuals helps to diagnose brain tumors, epilepsy, and other disorders.

Sometimes the patient's veins may be injected with a radioactive substance which will find its way to the brain and be detected by a radiation detector. A so-called scanner records the location of impulses from the radioactive material and maps out the outline of the brain on a film for study. Tumors, which have different degrees of ab-

sorption of radioactive materials, are thus located. (*See* SCANNING.) This method has proved more effective in many ways than the older means of photographing by X ray.

Another way of locating brain tumors is by ultrasonography. Sound waves above the range of human hearing are sent into the head and bounce back, much like radar; the echoing varies with the tissue reached by the sound wave. This method helps to locate any displacement of the midline of the brain due to pressure by a tumor. (*See also* MENTAL HEALTH; NERVOUS SYSTEM.)

Brain Tumors. Strictly speaking, any growth in the brain, whatever its cause, can be called a brain tumor. More commonly the term refers to a cancerous growth within the brain substance, and this is the definition we will use.

As in any other region of the body, a tumor involving the brain can be benign or malignant. (*See* MALIGNANT.) Tumors can arise from brain tissue (intrinsic tumors), or grow within the brain, after being spread there from another body region (metastatic tumors). Brain tumors, comprising 2 to 5 percent of all tumors, may occur at any age but are more common in children under ten. They reach peak incidence around the fifth and sixth decades of life. Contrary to popular belief, a history of head injury has never been shown to predispose a person to these tumors—nor has his race or occupation. Intrinsic brain tumors, though they rarely spread beyond the central nervous system (brain and spinal cord), are associated with a high degree of morbidity (sickness) and mortality (death rate).

The classification of brain tumors is based on the cell type from which the tumor originated. This can be determined by surgically removing the tumor and examining it under a microscope.

INTRINSIC TUMORS. *Gliomas*, tumors of the glial cells of the brain which normally act as supporting and repairing agents, constitute 50 percent of all primary brain tumors. They occur mostly in the cerebrum

(*See* BRAIN.) and have their highest incidence between the ages of forty and sixty. Because they tend to infiltrate other brain tissue so readily, all gliomas are considered to be malignant.

Medulloblastomas probably originate from a primitive cell formed early in the brain's development. They always occur in children and always grow in that region of the brain called the cerebellum. (*See* BRAIN.) Approximately 30 percent of all childhood brain tumors are of this type. They grow rapidly and spread readily. The child with a medulloblastoma has a very poor chance for recovery.

Meningiomas and *neurilemmomas* are tumors of the supporting structure of the brain. Meningiomas arise from cells of the pia-arachnoid, a tissue covering the outer surface of the brain, and constitute about 15 percent of all brain tumors. Because of their superficial location and slow growth, most meningiomas can be completely removed, and the patient cured.

Neurilemmomas develop from the Schwann cells, which encircle nerves. They commonly arise from the eighth cranial nerve (acoustic nerve) in a region at the base of the brain known as the cerebello-pontine *angle*. Deafness or ringing in the ears is often associated with this tumor.

Developmental tumors arise from cells once used in the brain's development that then became inactivated and served no useful function. Among these rather rare tumors are hemangioblastomas (growing in blood vessels), craniopharyngiomas, epidermoid and dermoid cysts, colloid cysts, and chordomas. These lesions gradually expand, taking up more and more space, but are usually benign.

Pituitary tumors are benign tumors of the pituitary gland. (*See* PITUITARY GLAND.) Since most arise from one of two cell types, chromophobes or eosinophils, they are accordingly termed chromophobic or eosinophilic adenomas. (*See* ADENOMA.) These slow-growing tumors cause neurological symptoms by pressing against the nearby optic nerve, the hypothalamus, the third ventricle, and the temporal lobe of the brain. (*See* BRAIN.)

METASTATIC TUMORS. It is stated in some medical studies that 40 percent of all brain tumors are metastatic; that is, they have spread to the brain after first developing elsewhere. About 50 percent of metastatic brain tumors come from primary tumors of the lung and breast. Also contributing are tumors originating in the pancreas, bowel, and kidney, as well as from malignant melanomas. (*See* MELANOMA.) These brain tumors are fast-growing, destructive, and highly likely to invade nearby brain tissue. When a tumor elsewhere in the body sends metastatic lesions to the brain, the outlook for the patient is poor indeed.

DIAGNOSIS. A brain tumor is not easy to diagnose because a tumor so often simulates some other neurological disease. As it grows, occupying more and more space within the cavity of the skull, pressure on the brain increases, causing generalized signs or symptoms. When the tumor presses on a specific region of the brain, however, the patient may have complaints about this particular area. General evidences of brain tumor include headache, nausea, vomiting, and a depressed state of consciousness (dullness). The patient may suffer partial blindness, double vision, seizures, or weakness; these symptoms may point to the presence of a brain tumor—as may a change in personality, impaired memory or judgment, and changes in speech.

A number of procedures can aid the physician in making his diagnosis. First and most important is a physical examination of the patient and his medical history, which may reveal some of the signs and symptoms of brain tumor. X rays of the skull are often useful, since certain tumors appear as various changes in position or density. A chest X ray can point out lung cancer, which could be the source of a metastatic brain tumor. Spinal taps are frequently helpful because some tumors alter the spinal fluid. A tracing of "brain waves" or electrical activity, called an electroencephalogram (EEG), can be valuable since in about 75 percent of brain tumor cases the EEG is abnormal. Radioactive materials which are picked up by the brain can be injected into a vein and then detected over the skull by a device resembling a Geiger counter. About 75 percent of tumor cases will show abnormalities here.

TREATMENT. Once the diagnosis of brain tumor has been made, some form of treatment must be started. There are three basic categories of treatment: surgery, radiation, and chemotherapy. (*See* CHEMOTHERAPY; RADIOTHERAPY.) As a general rule, surgery is the initial treatment for all brain tumors. The result depends on the location, type, and age of the tumor. Certain tumors (meningiomas, cystic astrocytomas) can almost always be completely removed. Other more malignant tumors (malignant astrocytomas) can virtually never be excised. In extensive malignant brain tumors the only operation which will benefit the patient is one which merely relieves the pressure that has built up inside the skull cavity.

Radiation therapy is very beneficial in treating certain tumors. It seldom cures a patient completely, but allows him to live longer and makes him more comfortable. Most malignant brain tumors respond very well to irradiation: their size decreases, and their growth rate slows down. When a tumor is located in areas of the brain which cannot be reached surgically it is generally treated by irradiation. Often radiation is used before or after surgery, when it is impossible to remove all of the tumor.

The chemotherapy of brain tumors is mostly experimental at this time. Various drugs have been injected into the tumor area, the space around the brain, and the blood vessels going to the brain. So far the results have been poor.

Brainwashing. An extreme method of persuading a person to change his beliefs by physical and mental deprivation is known as brainwashing. It is usually employed to compel a person to take up beliefs that may be directly opposed to what he now believes. Frequently an enemy attempts to force an interned victim to undergo a radical change of moral or political convictions or to commit treason.

Brainwashing is done in three stages. The victim is first disoriented and disillusioned by being deprived of regular meals, sleep, companionship, and reading material. Becoming depressed after several weeks of this, he begins to lose his sense of personal identity.

He is now ready for the second stage—interrogation. Questioning sessions take place at any time of the day or night. The victim first welcomes this chance for human contact, but he is so confused and anxious that he cannot concentrate on details. The interrogator, taking advantage of the victim's confusion and doubt, twists the victim's words so that eventually he cannot be sure of what is really true or false. Soon the victim will do or say anything to be released from mental torment. This is when he is presented with a prepared "confession."

The last stage of brainwashing is called conversion. The victim is treated with kindness and consideration and, knowing that his only hope for decent treatment is to agree with his tormentors, he will do just that.

Experience with Americans captured by the enemy during the Korean War has shown that they returned to their original ways of thinking after being released and sent home. (*See* BEHAVIOR; CHILD BEHAVIOR; MENTAL HEALTH.)

Breast Cancer, Female. When breast cancer in women is detected at an early stage, chances for successful treatment are good. (*See* BREAST EXAMINATION; BREAST TUMORS; BREASTS.)

Breast Cancer, Male. Although it is a far less frequent occurrence than in females, males can develop cancer of the breast. Those affected are generally older than females with the same problem, typically aged forty or older. Male and female breast cancer, with few exceptions, are identical.

Male tumors grow far more slowly than female tumors, and are usually not detected until late in their development. By the time the cancer is discovered, it has almost always extended into the underlying tissue. This is because the amount of gland tissue is smaller than in women. The cancer almost inevitably will have spread to the lymph nodes under the arm. Such a spread into the axillae (armpits) is termed metastasis.

Early symptoms, although slight and seldom heeded, are pain and swelling in the area. Ulcerations of the nipple occur later.

Treatment is, like that in the female, surgical removal of the affected tissue. But the outlook for males is poorer, owing to the advanced spread of the cancer. Irradiation following surgery helps improve the patient's chances for cure.

Breast Examination. Since early detection of breast lumps is important in the treatment of breast disease, breast examination is an especially valuable procedure. Gynecologists regularly check a woman's breasts as part of a thorough physical examination. (*See* BREAST TUMORS.)

Women should practice regular self-examination after each menstrual period. Increased nodularity that sometimes appears normally just before menstruation is no cause for concern.

Breast examination merits special attention from women over thirty—the group most vulnerable to various conditions. Examination of the breast should be meticulous, methodical, and gentle. A woman should test both breasts by lying on her back with one arm raised while the opposite hand examines the breast, and then again with the arm at her side. Both breasts should be examined this way. The entire

procedure should be repeated while the woman is standing in front of a mirror. Any masses discovered should be reported to a physician.

MAMMOGRAPHY. Women who have already lost a breast to cancer or who have a family history of breast cancer require more vigilant attention since they are a higher risk. For them and others who have a suspected growth, mammography is sometimes used. A mammogram is a radiologic examination of the soft breast tissue. Although it is a useful diagnostic procedure, special training and experience are required in taking and interpreting the films. It is also a useful examination procedure for women with heavy or pendulous breasts.

Breast Feeding. Milk from the mother's breast is the ideal food for a newborn child. Feeding a child from the breast, or nursing, can also provide psychological rewards for both the mother and the child. Nursing can also hasten the return of the uterus to its nonpregnant state, thus physically benefiting the mother.

Milk production begins in the breasts shortly after delivery. At times it may seem that the supply will be insufficient, but an infant's sucking will stimulate production and increase the supply sufficiently for his needs. Since the mother's attitude has a strong influence on her success with breast feeding, emotional upsets can sometimes diminish milk supply.

Nearly every mother is able to nurse her infant successfully. Only rarely will involuted nipples or her own or her child's illness prevent a mother from nursing. Infant formula, which closely approximates breast milk, can be fed from a baby bottle at such times. Formula can also be used as a supplement if the nursing mother will be away from home at a feeding and wants someone else to feed him. A doctor can advise on this.

The nursing mother has the advantage of

always having a supply of fresh, sterile milk available to fill her infant's needs. Additional equipment is unnecessary. Because breast milk digests so easily, the infant has few stomach or bowel problems.

Late in pregnancy, a woman can begin preparing her breasts for nursing by regular gentle massage of the nipples, getting them ready for the vigorous exercise they will receive from her infant's sucking. She should always keep her breasts clean and dry. If secretions are allowed to accumulate, infections can develop. A cream can be useful to prevent drying and cracking of the skin. A good supporting brassiere is essential, both during pregnancy and once a mother's milk has come in. Nursing bras, which not only support the breast but also can be opened to allow the infant to suckle, are particularly useful.

For the first few days following delivery the mother's breasts secrete only colostrum. This thick, yellowish fluid is not true milk, but the infant should be allowed to suckle for approximately three minutes, since this material contains antibodies

Self-examination of the breasts on a regular routine schedule is the best way to detect breast tumors or cysts quickly and prevent their developing into serious problems. Here are the steps:

(1) Examine your breasts visually with the aid of a mirror, first with your arms at the sides, next with them raised overhead. Watch for any changes in shape or size, or discharge from the nipples.

(2) Lie down and put a pillow under your left shoulder. Raise your left arm and put the hand under your head. Using small circular motions, gently feel the left breast with the right hand, keeping the fingers flat.

(3) The inner half of the breast should have a band of firmer tissue around the nipple, which is normal. Feel for other lumps from top to bottom of breast, and from nipple to ribs on each side.

(4) Move the pillow under your right shoulder, with your right hand under your head, and repeat steps (2) and (3) to examine your right breast.

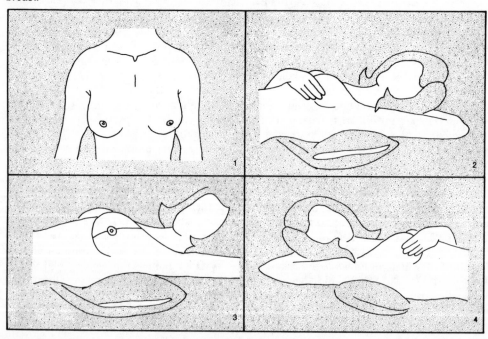

which help him resist infection. Also, the suckling will stimulate the mother's milk production.

After two or three days the mother's milk will come in. (Normal milk is thin and bluish.) The child can then be allowed to suck approximately five minutes at a breast for each regular feeding. When the child is about a week old, he can be allowed to suck for fifteen minutes or more to empty a breast completely. The mother can offer an alternate breast at each feeding or she can offer both breasts, beginning with the one used last at the previous feeding. The latter procedure will ensure that each breast is emptied completely.

Feedings can be scheduled either by the clock or on demand. At first the infant will need to be fed every three or four hours. The number of feedings will gradually diminish as he sleeps through the night and finally when he receives solid foods. During feeding the child can be cradled in the mother's arms or nestled on a bed beside her. Both mother and child should be comfortable.

Part way through each feeding and again at the end the child should be burped to dislodge any air bubbles that he might have swallowed. Overfeeding a nursing baby is quite rare.

The nursing mother should pay special attention to maintaining a well-balanced diet rich in calcium, protein, and vitamins A and C. Milk, meat, eggs, and green leafy vegetables are particularly important. Since drugs (including laxatives) can appear in the woman's milk and affect the infant, only those prescribed by a physician should be taken. Substances such as alcohol and chocolate can also sometimes affect the infant.

The mother should always be alert to any cracks or fissures on the nipples since these can lead to infection, and if an infection should develop, she might have to discontinue nursing. (*See* MASTITIS.) If the breasts are not emptied regularly, the result may be engorgement—a painful condition that can be relieved by manually expressing some of the milk or by using a breast pump.

Some mothers breast feed until their child is six months old or until he can drink from a cup. Others continue nursing for more than a year. Much of this depends on the prevailing culture and the mother's wishes. Her milk is often the best source of nutrition available, although modern formulas now give most women a choice. No mother should feel guilty if she breast feeds her child for only a short time—or not at all.

The doctor can give valuable advice on how to wean the baby. Weaning can be done by gradually decreasing the number of times the infant is put to the breast or by stopping all at once. Engorgement of the breasts will subside after about seventy-two hours if they are not stimulated. Lactation will cease. Binding the breasts, or otherwise providing good support, is essential. If they become painful, aspirin will help.

If a mother has any doubts about breast feeding or is having any difficulty, she might contact a local chapter of La Leche League, an organization interested in promoting breast feeding. (*See* LA LECHE LEAGUE.)

Breasts. Characteristic of all mammals, breasts provide the means by which a mother suckles her young. (*See* BREAST FEEDING.) In the human being, the breasts are paired and located on the chest between the arms. In lower mammals, breasts can vary in number, size, shape, and location, though all have some form of nipple which the young can suck.

Immature children of both sexes have flat breasts characterized only by the presence of nipples and surrounding pigmented areola. In the human male the breasts remain relatively flat except for a year or so around puberty. In the female, however, breasts develop as a secondary sex characteristic, assuming a round, firm contour at

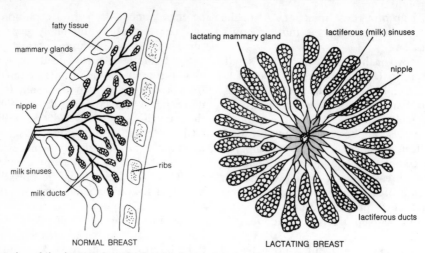

NORMAL BREAST   LACTATING BREAST

The interior of the breast, front and side views, showing the mammary glands, sinuses, and ducts through which the milk passes. The side view shows the normal breast; the front view shows the beginnings of enlargement during pregnancy to prepare for lactation.

maturity. Their size is frequently linked with a woman's heredity, though it can be altered by cosmetic surgery.

Breasts often provide a focus for sex play preceding intercourse. (*See* SEXUAL RELATIONS.) The nipples are particularly sensitive to stimulation and can become firm and erect in both female and male.

As the woman grows older, the tissue of the breasts loses its firmness and they begin to sag. Since breast tissue is spongy rather than muscular, it requires external support, usually in the form of a brassiere, if firmness is to be maintained.

During pregnancy a woman's breasts undergo marked changes. In the early weeks, they are often tender and will tingle. The nipples become characteristically larger, darker, and more erect. After about the second month of pregnancy, the breasts enlarge, and gentle massage will sometimes produce the thick yellowish fluid known as colostrum. If the breast enlargement is extensive, striae or stretch marks will be noted.

The flow of blood to the breasts increases markedly during pregnancy and continues throughout lactation. For this reason the

veins become quite prominent. When a woman is lactating, the spongy lobes of the breasts fill with milk, which then drains through the ducts to the numerous individual openings located on the nipples.

Diseases of the breast are not uncommon. (*See* BREAST TUMORS; MASTECTOMY; MASTITIS.)

Breast Tumors. Not all lumps or masses within the breast are tumors, though nearly all breast tumors begin as lumps or masses. A variety of breast tumors and cysts is possible.

Cystic disease is the most frequent type of breast mass. It usually appears as separate and tender breast masses. A cyst is a sac filled with liquid, and pain or tenderness often calls attention to it. Just before menstruation the pain may occur or intensify and the masses increase in size. This disease of the breast is most common among women between thirty and fifty years of age; it is rare in women after the menopause.

Frequently several masses can appear in both breasts, and an operation is usually performed to determine whether a mass is performed to determine whether a mass is cancerous. If it is not, the cysts are removed with as little irritation of surrounding tissue as possible. Since they can reappear, the woman should examine her breasts monthly just after her period and notify her physician if she finds any lumps. (*See* BREAST EXAMINATION.)

Adenofibroma of the breast is the name for a round, firm, discrete (separate), relatively movable, nontender mass. It is found in young white women usually within twenty years after puberty, and more often, and at a younger age, in Negro women. Once the growth is discovered, it should be removed surgically.

Breast cancer, the most common fatal malignancy in women, generally appears as a single, nontender, firm-to-hard breast mass with poorly defined margins. Because early detection can help alter the course of the disease, all women over thirty should examine their breasts monthly after each menstrual period.

Removal of the affected breast is the most common treatment. (*See* MASTECTOMY.) When treated by radical mastectomy, 40 to 60 percent of the patients have been reported cured after five years. When there is no evidence of spreading at the time of mastectomy, the five-year cure rate approaches 75 to 85 percent.

Radical mastectomy, however, is usually limited to those patients who stand some chance of cure. If the carcinoma is inflammatory (*see* CARCINOMA), or if the cancer has already spread to nodes and other parts of the body, or if there is swelling, the doctor probably will not remove the breast. Instead he may recommend treatment with radiotherapy or chemicals, which is sometimes helpful, or prescribe the addition or removal of hormones.

If other members of a woman's family have developed breast cancer, she is at least twice as likely to develop the disease. Also, women who have had cancer in one breast stand a greater chance of developing cancer in the remaining breast. Male breast cancer can also occur, though this condition is quite rare. (*See* CANCER.)

Breath Analyzer. The instrument that measures the amount of alcohol in a person's blood is a breath analyzer. The person being tested exhales into a tube that conducts the gas through a liquid containing a chemical sensitive to alcohol.

The breath analyzer has been valuable in studying the relationship between car accidents and particular percentages of alcohol in drivers' blood. It has also been used in studies of the effects of alcohol on visual perception and acuity, reaction times, memory, motor coordination, and concentration power. These studies indicate that all drivers are impaired at the 0.10 percent blood alcohol level.

Breath Holding. When a young child has a fit of anger or extreme anxiety, he may have periods of holding his breath. Sometimes this can happen after he has been suddenly startled. He may first hold his breath, then breathe deeply and rapidly for a moment, then later hold his breath again. Children learn early that if they stop breathing they will get whatever they want from their frightened parents.

In severe cases the child may turn pale and lose consciousness. But fortunately the respiratory system is under dual control, voluntary and involuntary. Thus when the child is unconscious he will automatically relax and begin to breathe. Although this whole procedure may be very alarming to parents, the problem is never as serious as they fear.

As with all other childhood disturbances, love and understanding are the best remedies for breath holding. Do not underestimate a child's fears; rather, give him reassurance that he is loved and protected. However, do not become permissive to the point that a child knows he can always get the upper hand by holding his breath.

Breathing. The process of drawing air into the lungs and then expelling it after the oxygen has been removed is breathing. Intake of air is called inspiration, or inhaling; expulsion of air is expiration, or exhaling. This is the first step in the total process of respiration by which oxygen is taken from the air, pulled down into the individual units of the lungs, the alveoli, and transported via the blood to provide oxygen to the tissues. Finally carbon dioxide and other waste gases are removed from the blood and expelled from the body. Thus breathing is the mechanical, initial stage in this process. (*See* RESPIRATION.)

The intake of air is brought about chiefly through contraction of the diaphragm, which is the muscular membrane separating the chest from the abdomen. The contraction pulls it downward and causes air to flow into the lungs. Three groups of external muscles also contribute to inspiration by raising and lowering the chest cage. Raising the cage reduces pressure in the chest cavity and air flows in; lowering it increases pressure and forces air out of the lungs.

Normally, the expiration of air is a passive process, a natural result of relaxing the diaphragm and the muscles of the chest cage. But forceful expulsion of air can be achieved by a contraction of the abdominal muscles. This forces the abdominal contents upward against the diaphragm, which is forced upward and produces expiration. This is why we whoosh out air when we are struck in the abdomen.

Breathing is both a voluntary and an involuntary process. We can breathe when we want to, hold our breath, or breathe faster than normally. But even during sleep and when we are not thinking about it, we continue to breathe. Certain stimuli will increase the normal amount of breathing: anxiety, infection, exposure to heat, and exercise. In all cases, nervous impulses to the brain are in control.

Before birth there is a small amount of fluid in the lungs, the thorax is unexpanded, and the chest is filled with the airless lungs.

At birth, the diaphragm descends, the size of the chest cavity increases, and air is pulled into the lungs. The obstetrician's slap on the newborn baby's bottom helps him to take his first breath.

Bright's Disease. Several kidney diseases characterized by edema and an excess of albumin in the urine and diminished excretory function are also known as Bright's disease. (*See* GLOMERULONEPHRITIS; KIDNEY.)

Bromide. One of the group of depressant drugs which is as old and as easy to use as alcohol is potassium bromide. Popular in the late nineteenth century for treating "nerves," it is now rarely prescribed by physicians. Instead, it is a widely used ingredient in headache and nerve compounds which may be purchased without a prescription.

Although given in small daily doses of three to five grams, potassium bromide cannot be voided from the body quickly enough to rid it of three to five grams in one day. The drug accumulates in the body and causes chronic intoxication, leading to faulty thought and memory processes, tiredness, emotional problems, and death. Along with these signs are skin rashes, appetite loss, constipation, and loss of coordination. (*See* DRUG ABUSE.)

Bronchial Asthma. A respiratory ailment usually brought on when an allergy to airborne substances leads to swelling of the bronchioles and an inability to exhale air from the lungs is bronchial asthma. The most common allergenic substance is plant pollen. (*See* ALLERGY; BREATHING; LUNGS.)

In a person afflicted by bronchial asthma, such substances cause swelling, or edema, of the tiny ends of the air passages in the respiratory system, the bronchioles. In addition, there is a spasm of the smooth muscle walls of the bronchioles. When the pa-

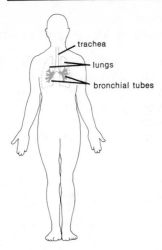

trachea

lungs

bronchial tubes

tient inhales, the air passes adequately through the bronchioles, but he has trouble exhaling because they have become occluded. This in turn leads to air hunger or air starvation.

As time goes on, and the patient continues to breathe in deeply but is unable to breathe out, air will be left in the lungs and the chest will become permanently expanded. The amount of air that cannot be exhaled keeps increasing and the condition is self-perpetuating.

Bronchial asthma can be treated by removing the patient from the allergens which bring on attacks. If he is allergic to specific plant pollens, his attacks will of course increase when the plants bloom. This is the reason some people are troubled only at certain times of the year. In some instances, the seasonal attacks are so severe that the patient's well-being demands that he move to an environment where the pollens are entirely absent.

Medication is also available to combat the allergic reaction. Such drugs are antihistaminic; that is, they attack the histamine formation in the body which brings out the allergic reaction. Various drugs work better for some patients than others, and an individual may have to try one after another to find out which is best for him.

The strongest medications for treatment of allergy are available only by prescription.

Bronchial Tubes. The passages that convey air into the lungs are the bronchial tubes. Air is breathed in through the nose or mouth into the trachea, which transmits the gases into the chest and extends as two forked bronchi, one going to each lung. The bronchi in turn divide and distribute air to the lobes of the lungs. The bronchi finally end as minute bronchioles which pass air into the alveoli, the working units of the lungs. All transmission of oxygen takes place at the alveoli. These are surrounded by capillaries which then pick up the oxygen, leave off waste gases such as carbon dioxide, and take the freshened blood to the body tissues.

Since the bronchial tubes transmit all the air a person breathes, they also come in contact with disease-causing organisms and substances. Occasionally they may become irritated by dust or infected by bacteria or viruses. (*See* BRONCHIAL ASTHMA.)

Bronchiectasis. In the lung problem called bronchiectasis, there is dilatation of the air passages called bronchi. In other words, the bronchi tend to stretch out or bulge. They lose their normal elasticity, and the functioning of associated muscles is impaired.

The outward symptoms of bronchiectasis include coughing and spitting up of large volumes of pus-filled phlegm, sometimes foul-smelling or bloody. Fever, loss of weight, and other signs of general illness may occur.

The physician who suspects bronchiectasis uses a stethoscope to detect sounds (rales) of air blockage in the bronchi. He will look for problems that may have brought on bronchiectasis, such as pneumonia, tuberculosis, other infections, or bronchial obstruction by tumors or substances that may have been accidentally inhaled by the patient. A chest X ray may disclose useful information, but in some cases the precise cause of bronchiectasis cannot be found.

Drainage of the thick fluid that collects in the lungs helps relieve the symptoms of the disease. Drugs taken by mouth or given in a nasal aerosol spray are used to loosen the phlegm. The patient then lies on his stomach with his shoulders over the edge of the bed and his folded elbows resting on a pillow on the floor. This places the head and shoulders below the chest and aids the outward flow of the fluid. The routine is followed for up to fifteen minutes at intervals of several hours.

Infections are treated with antibiotics. Surgery to open obstructed passages in the lungs is sometimes necessary. In chronic forms of the disease, the patient usually feels better if he avoids polluted air and refrains from smoking. He will also feel better in dry, warm climate. (*See* BRONCHITIS.)

Bronchitis. There are two general forms of bronchitis, both marked by inflammation of the bronchial tubes of the lungs, coughing, spitting up of phlegm and mucus, and breathing difficulty.

One form is acute bronchitis. This is a complication of a respiratory or other viral infection. There may also be fever. In adults, acute bronchitis usually is not dangerous, but in infants and younger children it may be quite serious. Acute bronchitis is treated with bed rest, steam inhalation to help clear air passages, antihistamines, codeine products for coughing, and antibiotics for infection.

The second form, chronic bronchitis, lingers on and on, sometimes for a lifetime. Most people who develop this disease are heavy smokers. It is also common in areas of high air pollution. Sometimes the attacks of coughing and difficult breathing may be seasonal or may come and go for no clear reason, but if neglected, change gradually to a constant problem. Many sufferers from chronic bronchitis come to accept the coughing, wheezing, and spitting as part of their daily life.

Chronic bronchitis is often a symptom of other problems such as emphysema or cor pulmonale. (*See* EMPHYSEMA; PULMONARY HEART DISEASE.) If any line can be drawn between the early stages of bronchitis and other lung disorders, it is a fine one indeed.

Colds and other infections cause much discomfort and sickness among persons who already have chronic bronchitis. The patient should follow a regimen of plenty of rest, good nutrition, and other general health measures to avoid these complications.

Above all, the person with chronic bronchitis should avoid smoking. He should also keep himself removed from polluted air, dust, or fumes that provoke attacks. Remedies similar to those used for acute bronchitis are useful for relieving the chronic form. However, no way is known to clear up chronic bronchitis except to eliminate the primary irritant, whether cigarette smoke, polluted air, or a stubborn infection.

Tests may be made to determine if the cause could be a particular irritant (allergen) to which the individual may react. (*See* ALLERGEN; ALLERGY.) For information on related diseases, see LUNGS.

Bronchopneumonia. A condition including inflammation of the lungs, which sometimes follows infections of the upper respiratory tract, specific infectious fevers, and diseases, is called bronchopneumonia. It is also known as catarrhal pneumonia, lobular pneumonia, and capillary bronchitis. (*See* BRONCHIAL TUBES; PNEUMONIA.)

Bronchoscope. An instrument used to examine the inside of the bronchial tubes is called a bronchoscope. The examination itself is referred to as a bronchoscopy. (*See* BRONCHIAL TUBES.)

Brown Recluse Spider Bite. Formerly rare in the United States, the brown recluse spider, *Loxosceles reclusa,* is now so common and dangerous that public health services give periodic warnings through the news media. As poisonous as the black widow spider, it may be found in every state.

It may be recognized by the same hourglass marking on its underside that the black widow spider bears. It is brownish in color, less than ½ inch in size, and has very long legs. The brown recluse weaves a large, irregular web and may be found under stones, in dark, moist places, and in stored clothes—its favorite indoor hiding place.

Its bite is extremely painful and its poison is a neurotoxin, for which there is no antivenin available. The symptoms of the bite are similar to those caused by the black widow spider. (*See* BLACK WIDOW SPIDER BITE.) Victims should be hospitalized immediately.

Brucellosis. Frequently called Bang's disease, brucellosis is an infection of cattle which causes abortion and sterility. The diseased animals are detected by blood and milk tests, and quarantine measures and vaccines provide effective control. This is a zoonotic disease which man gets from contact with cattle, swine, or goats. (*See* ZOONOSES.) In man, the disease is called undulant fever. (*See* UNDULANT FEVER.)

Bruise. The dark discoloration beneath the skin indicating blood accumulation in the tissues after injury to that area is called a bruise. The injury damages the small blood vessels (capillaries) in the area, and blood is released from these vessels into the surrounding tissues. At first the bruise is red or purple, which means that fresh blood is present. In time, the hemoglobin in the red blood cells begins to break down and change color. (*See* BLOOD.) The bruise reflects this by changing first to a brownish color and then to a yellow-green before it disappears.

Some people bruise very easily, because of having very fragile blood vessels which rupture easily, or a diminished number of the blood platelets required for blood clotting, or blood disorders such as leukemia and hemophilia.

Bubo. This is a loose term used in two different senses: (1) In general, bubo means a lymph node, especially in the axillary or the inguinal region (groin), that has swollen because of some acute or chronic infection, particularly if it goes on to form and discharge pus. The buboes seen in typical cases of bubonic plague appear especially in the inguinal region and are painful. In untreated cases of syphilis, buboes may appear two or three weeks after the primary lesion. (2) Bubo is also used more specifically to mean a distinct, generalized infectious disease caused by a particular virus and transmitted by sexual contact. Also called *lymphogranuloma venereum,* it is widely distributed through the world, but in 1964 only 543 new cases were reported in the United States.

Bubonic Plague. The acute and severe infectious disease characterized by high fever, lymph node enlargement, and bacteria in the blood and caused by a bacterium named *Pasteurella pestis* is called bubonic plague. This centuries-old disease was first accurately described in 542 A.D. when plague devastated the Egyptian port of Pelusium. During the fourteenth century the illness spread through Europe, the Middle East, China, and India and was known as the "Black Death." In Europe alone, one-fourth of the population died as a result of this plague epidemic. Although cases of bubonic plague have recently been reported in many parts of the world, only about ninety cases were reported in the United States during the first half of this century.

The bacterial organism which causes bubonic plague is quickly destroyed by sunlight, heat, and chemical disinfectants. This bacterium usually lives in the common rat. The flea which inhabits the rat's fur takes the organism into its system and then transmits it to man. The lymph nodes near the site of the flea bite become full of the bacteria and are enlarged and painful. The bacteria then may enter the bloodstream, causing fever and involvement of other organs. Plague pneumonia (lung infection) commonly occurs and can be spread to other people via the droplets produced in sneezing or coughing.

Bubonic plague usually affects a person quite rapidly, producing a sudden high fever (103° to 104° F.), rapid pulse, fatigue, and muscle ache. Mental symptoms and delirium occur in the later stages of the disease. (*See* DELIRIUM.) In nearly every case enlarged and very painful lymph nodes are found in the groin, armpit, or neck. In severe cases the bacteria enter the bloodstream, resulting in severe illness and death within three to five days of the beginning of the illness.

Even more serious is the development of plague pneumonia, which can be spread directly from patient to patient. Fever, rapid pulse, and breathing problems occur very quickly. Headache, muscle ache, and cough develop in a few hours and soon the patient is gravely ill. The production of frothy, bloody sputum is typical of plague pneumonia.

In order to prevent death, plague pneumonia must be treated very early and this stage responds well to the antibiotic drugs streptomycin, chloramphenicol, and tetracycline. But plague pneumonia is almost always fatal unless treated within twelve hours of its onset.

The prevention of bubonic plague requires the elimination of the common rat or its flea by means of rat poisons or flea poisons (DDT). Improved living conditions almost always stop outbreaks of plague.

Vaccines which protect humans against *Pasteurella pestis* have been used, but their effectiveness has not been well studied. (*See* VACCINATION.)

Bug Bites. Although a group of true bugs (hemipterous insects) does exist within the class Insecta, the use of the word "bug" is both slang and informal. Any animal whose body is divided into three parts and has three pairs of legs and two pairs of wings is correctly called an insect. (*See* INSECT BITES.)

Buerger's Disease. *Thromboangiitis obliterans,* another name for Buerger's disease, describes the problem scientifically. Clot formation *(thrombo-),* with inflammation of the arteries and veins *(angiitis),* causes blockage of blood flow and destruction (obliterans) of tissue.

In some diseases, the harmful role of smoking is vague and difficult to prove. However, this is not the case in Buerger's disease, because it rarely occurs among persons who do not smoke. Also, it is almost impossible to cure Buerger's disease if the patient continues smoking. If he stops the habit, his chances of recovery are usually good unless the disease has progressed too far and the person has smoked too long before corrective measures are taken.

Buerger's disease is most common among men smokers from ages twenty to thirty-five or forty. It affects the limbs, and its symptoms closely resemble those of other blood vessel disorders which may be confined to the arms and legs, such as atherosclerosis and *arteriosclerosis obliterans.* (*See* ARTERIOSCLEROSIS; ATHEROSCLEROSIS.)

The person with Buerger's disease gets insufficient nourishment because of lack of sufficient blood flow (ischemia), and body cells cannot live without receiving oxygen and other essentials carried by blood.

In Buerger's disease the first symptoms may be aching and lameness of the undernourished muscles of the legs, arms, hands, and feet. (*See* CLAUDICATION.) These extremities may be cold or numb, or they may have varied sensations such as tingling, prickling, or even burning. Such symptoms may not be continuous, but may come and go as the disease runs its typical course of remission (disappearance of symptoms) and recurrence over periods of days, weeks, months, or even years.

It is not known why the disease should get better or worse in this way, but this characteristic is a threat to the smoker: *quit smoking.* He may use the disappearance of the symptoms as an excuse to keep on smoking.

With the continued use of tobacco, the disease may so severely block the flow of blood that tissue death is extensive and gangrene results. When this occurs, amputation of toes, fingers, legs, or arms may be the only measure left to save the person's life.

Efforts to improve circulation with the use of grafts of artificial arteries have had limited success. In some cases, nerves are cut (sympathectomy) to eliminate the spasms or contractions of the arteries that may complicate the disease.

Persons with Buerger's disease, like all persons with circulatory problems in the limbs, must be very careful to keep their feet clean and free from bruises or cuts. These measures are important because infections are difficult to clear up when the circulation is not normal.

Antibiotics should be used at the first sign of infection in the limbs of the patient with Buerger's disease. Otherwise the problem could quickly progress to gangrene and require emergency amputation.

The only really effective mild treatment for Buerger's disease is abstinence from smoking in its early stages. If a patient neglects this measure, he may well face the drastic emergency measures noted above. There seems to be no middle road.

Actually, few persons die from Buerger's disease. Once they have lost their toes, fingers, or a leg by amputation, they have usually learned their bitter lesson and will refrain from smoking. By comparison, many other diseases which obstruct the circulation have a relatively high death rate, due to complications.

Sometimes the symptoms of Buerger's disease may be confused with those of Raynaud's disease, a problem chiefly of women and not definitely known to be associated with smoking. (*See* RAYNAUD'S DISEASE.)

Bulla.　A large blister inside or under the skin and filled with fluid is a bulla. (*See* BLISTERS; SKIN.)

Bunion.　A swelling at the ball of the big toe, involving inflammation of the mucosal tissue underlying the toe and hardening and thickening of the outside layer of tissue, is a bunion. The swelling may be so large as to force the toe toward the outside of the foot. There is considerable pain, especially when a person wears shoes and walks.

Treatment of bunions depends almost entirely on the severity of the problem. Small bunions may subside if a pad is worn in such a way as to remove pressure from the area. Larger bunions that affect the joints of the toe may require surgical removal.

The general appearance of bunions may be similar to the swelling due to gout, but the bunion, unlike gout, is not transient.

Burns.　There are three standard classes of burns, depending on how deeply the skin is burned.

First-degree burns cause only a reddening of the skin (erythema), with no blistering or destruction of flesh. These burns affect only the outer layer of skin (the epidermis); they heal rapidly and seldom require any treatment.

Second-degree burns damage the epidermis and may penetrate slightly into the dermis (corium), the layer of skin below the epidermis. There is much pain, with destruction of hair follicles and sweat glands. Infection is a dangerous and frequent complication.

Third-degree burns destroy the full thickness of the skin down through the innermost (subcutaneous) layer. The burning will either whiten the skin or char it black. The destroyed skin sloughs off, leaving the area raw and red. The skin that is shed is called slough, or eschar. When the area of a third-degree burn is larger than about an inch in diameter (2.5 cm.), it will not heal satisfactorily without a skin graft.

Sometimes burns may penetrate into muscle, bones, or other tissue below the skin. These are usually classed as severe third-degree burns, but sometimes are called fourth-degree, or char burns.

The risk of burns to the patient is related to not only the degree but also to the specific areas burned, the amount of the body burned, the age and health of the patient, other injuries (such as smoke inhalation), and individual differences in response to treatment. All these factors determine whether a person should be hospitalized or treated at home. Most persons with second- or third-degree burns over 15 to 20 percent of their body area must be hospitalized. If the person is very young or very old, has very deep burns, or is burned on the face, neck, hands, or feet, he may need to be taken to a hospital, even if as little as 2 or 3 percent of his body is burned.

FIRST AID. If someone's clothes catch on fire, tear them off or smother the flames with a wet towel or a blanket, rug, or coat. If one of these is not immediately available, roll the person against the ground.

Cold water is the best emergency treatment for burns. When someone in a restaurant is scalded with hot coffee or other food, grab the nearest pitcher or glass of ice water and pour it on the burned skin immediately. This will reduce the amount of tissue damaged by the burn.

If someone is severely burned, call a doctor at once. He will tell you to move the patient to his office or to a hospital. Or you may, of course, drive immediately to the emergency room of the nearest hospital, but

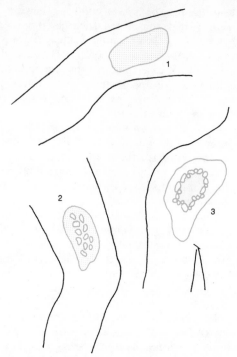

Three classes of burns. In a first-degree burn (1) the skin is reddened and painful to the touch. In a second-degree burn (2) the skin is blistered. In a third-degree burn (3) some skin and deeper tissues are burned away or charred.

you will be sure of faster care if you telephone in advance.

If you are forced to wait for transportation or for the arrival of the doctor, have the victim submerge the burned area in a sink or basin of cold water. If the area is large, get him into a tub of cold water at once, then remove the clothing from over the burned areas. If any is stuck to the burned tissue, cut off that part of the garment and leave it for a doctor to remove.

When transportation arrives, do not dress the patient, but cover him with clean sheets or a blanket. If there is any delay in getting him to the doctor, give him water, soft drinks, or similar beverages to prevent dehydration of his system.

Do *not* give the patient alcohol in any

form. Do not force liquids into him if he is unconscious.

Petrolatum and some ointments have practically no value in first aid to the seriously burned individual. Leave such medication to the doctor. Great harm has been done by smearing badly burned areas with butter, grease, and ointments. This can make treatment difficult for the doctor and even promote infection.

Home remedies for burns are handy but only for minor first-degree burns or second-degree burns of a very tiny area. These small minor burns should be cleaned of any dirt with mild soap and water. But leave any washing of more serious burns to the physician. Some burn wounds should not be washed at all, or treated with medication of any kind.

Remember that infection is the greatest risk in burns. Part of your first aid is to avoid touching the burns with dirty hands or any other soiled material. Bacterial infection is the cause of most deaths of burn patients.

If someone has been burned by a chemical, flush it off with water. If a large area of the body is involved, the chemical should be rinsed off under a cold shower. Many industrial plants have emergency showers for this very purpose.

If an eye has been burned with a chemical, rinse it out with a weak solution of sodium bicarbonate (baking soda), then place a cotton or some other soft pad over the closed eye and get the patient to a doctor or hospital at once.

For first aid in ultraviolet lamp burns, *see* SUNBURNS.

If there is a delay in getting the severely burned victim to the doctor, you should also treat the patient for possible shock. (*See* SHOCK.)

HOW DOCTORS TREAT BURNS. When the burn patient reaches a medical office, clinic, or hospital, the doctor—or often a team of doctors and nurses—continues emergency care to make sure that the patient does not succumb to shock and that he gets enough fluids to prevent dehydration.

Persons with burns of the head or neck, or with smoke inhalation injuries to the lungs and respiratory passages, may not be able to breathe properly, and tracheotomy may be needed. This surgery opens a passage in the throat so that air can get through.

Only after measures are taken to deal with life-threatening complications does the doctor or medical team turn to the burn itself. It will be cleaned and any loose dead tissue removed, then treated either by a closed or an exposed method.

In closed treatment, petrolatum and gauze are used to cover the wound. Over this is placed cushioning and absorbent dressings and a final bandage to keep them in place.

Silver nitrate solutions are used in one closed treatment method. These saturate the gauze bandages and help destroy bacteria. Other agents which have achieved dramatic success in preventing infections have been combinations of anti-infective drugs.

Liquid silicone has been used to cover burns of the hands. It aids recovery of the burn itself and helps prevent crippling of the fingers, but it is *not* a first-aid measure.

In the exposed treatment, the wounds are left open to the air. Fluid (serum) naturally develops and solidifies to seal the burn. Sometimes temperature-controlled enclosures are used over patients' beds to keep them comfortable when they have exposed burns.

Several beds have been developed to support patients who have burns on both sides of their bodies. One uses air jets to hold up the patient in a manner similar to that used to lift hovercraft vehicles over land and water. Another has tiny beads floating in air to form a soft mattress.

Patients in regular hospital beds must be turned often so that they do not lie too long on injured parts.

SKIN GRAFTS. The first skin grafting is usually performed within a few weeks after the burns occur. It is essential to replace skin which cannot grow back by itself, close up the wounds against infection, and help the person regain normal body functions.

These first grafts are usually homografts—that is, skin from another person. Skin may be taken from a live person for this purpose, but most homografts are made with skin from a cadaver (dead person). Heterografts—skin from an animal other than man—may also be used: pig or dog skin. Both homografts and heterografts are temporary, serving to protect the area and condition the tissues to receive a permanent graft.

The homograft or heterograft is generally rejected by the recipient within ten to twenty days. This rejection is a normal tendency of the body to refuse to accept parts of another person or animal as its own.

When the permanent grafts are rejected, they are removed and the areas covered with autografts—skin taken from other parts of the patient's own body, such as the thigh. Needless to say, the tissue of this skin must be capable of healthy growth, so it will readily cover the portion from which the graft has been taken.

The skin is removed for transplant with a mechanical cutter, called a dermatome, which can be adjusted to take various thicknesses of skin. When there is need for extensive grafting, a special type of dermatome is sometimes used. This cuts small slits into the skin, so it can be stretched until it is in the form of a mesh. Thus stretched, it can cover an area up to twice its original size. The tissue of the person's body gradually grows to join permanently with the graft and fill in the spaces between the mesh.

A year or more after the graft has "taken," reconstructive surgery may be performed to remove scar tissue and use plastic material to improve the appearance of the patient. (*See* PLASTIC SURGERY.)

Good diet, perhaps with additions of certain minerals and vitamins, is necessary for burn patients. Infections and loss of body protein and potassium during the sloughing of dead skin may contribute to malnutrition, disorders of metabolism (conversion of food to energy), anemia, and other complications.

Bursa. Between most moving surfaces in the body there is a small fluid-filled sac, called a bursa, which is rather like a balloon containing a little water. Bursas are most frequently found between bone and muscle. They help reduce friction, making it easier for the surfaces to move across each other.

The only time a person notices a bursa is when it becomes distended with liquid or becomes hot, swollen, and painful from some sort of injury. The condition of such an inflamed bursa is called bursitis. (*See* BURSITIS.) When this happens, movement becomes painful. In fact, the bursitis sufferer feels pain even when the affected joint is not moved.

Bursitis. A synovial bursa is an enclosure, or sac, of fluid which serves to prevent friction between parts of a joint. Bursitis means an inflammation of a bursa. (*See* JOINT.)

Bursitis usually follows an injury, strenuous exercise, a chill, or an infection. It may occur on just one or two occasions (acute bursitis) or may flare up many times during a person's lifetime (chronic bursitis). During an attack, there is a sharp pain in the bursa and nearby tendons. On taking an X ray of the joint, the physician usually finds calcium deposits there. These deposits cause much of the pain and discomfort of bursitis. Just why they develop is not known.

Bursitis is most common in the shoulder joint—a part of the body often subject to

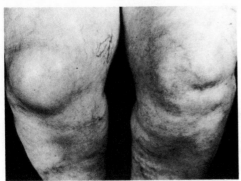

Water on the right knee of a man suffering from bursitis.

abuse by athletes, weekend handymen, and housewives. But sometimes an attack will occur for no obvious reason.

When an attack occurs the patient should rest his shoulder and arm, although in mild cases he may be able to gently move his arm to "work out" the pain. A physician or a physical therapist may manipulate the arm, asking the patient to let it "go limp" during the process.

Before such manipulation is possible it may be necessary to inject procaine, lidocaine, or another pain-blocking drug into the bursa. Injection of hydrocortisone or other corticosteroid preparation is almost standard treatment to reduce the swelling in bursitis. Phenylbutazone may also be used. (All these drugs require cautious administration, as there may be side effects.) X-ray therapy is often helpful. In long-standing or severe cases, the calcium deposits may have to be removed by surgery.

Bursitis, although usually in the shoulder, sometimes appears in the knee or elbow joints, and less often elsewhere. Wherever it occurs, the patient must be careful not to strain the affected limb for some time after the attack itself has subsided. Simple non-strenuous exercises will help build up the ability of the joint to work normally again, without pain.

Warm wet dressings may serve as a good first-aid measure during an attack. Aspirin or other household pain remedies also help.

The pains and other symptoms of bursitis may be confused with those of arthritis, the most common joint disease. (*See* ARTHRITIS.)

Buttock. The muscular region of the upper thigh in the back is called the buttock. The major portion of this structure is formed by a muscle called the gluteus maximus. In addition, there is much fat in the buttock, which serves as padding when a person sits.

The buttock, since it is largely muscle, is often used for intramuscular injections. (*See* INJECTIONS.)

C

Cachexia. Weakness, emaciation, and general ill health caused by a serious disease is called cachexia. The word is derived from two Greek words meaning "bad state." (*See* MALNUTRITION.)

Cadmium. After mercury and lead, cadmium is considered the worst environmental pollutant. Exhaustive surveys have shown that cadmium exists in detectable concentrations in soils, plants, foods, animals, and several kinds of human tissues. Seafood and meats have higher concentrations than vegetables and food grains. An analysis of cadmium in the blood of men in nineteen American cities showed small, but detectable levels in about half of the sample. The sources of cadmium are many, including smelting and plating operations, printing operations, soldering, and welding.

Concern over cadmium stems from the fact that scientists have linked cadmium with hypertension in rats. Cadmium levels in the air of twenty-eight American cities have been closely correlated with the incidence of death from hypertension and arteriosclerotic heart disease. Other maladies caused by higher levels of cadmium include proteinuria, kidney damage, and early testicular atrophy. (*See* TRACE ELEMENTS.)

Caffeine. A bitter alkaloid extracted from coffee or tea is called caffeine. It is used as a stimulant and a diuretic. Listed under a drug grouping called "mind-altering drugs," caffeine is one of the most widely used legal drugs, being found in coffee, tea, chocolate, and cola drinks.

Caffeine has been used since the fifth century A.D., when it was a trading item whose effects formed the basis for the Oriental tea ritual of Buddhism-Shinto. The *Thea sinensis,* a plant containing caffeine and related

to the camellia, reached American shores in 1665. While most countries are fighting drug consumption in all forms, they forget that the drinking of tea and coffee is one of the truest types of addiction, as caffeine is a mental stimulant. England was and still is considered the country with the highest annual tea consumption.

Chocolate, known for providing quick energy, cola drinks, and several lesser known substances such as guarana, the betel nut (Asia), khat (Africa), and the kava (Pacific Islands), are stimulants containing caffeine. They have been a part of religious and marriage ceremonies throughout the world since the beginning of time.

Research conducted into the side-effects of caffeine on the nervous system has shown that heart palpitations, dizziness, sweating, and anxiety are normal symptoms of excessive caffeine consumption.

Caisson Disease. Painful sensations in the limbs and abdomen which occur as a result of rapid reduction of air pressure are sometimes referred to as caisson disease, decompression sickness, or bends. (*See* BENDS.)

Calamine Lotion. One of the most familiar, simple remedies for the temporary relief of various skin disorders is calamine lotion. It is most commonly used for the relief of poison ivy rash and sunburn. It helps to relieve itching, dry up blisters, and cool the skin.

Calamine is a pink powder consisting of zinc oxide and some ferric (iron) oxide. The product is a shake lotion containing a suspension of calamine and other ingredients. Sometimes a small amount of phenol is added to enhance the anti-itching effect, and the product is called phenolated calamine lotion. A small amount of salicylic acid may be added for a mild peeling effect. To combat infection, antibiotics may be incorporated singly or in combination. These ingredients are usually added to basic calamine lotion at a doctor's request, by prescription. Simple calamine lotion does not require a prescription.

When calamine lotion is applied to the skin, the liquid part of the product evaporates and produces a cooling effect on the skin. This makes burns feel better. A layer of pink powder remains to form an adherent, protective layer on the skin which helps to dry up blisters and relieve itching. Some people and certain areas of the skin do not tolerate calamine lotion. Sometimes it proves to be too drying or irritating because it may become crumbly and gritty in moist areas of the body. The pink powdery deposit may be a disadvantage in using the product on exposed areas during the day.

Calcitonin. The thyroid gland secretes, in addition to thyroid hormones, a newly discovered hormone which lowers the serum calcium concentration. This hormone was originally believed to be secreted by the parathyroid gland. First called calcitonin, its name was changed to thyroidcitonin, then back to calcitonin—even though everyone now agrees that it is secreted by special cells in the thyroid gland. It acts in opposition to the parathyroid hormone when the latter has raised the serum calcium level above normal. It does this by limiting the amount of calcium released by bone. The two hormones thus offer a tight control of serum calcium concentration. (*See* PARATHYROID GLAND; THYROID.)

Calcitonin is not yet available for clinical use. When it is it may be of great value in the treatment of hyperparathyroidism and other diseases associated with high serum calcium levels.

Calcium. One of the nutrients that is necessary to satisfy the needs of the body is the mineral calcium. Because it is both a body builder and a body regulator, it is of great nutritional significance. (*See* MINERALS; NUTRITION.)

The calcium we eat in foods is necessary for skeletal growth, the development of dental tissue, maintenance of bone and tooth structure throughout life, and the regulation and maintenance of body processes.

Some experts recommend diets with large amounts of calcium. Others feel that body needs can be met by relatively small quantities of food calcium. But all agree that during periods of growth, as in childhood, pregnancy, and lactation, greater amounts are needed.

Milk and milk products are our greatest sources of calcium. They provide three-fourths of the calcium in our food supply. One cup of milk contains 285 milligrams of calcium. The calcium in two cups meets about three-fourths of the daily recommended allowances for adults. Various technological processes used in the production of different milk products may result in concentration of milk calcium. One cup of evaporated milk, for example, contains 635 milligrams of calcium. Evaporated, condensed, dry whole, and nonfat dry milk, when used in the preparation of mashed potatoes, puddings, cooked cereals, and breads, substantially increase their calcium content.

Cheeses and ice cream are also good sources of calcium. One-third of a pint of ice cream, a medium serving, has about 115 milligrams of calcium.

Vegetables and fruits are the second-best source of calcium in our diets. (*See* DIETS.)

Calculi. When calcium and phosphorus or other chemicals occur in the blood at abnormally elevated levels, they may form calcium phosphate which crystallizes as pebbles or calculi. Most often, these calculi develop in the kidney or bladder and are called kidney or bladder stones.

Increased levels of calcium may be due

to a number of causes, generally associated with increased phosphorus. (*See* HYPER-CALCEMIA; HYPERPARATHYROIDISM.) Since the body tries to rid itself of the elements and the phosphate through the urine, most calculi are found either in the bladder or kidney. Also, there is a normally high level of oxalate in the urine, and this can combine with calcium to form calcium oxalate stones.

Such calculi are insoluble in alkaline urine, and thus physicians prescribe acidic diets and drugs to produce acidic urine to dissolve the stones. If this fails, surgery is used to remove them.

Calluses. Areas of skin that are subjected to chronic pressure and friction may thicken and develop calluses. (*See* CORNS AND CALLUSES.)

Another kind of callus is a temporary structure that forms between the two parts of a fractured bone.

Calories. The human body is a work machine; food is its fuel. The food when consumed gives energy. The amount of energy is measured in calories, or units of heat. The word *calories* comes from the Latin word *calor,* meaning "heat."

The individual's daily caloric consumption should be high enough to keep body weight or rate of growth at a level for good health and well-being. Calories are stored in the body, and when all of them are not used, additional weight results. A person who habitually consumes more calories than he expends will store the extra units as body fat, or adipose tissue.

Caloric needs of individuals differ. Energy requirements depend on physical activity, body size, age, climate, and environment. Growing children, adolescents, pregnant women, and nursing mothers have special needs.

Generally, the caloric value of the food eaten should equal the energy used by the body. For example, only a moderate amount of energy is needed for walking. On the other hand, a laborer digging a ditch or an active tennis player needs more calories. A man doing sedentary work may require 2,500 calories each day. A man doing exceedingly hard manual labor may require as many as 5,000 calories.

The range for men engaged in moderate physical activity is 2,200 to 2,900 calories; for women, 1,600 to 2,100. Older persons usually require fewer calories than middle-aged persons. In all age groups, caloric requirements depend on the amount of physical activity.

Physicians sometimes order a high-calorie diet for patients who are underweight. These persons may be recovering from disease or, for some other reasons, have been unable to obtain and eat enough food for their energy needs. Fats and carbohydrates are high-calorie foods and are usually recommended for this purpose. Foods for a high-calorie diet should be carefully chosen and adapted to the patient's needs.

When a low-calorie diet is advised, the diet should be adequate in all nutrients. To encourage weight loss, the diet should include a variety of readily available foods and provide enough substance to be satisfying. (*See* DIETS.)

Methods of cooking meat, fish, poultry, eggs, and vegetables, as well as the sauces and dressings used with desserts and salads, affect the total caloric level of a menu.

Pregnant women should give special attention to diet because some extra calories are required for the growth of the fetus. Sometimes, if a woman restricts her activities, extra calories will be stored even if she does not increase her intake of food. Many women, especially those caring for young children, lead very active lives while pregnant. Others, who reduce their normal physical activity, might be advised to eat less.

Caloric requirements of elderly people are difficult to predict because of the variations in their physical activity.

If their weight remains constant, their caloric intake is probably correct.

Nutritionally speaking, the term "empty calories" applies to foods lacking in proteins, minerals, and vitamins. (*See* VITAMINS.) Sources of empty calories are sugar, some cooking fats, some baked goods, and alcohol.

Camphor. This product, widely used many years ago, is made from the bark and wood of an evergreen tree of Southeastern Asia. A synthetic camphor is also made from oil of turpentine.

Camphor salicylate is a medicinal white powder used as an antiseptic and astringent. When diluted and compounded, it is given internally for diarrhea. Camphor menthol is used externally as an antiseptic and deodorant; diluted, it is used as a nose and throat spray.

Many children are poisoned by overdoses of camphor products, which are highly toxic if misused. Signs are a burning in the throat and stomach, nausea, thirst, vomiting, headaches, and convulsions. After a few hours, the breath and urine smell of camphor. Treatment begins with washing out the stomach, followed by a large dose of magnesium sulfate. The victim should be kept warm until medical aid arrives.

Canal. Any tubular, narrow passageway forming a tunnel through the body proper or through specific tissues or organs is termed a canal. For example, the entire passageway by which food travels through the gastrointestinal tract is known as the alimentary canal. This canal extends from the opening at the mouth all the way through the intestines, opening again at the anus. There are canals passing through bone tissue, through the eye, and through glands. Also, the channel through which an individual hair grows is called the hair canal.

Cancer. Some people are so terrified by cancer that they avoid even mentioning the disease. Unfortunately, this attitude leads many to cling to an "It can't happen to me" attitude, and they neglect to heed the early warning signs.

Deaths from cancer are second only to those from heart disease. At the present time, in the United States alone, close to one million persons are under treatment for cancer. New cases number 750,000 yearly. Every year about 250,000 cancer patients are cured. Another 500,000 die, but one out of every two die needlessly. Their cancers could have been cured if they had seen their doctors when the first danger signs appeared. (*See* CANCER DETECTION.)

Undoubtedly, many victims could also have avoided cancer if only they had stopped flirting with the disease by smoking heavily, overexposing themselves to the sun, or abusing their bodies in other ways. And more cancer patients would live, too, if man concerned himself more with stopping pollution of the air. (*See* CANCER PREVENTION.)

Of course, it is impossible to forecast just how long a person may have good health after surviving a bout with cancer. But this is just as true of recovery from any other disease. For statistical purposes, we regard a person as "cured" of cancer if he remains free of the disease for at least five years after treatment. Many who heeded the early signs of cancer have been fully cured and lived an average lifetime.

One of the fictions about cancer is that it is pretty much a disease of old age. Yes, many of the aged do succumb to it, but about 50 percent of all cases occur among people under sixty-five. And more schoolchildren die of cancer than from any other disease.

WHAT IS CANCER? Cancer is a disorder of the cells of the body. Normal cells have a built-in control mechanism. They are coded so that they develop in an orderly fashion, and adjust themselves constantly to the part of the body in which they are located. (*See* CELL.)

In the cancer cell something happens to the built-in mechanism. The cell no longer

Know Cancer's Warning Signals!

• Change in bowel or bladder habits

• A sore that does not heal

• Unusual bleeding or discharge

• Thickening or lump in breast or elsewhere

• Indigestion or difficulty in swallowing

• Obvious change in wart or mole

• Nagging cough or hoarseness

*If you have a warning signal, see your
doctor.*

American Cancer Society

responds in terms of the body environment, but reproduces itself wildly. More and more cells develop, but they are useless at best, and often grow to choke off the functions of normal cells, tissues, and organs.

The unhealthy cell colonies are called neoplasms, which simply means new growths. Some neoplasms, while not normal growths, are not cancers but are called benign tumors. These grow within a confined area of the body, are somewhat similar to the normal cells about them, and seldom cause death. Often benign tumors are removed by surgery because they press on vital organs or tissues. But if excised (cut out), they seldom return. (*See* TUMORS.)

Metastasis. On the other hand, malignant neoplasms, or cancer, may consist of cells far different from those nearby. The cells, as they multiply, tend to spread in various directions, very often through lymph vessels. They also exhibit metastasis, which means that they can travel through the body to take root in other organs and tissues to start new pockets of cancer. This is why early detection is important. If possible, the cancer should be destroyed while it is still confined to a small area and has not started metastasis.

The cancer cells, in metastasis, may travel through the blood and lymph or in other liquids such as that in the abdominal cavity. The secondary growths, or metastases, may particularly take hold in the lungs, the liver, or the bones, greatly complicating treatment.

Normal cells reproduce by dividing at a rate required by the body. They also die off from time to time, so that there never are more than the system requires. Cancer cells in some cases may even reproduce at a slower rate than normal cells but appear to die off more slowly. This leads to a gradual accumulation of useless, and dangerous, cancerous tissue.

The enlarging mass of cancer cells takes nourishment from the bloodstream which should go to normal cells. When the tumor grows so large that there is not enough nourishment for all its cells, then necrosis (tissue or cell death) occurs. Some of the cancerous cells die, resulting in ulcers and bleeding. There may be no pain until the cancer presses on or attacks nerve tissue.

Types of Cancer. There are two general classes of cancer. One, carcinoma, develops from epithelial tissue, which lines the inner passages of the body or composes the outer covering called skin. The other, sarcoma, originates in connective tissue. There are also many variations of these two types, usually named for the specific tissue involved—for example, adenocarcinoma, from the epithelium of glands; lymphosarcoma, cancer of the lymphatic glands and vessels; myeloma, cancer of the bone marrow; and rhabdomyosarcoma, cancer of the voluntary muscle tissue.

WHY DOES CANCER START? Usually it is difficult or impossible to determine, or even guess, why cancer started in an individual. But some causes are well established. We know that soot, tar, pitch, asbestos, radiation, and a long list of other agents may be cancer causing. We call them carcinogens. (*See* CARCINOGENS.)

In addition to known carcinogens, there are many borderline substances which are somehow connected with cancer, but we are not quite sure that they actually cause it. The best known example is the tobacco of cigarettes. It is well established that more smokers get lung cancer, but is the tobacco merely a trigger of some sort which makes existing cancer flare up? We do not know. Pipe smokers may get cancer of the mouth or lip, but we are not sure whether the tobacco does it, or just the heat of the pipe. (*See* SMOKING.)

Ultraviolet and other forms of radiation are known to cause cancer of the skin. (*See* RADIATION.) We also know that cancer may result from a mole or start at the site of a burn.

From an examination of known and suspected carcinogens, it appears that at least some forms of cancer are the result of continued irritation of body cells or tissues, whether the irritation comes from an obviously physical act—such as picking at a mole—or from chemicals, invisible rays, or heat.

Damage to the Cells. Just how does this irritation damage the cell and make it change into a monster which persists in producing more of the deadly cancer cells? This question has not yet been completely answered. The defect is at least partly in the cancer cell's reproductive process. Thus, researchers have been looking to the chromosomes of the cells. Chromosomes are bodies in the cells which carry the genetic messages as the cell divides and duplicates itself. The chromosomes determine just what type of a cell will result, and what combinations of cells (a whole man, for example) will develop.

The chromosomes are made up of nucleic acid. They may have an almost unlimited variation in the form of chains of molecules (called DNA or RNA) which carry the genetic messages for every form of life. (*See* DNA.) There is good evidence that carcinogens damage these molecular chains and start the cells producing defective copies of themselves instead of normal cells.

Viruses and Cancer. The microorganisms (or germs) called viruses are definitely associated with some cancers of plants and animals. They appear to damage the molecular chains of the cell nucleic acids. But evidence that viruses may cause cancer in humans has been hard to gather. If viruses do cause cancer in humans, they must be only certain specific viruses, for every person is exposed to viruses all his life, and not everyone gets cancer. (*See* VIRUSES.)

Hormones and Cancer. Hormones flow through the bloodstream, giving us male or female characteristics and adjusting other bodily processes. Hormones are also related to cancer, but just how is unknown. Certain malignant tumors, however, enlarge more rapidly if the patient takes certain hormones, or less rapidly if he takes other hormones.

It seems quite clear that hormonal imbalances do not cause cancer, but rather have an effect on cancer if it already exists. In fact, one theory holds that we all have cancer cells within our bodies and that they lie dormant (inactive) until something—a chemical, radiation, a hormone, or some other irritant—sets them off on their runaway reproductive cycles.

FOODS, DRUGS, AND CANCER. Quite often scientists have demonstrated that certain common chemicals used in drugs and prepared foods can actually cause cancer in mice or other laboratory animals. This evidence may serve as a warning of possible danger, but is difficult to interpret. What may be toxic (poisonous) to some forms of life is safe for others. In fact, when small doses of known carcinogens are given to mice from the same litter, only some of them develop cancer. There seem to be individual differences even in the same species of plant or animal life, including man. Some successfully resist cancer; others do not. When science finds out why certain individuals seem more susceptible to cancer than others, we may be on the way to resolving controversies regarding whether certain substances are carcinogenic.

Immunity and Cancer. Man is known to develop an immunity to many diseases—measles, rabies, and smallpox, for example. There is some evidence to suggest that we may also develop an immunity against some types of cancer. To become immune, a person must have in his body certain substances called antibodies. There are many types of antibodies, and each fights a specific disease.

To become immune to a disease, you must either have the related antibody in your system (natural immunity) or have the capacity to develop the antibody (acquired immunity). The antibodies usually develop in quantity when a person acquires a disease, or is injected with a small amount of live or dead disease particles, as in a vaccination.

Some researchers believe that the thymus gland, and possibly the appendix, may release antibodies or other substances that protect against cancer.

Hopefully, man will some day be immunized against cancer by vaccination. (*See* IMMUNIZATION.)

HOW CANCER IS TRANSMITTED. Can you "catch" cancer from someone else? All the evidence we have to date supports the theory that you cannot. But scientists have been studying so-called pockets of cancer—that is, an unusually large number of cases which appear within a community or the same family.

The most likely explanation for the occasional "pockets" is that there was a local cancer-causing agent or circumstance in the environment. People in the same family who get cancer may also have eaten or been exposed to something which was carcinogenic. There is evidence that while cancer probably cannot be inherited, the tendency toward getting the disease may be higher in some families than others.

The world distribution of cancer is puzzling. Why, for example, is there more stomach cancer in Japan and the Scandinavian nations than in the United States? Or why is cancer of the liver more common in certain specific areas of Africa, Asia, and other warm climates? It is easier to guess why there is more cancer of the lungs in areas of high air pollution, or more cancer of the scrotum among chimney sweeps and workers in industries using gas, tar, pitch, and creosote, all known carcinogens.

In experiments with animals, malignant tumors have been transplanted from one laboratory animal to another and have produced cancer in the second animal. A type of cancer has also been transmitted from one laboratory hamster to another through the bite of a mosquito. You should remember, however, that we do not yet know whether similar transmission can occur among humans.

TREATMENT FOR CANCER. When cancer is confined to a small area, relatively simple surgery can often entirely eliminate the disease. But when the cancer has begun to spread, radical (extensive) surgery may be necessary. This usually will include excision (cutting out) of nearby lymph glands, a frequent route of spreading cancer. (*See* LYMPH.) It is better to do too much surgery rather than too little, for apparently even a single live cancerous cell left in the body can divide and start up a new cycle of the disease.

In advanced cancer, some surgery may involve cutting nerve roots (rhizotomy) to relieve pain. Cryosurgery (operating at very low temperatures or freezing of tissues) and laser surgery (using a powerful light beam to cut or destroy tissue) are also employed. (*See* CRYOTHERAPY; LASER.)

Radiation Treatment. While exposure to uncontrolled radiation may cause cancer, controlled radiation (irradiation or radiotherapy) is one of the most effective methods of treating the disease. The same X rays that are used for examination are valuable for therapy. Other irradiation may use radium or artificial radioisotopes as a source. The radioactive rays can destroy cancer cells, but may affect normal cells as

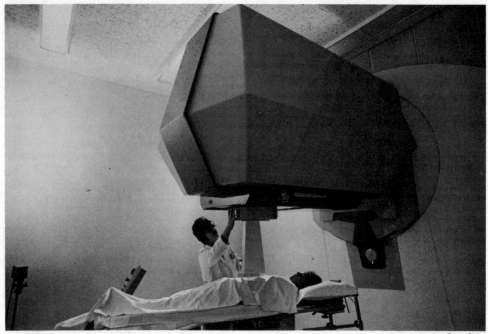

American Cancer Society

A betatron, like the one shown above, produces powerful radiation by
accelerating electrons to velocities close to the speed of light. It
was developed in 1940 and was first used mostly by physicists and
engineers; for some years medical researchers have been developing
techniques to use the betatron in the treatment of cancer. The machine
in the photograph is one of the most powerful in the United States
and is located at the University of Maryland.

well. The irradiation must be carefully controlled so that as many as possible of the
cancer cells are destroyed, with a minimum
of damage to normal tissue.

Irradiation may be from outside the
body, from radioactive fluids injected into
the body, or in the form of so-called seeds
or needles, small particles containing radioactive material which are inserted into parts
of the body. (*See* RADIOTHERAPY.)

Chemotherapy. A third method of treating cancer is chemotherapy, the administering of drug products, by mouth or injection, which either destroy cancer cells or
inhibit their growth.

Some of these products are anti-
metabolites—that is, they act against metabolism, the process by which chemicals
in the bloodstream are converted and used

for the nutrition of cells. The aim is to block
the nourishment of the cancer cells with
little effect on normal cells. This, however,
is difficult to achieve, and careful attention
must be paid to the amount of antimetabolites used, lest they do extensive harm to
healthy cells.

An alkylating agent is one that is used to
affect the DNA of cells so that reproduction
of the cancer cells is stopped. As in the case
of the antimetabolites, the alkylating agents
have limitations because of their toxic effect
on noncancerous tissue.

Despite the ever-present danger of side
effects, chemotherapeutic agents have been
very effective against certain malignancies.
They may well become the primary treatment for cancer.

To reduce exposure of the entire body to

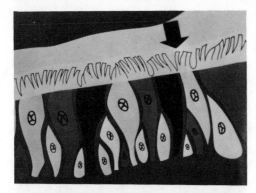

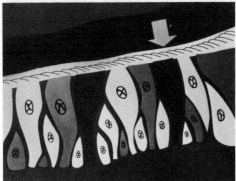

American Cancer Society

Bronchial cilia (hairlike structures which line the inner surface of the bronchial tubes) are an important part of the body's filtering mechanism. They are immobilized by continued cigarette smoking, as these drawings illustrate. At top, the arrow points to the normal appearance of cilia, which keep foreign particles from entering the lungs. At bottom, cilia are weakened and the bronchus has difficulty getting rid of mucus, which builds up. This produces the well-known "smoker's cough" as the bronchus is forced to exert unusual effort to expel the mucus.

chemotherapeutic drugs injected into the bloodstream, a technique called isolated perfusion (or infusion) is used. By means of a pump and tubes attached to two places in the blood vessels, the chemotherapeutic agent is circulated only through that part of the system where the tumor is located. (*See* CHEMOTHERAPY.)

Other Cancer Treatments. Cancer cells, like normal cells, must receive nourishment if they are to exist and multiply. They also need various amino acids to build up their own proteins. One such amino acid is phenylalanine. Research has shown that if the body's intake of phenylalanine is cut down, then cancer cells will die. However, there is a problem in using a diet low in phenylalanine for cancer therapy, because this amino acid is also needed for normal cell growth.

Little success has been achieved in trying to cure cancer by changes in diet. Among laboratory animals, however, extra vitamin A has been found to slow down the growth of some tumors, both benign and malignant.

Sadly, many people with cancer have been victims of money-making schemes built around unproved cures for the disease. There are special diets, magic capsules, magnetic gadgets, mystic bracelets, and countless other devices and pills. All of these have no effect on the cancer whatever. While the "treatment" continues, the tumors keep on growing, unwatched and untreated, until they are beyond cure by surgery, radiation, chemotherapy, or any other accepted therapy. Be wary of exaggerated claims for cures by alleged doctors who have not had formal M.D. or D.O. training. (*See* QUACKERY.)

There is little doubt that a person with faith and a real desire to get well has a much higher chance of recovery than the despondent patient who is sure he will die. But there is no proof that so-called faith-healers can cure cancer. Any of their apparent cures may merely be remissions (temporary relief from symptoms), which do occur spontaneously among some patients for unexplained reasons.

CANCER OF THE LUNG. Carcinoma of the lung is the most common cancer among males. It has become more frequent with the use of tobacco and the earlier average age at which people start smoking. It is also becoming more common among women smokers. Some researchers, particularly those sponsored by the tobacco industry, insist that there is "no causative relation-

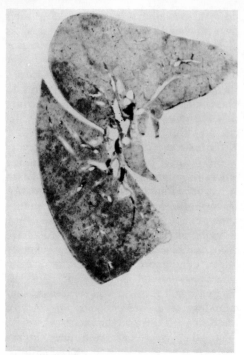 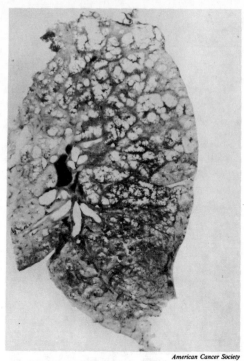

The photograph at left shows normal lung tissue. The air sacs are too fine to be visible. At right is the lung tissue of a heavy smoker, showing an abundance of greatly enlarged air sacs.

ship of smoking to cancer." We may not yet know why it happens, but study after study has proved that your chances of getting lung cancer are tremendously increased if you smoke heavily. And your chances are smaller if you have never smoked. (*See* SMOKING.)

Air pollution and exposure to radioactive materials are also known to cause cancer. In fact, if you live out in the country, away from industrial air pollution, and do not smoke, then it is very unlikely that you will develop lung cancer.

Most lung cancer begins in the bronchial passages. From there it may metastasize to the liver, the outer lining (pleura) of the lung, the bones, the lymph nodes (cervical glands) of the neck, the adrenal glands, the brain, the skin, and less frequently elsewhere in the body. Such metastasis is the

rule, rather than the exception, in lung cancer which has not been caught at its very beginning. When mass surveys have been made in attempts to find cancer cases, only about 10 percent of those lung cancers detected can be cured. This is because so many are far advanced.

The message of the above paragraphs is this: Don't smoke. If you do, you are gambling with death unless you have frequent examinations of your lungs.

Among the signs of lung cancer are coughing, spitting up of blood (hemoptysis), chest pain, and dyspnea (difficulty in breathing). But the cancer may be well developed before any of these appear. Sometimes the signs of lung cancer are absent until the disease has metastasized to a distant part of the body. For example, leg pains may be found to be caused by thrombophlebitis (inflammation of the veins due to a blocking), and the latter may then be found to be a complication of lung cancer.

X rays, examination of sputum, washings from the lungs, bronchoscopy (examination of the lung by an inserted instrument), or needle biopsy (taking of a sample of lung tissue with a hollow needle) are used by the physician to diagnose lung cancer.

Removal of the tumor by surgery is often necessary. Usually a large part of a lung, or one entire lung, must be cut out in an effort —often unsuccessful—to stop the spread of the cancer.

Radiation and chemotherapy are also used, but usually tend to slow down the progress of the disease or relieve symptoms, rather than effect a cure.

Bronchial adenoma is a less common type of lung tumor in which the cells have characteristics of those of glandular tissue. They may or may not be malignant, and only in a small percentage of cases do they tend to metastasize. Because of the slower growth of bronchial adenomas, they can be completely cleared up with surgery more often than can lung carcinoma.

CANCER OF THE BREAST. Breast cancer is the most common malignancy among women. It seldom appears before the teens, and becomes more frequent as the woman grows older. It is more common among women who do not nurse their own babies, as well as among unmarried women and those who have passed the menopause (change of life). Breast carcinoma usually starts in the ducts which lead from the milk glands. If undetected, it may then spread via the lymph nodes. Metastases to the lung, liver, and bone are quite common.

The first sign of breast cancer is a painless lump in the breast. It appears most often on the upper, forward part of the breast, but may start elsewhere, including the inner portions. Early detection is so important in breast cancer that the lives of untold thousands of women probably could be saved each year if they had followed simple breast self-examination techniques. (*See* BREAST EXAMINATION.) Other signs of possible cancer of the breast are a rash around the nipples, a bloody discharge from the nipples, or retraction of the nipple. Sometimes dimple-like depressions may be found elsewhere on the breast.

Many lumps found in the breast may not be cancerous, but rather one of two benign conditions: (1) fibroadenoma, in which there is a firm, movable lump, usually occurring in women under thirty-five; (2) cystic disease of the breast, more commonly found in women over thirty and sometimes painful in the premenstrual period. (*See* BREASTS.)

Often the surgery performed for breast cancer must be radical—removal of the entire breast, associated muscular structure, and nearby lymph nodes. Such extensive surgery may distress some women, who fear they will lose their feminine figure and attractiveness. But this surgery often arrests the cancer completely, whereas avoidance of it may carry a risk that the malignancy will reappear in the other breast or elsewhere in the body.

Women who have lost one or both breasts to cancer surgery can make good adjustments by being fitted with special padded bras (prostheses). Sometimes these former cancer patients join clubs whose aim is to assure more recent surgery patients that the loss of the breast does not affect one's femininity or normal living.

Hormonal treatment and radiation are helpful in many cases of breast cancer and may be combined with surgical treatment.

When breast surgery is impractical, an oophorectomy (removal of the ovaries) may be performed. The purpose is to reduce the production of estrogen, a hormone manufactured by the ovaries. Estrogen reduction often depresses the growth of malignant breast tumors. An adrenalectomy (removal of adrenal glands) and a hypophysectomy (removal of the pituitary gland) are other means of reducing estrogen output. These three types of surgery are usually confined to women who have not yet reached the menopause. They may also be given testosterone, a male hormone which reduces production of estrogen in the female.

After the menopause, the body's production of estrogen is reduced gradually. Thus, other types of hormonal treatment for breast cancer may be needed for older patients.

Cortisone and other chemotherapeutic agents also have some value in treating breast cancer.

CARCINOMA OF THE CERVIX. Ranking second to breast cancer in frequency of malignancies among women is carcinoma of the cervix (the opening from the uterus to the vagina).

One form of cancer of the cervix is called carcinoma in situ (i.e., cancer in place). This means that a nidus (small area where the disease begins) exists, but it has not spread widely. Sometimes the nidus may be present for years and not be visible, but it is relatively easy to determine if such hidden cancer exists. This is done by gently scraping off some tissue from the cervix in a procedure called a Papanicolaou smear (Pap test). The tissue is examined under a microscope for evidence of cancer cells. (*See* PAP SMEAR TEST.)

If caught early, nearly every case of cancer of the cervix in situ can be completely cured. This is why women should have a Pap smear taken regularly—at least once a year and more often if they have any reason to suspect a problem in the cervix. If neglected, however, this type of cancer may develop into invasive carcinoma of the cervix, which, as the name implies, invades nearby tissue and may metastasize into the vagina, pelvic wall, bladder, rectum, and elsewhere. Thus, a regular physical examination of the cervix is important. Cancer there may become very advanced before any obvious signs appear.

When the carcinoma is of the invasive type, there may be spotting, bleeding, or changes in the pattern or character of other female discharges. When it is advanced there will be, of course, symptoms of disorders of whatever part of the body may be affected by the metastasis. For example, blocking of urination and uremia (urine products in the blood) is a common and often fatal complication of cancer of the cervix.

Removal of a portion of the female organs by surgery (hysterectomy) can end the threat of cancer in situ. (*See* HYSTERECTOMY.) But treatment of the invasive form is more difficult, and may require both surgery and radiation. Nitrogen mustard, one of the alkylating drugs, may be of some value.

The in situ type of carcinoma of the cer-

Left: Normal cells of the cervix. *Right:* Cancerous cells of the cervix.

American Cancer Society

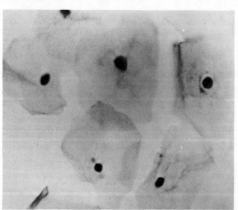
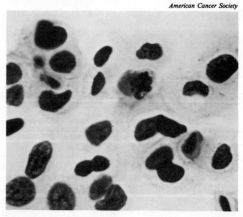

vix most often occurs in women between the ages of thirty and thirty-five years. The invasive type usually appears later, at an average age of forty-nine, probably because many women harbor the cancer for many years before it is discovered.

CANCER OF THE UTERUS. Carcinoma of the uterus is about as common as cervical cancer in postmenopausal women, although not as frequent among younger women.

Most uterine cancer originates in the mucous membrane lining the uterus and hence is called endometrial cancer. Bleeding after the menopause is an important sign. In fact, as much as 40 percent of all bleeding in postmenopausal women is the result of cancer of the uterus. Many women with this cancer have had a history of various female difficulties, such as infertility, irregularities of menstruation, or an excessive flow during menstruation (menorrhagia). Panhysterectomy (complete removal of the uterus) and irradiation are used in treatment.

CANCER OF THE OVARIES. Tumors of the ovaries are generally benign, although some may be malignant, particularly among older women.

There may be an obvious enlargement in this area, general loss of weight, and pain in the abdominal region. There may also be problems of elimination from the urinary or intestinal systems, and ascites (collection of fluid in the abdominal region). Bleeding from the vagina can occur sometimes, although this is not too common a sign of ovarian cancer. Once in a while the tumor may result in changes in female characteristics—either masculinization or feminization.

Surgery is the most successful treatment. This includes removal of the whole uterus and both ovaries. Radiation and chemotherapy are also used, sometimes to relieve suffering in difficult cases.

CANCER OF THE VULVA. Malignancies of the vulva, the outer portion of the female organs, is often preceded by leukoplakia, white ulcerlike areas such as also frequently appear on the mucous membrane of the mouth. (*See* LEUKOPLAKIA.)

Most cancer of the vulva can be seen and recognized early and prompt surgical treatment brings excellent results. If the cancer has spread, the surgery may include excision (cutting out) of the vulva and parts of the vagina.

CANCER OF THE PROSTATE. Among elderly men, cancer of the prostate is quite common. Autopsy statistics have shown that a large percentage of older men and 15 to 45 percent of all men have had some evidence of prostatic carcinoma, even though death may have been due to another disorder.

The prostate is a male gland that secretes a fluid added to semen during sexual ejaculation. (*See* PROSTATE GLAND.) It surrounds the duct (urethra) which carries the urine from the bladder. Thus, cancer or any other enlargement of the prostate produces difficulty in urination. Other symptoms of prostatic cancer may be frequent urination, urinating at night (nocturia), blood in the urine, pain in the lower back (sciatica), and loss of weight. Metastases from prostatic cancer may first appear in the lymph glands close by, then in the bones of the pelvis.

Frequent examination of the prostate in men over fifty is important, as cancer is much easier to treat when confined to this organ. Radical prostatectomy (removal of the prostate and nearby tissue) is the usual treatment.

As the prostate is dependent upon stimulation by male hormones, removal of the testes (or testicles), a source of hormones, often slows down the development or metastases of cancer of the prostate. Female sex hormones have, in a large percentage of cases, prolonged the life of the patients.

CANCER OF THE TESTES. Cancer of the testes is much less common than that of the prostate. It is a disorder of younger adult men, usually under the age of thirty-five. The first signs may be a painless enlargement of the testes or an aching in the perineum, the area between the scrotum (sac containing the testes) and the anus (the opening through which solid matter is eliminated from the body). The cancer may metastasize along the lymph nodes or to the liver or lungs. Treatment is by orchiectomy (removal of the affected testis or both testes) and irradiation.

CANCER OF THE STOMACH. The early symptoms of cancer of the stomach are usually similar to those of other stomach problems, such as mild indigestion and nausea.

Later there may be blood in the feces, anorexia (loss of appetite), stomach pain, weight loss, and an obvious lump which can be felt with the fingers. Other symptoms are anemia and an absence of hydrochloric acid in the gastric juices (achlorhydria, or hypochlorhydria). The cancer may metastasize to the lymph nodes nearby, to the peritoneum (membrane lining the abdominal walls), to the liver, and elsewhere, with a wide variety of symptoms. Ulcers often appear, with pain and discomfort similar to that caused by nonmalignant ulcers. (*See* ULCERS.)

The malignancy is usually confirmed by X ray and biopsy and treated by removal of part or all of the stomach (gastrectomy). In order to get at all of the possible "roots," or spreading cancerous cells, the surgeon may need to remove other organs close by, such as part of the esophagus, part of the pancreas, spleen, etc.

Early detection is important in stomach cancer, as it is in other types. By the time carcinoma of the stomach is found in the average group of patients, half of the tumors are so far advanced that they cannot be resected (removed by surgery).

Sometimes a subtotal (partial) gastrectomy is performed. Then a new passage is made from the remaining part of the stomach to the jejunal portion of the intestines. This is called a gastrojejunal anastomosis. In other cases, a total gastrectomy may be necessary. Then the esophagus is connected directly to the jejunum—an esophagojejunal anastomosis.

CANCER OF THE INTESTINAL TRACT. Cancer of the colon and the rectum have similar symptoms: bleeding from the rectum, constipation or some other sudden change in bowel habits, diarrhea, and frequent passing of gas (flatus). Polyps (benign growths from the inner linings of the intestines) are often premalignant; that is, they may appear before the actual cancer develops. Hemorrhoids may occur at the same time as cancer and contribute to the bleeding, but they are not usually premalignant. (*See* HEMORRHOIDS.)

Ulcerative colitis is nonmalignant, although persons with chronic ulcerative colitis are more likely to develop carcinoma of the colon than are persons with no history of intestinal problems. Tumors of the upper intestinal tract—the small intestines —are less common than those of the large colon and rectum.

Many tumors of the rectum are located by the physician, using a rubber-gloved finger. Internal visualizing devices (a sigmoidoscope or a proctosigmoidoscope) can detect cancer farther back in the rectum and colon. By looking into one end of these instruments, the doctor actually can see the tumor.

The tumors are removed by surgery, along with a portion of the intestines to which they are attached. In addition, nitrogen mustard or other chemotherapy may be employed.

Sometimes, when an extensive portion of the intestines has been removed, it is necessary to make an artificial external passage (colostomy) for the removal of feces (waste solids). (*See* COLOSTOMY.)

CANCER OF THE ESOPHAGUS. About four out of five malignancies of the esophagus occur in men. They are more common in Oriental countries than in the Western world, possibly because of different dietary habits.

The esophagus is the passage from the throat to the stomach. Cancer here produces difficult swallowing, pain under the sternum (breastbone), pain or discomfort during or after eating solids, and regurgitation (coughing up of food). If the cancer is in the upper part of the esophagus, the symptoms may be confused with those of tonsillitis or laryngitis. If in the lower part, the signs may be similar to those of hiatus hernia or angina pectoris. (*See* ANGINA PECTORIS; HIATUS HERNIA.)

Cancer of the esophagus may spread to the air passages, lungs, or lymph nodes. It is treated by removing the affected portions and drawing up a section of the stomach, by surgery, to bridge the gap. Radiation is used as an adjunct to, not as a substitute for, surgery. In advanced cases, the radiation may help relieve pain or slow the progress of the malignancy.

CANCER OF THE PANCREAS. Most of the malignancies of the pancreas occur at the head (larger end) of the organ; only about one-quarter of the cases affect the body or tail (small end). As with cancer of the esophagus, four of five victims are men.

This type of cancer is hard to cure. The pancreas is involved with the vital function of helping keep the blood sugar in proper chemical balance, as well as providing juices for digestion. When the organ is the site of adenocarcinoma—the most common malignancy here—the normal functioning of the pancreas is affected. But metastases are also common to lymph nodes, nearby structures, and the liver. Cancer particularly of the body and tail of the pancreas may soon metastasize widely through the body.

Symptoms of cancer of the pancreas include jaundice (yellowing of the skin), anorexia, loss of weight, and pain in the upper abdomen and the back. There also can be a painful and enlarged gallbladder, and thrombophlebitis (a disorder of blood circulation) in the legs or arms.

Surgery is used to remove the malignancies from the pancreas and surrounding tissues. Unfortunately, pancreatic cancer usually has progressed quite far by the time it is discovered, so cures are infrequent.

CANCER OF THE GALLBLADDER. Adenocarcinomas of the gallbladder are likewise difficult to cure because they too are generally well advanced before discovery. Unlike pancreatic cancers, the number of cases of gallbladder malignancies among women outnumber those of men by at least two or three to one. The reason for this difference between the sexes is not known.

The symptoms of cancer of the gallbladder are similar to those for other diseases of this organ: inflammation, tenderness, pain (often severe), chills, fever, and jaundice. (*See* GALLBLADDER; GALLSTONES.) Gallstones are not usually blamed for the development of cancer, although the stones are present in as many as nine out of ten cases of gallbladder malignancies. Most of the cancer is found during examination for stones or other nonmalignant blocking of the bile ducts.

Surgery is advocated for cancer of the gallbladder, although many cases are so extensive when they are found that it may be of little value.

CANCER OF THE LIVER. Only some 1 to 2 percent of all cancers in the United States start in the liver, but up to 50 percent of all cancers eventually metastasize to the liver.

Hepatomas (liver tumors) are much more common in the Orient and in East Africa than elsewhere. About three out of four cases are found in males. Studies have shown that carcinoma of the liver seems related in many cases to cirrhosis of the liver, a disorder caused by varied factors including alcoholism, dietary insufficiencies, and the intake of certain chemical agents. (*See* CIRRHOSIS OF THE LIVER.)

The signs of cancer of the liver include inflammation, pain, weight loss, jaundice, and general weakness. Metastases to distant parts of the body are not too frequent in liver cancers, but the disease may spread to the lymph nodes and lungs.

Sometimes the disease is caught early and affects only part of the liver. Then only one of the two lobes of the organ may be removed, the remaining one often serving almost as well as two. In advanced cases radiation is of some value.

CANCER OF THE KIDNEY. Adenocarcinoma of the kidney, also called hypernephroma, is most common among males. The first sign may be hematuria (blood in the urine), without any pain. As the tumor grows, various other signs may appear—anemia, liver disorders, fever, and neuropathy (nervous system problems)—which can easily be confused with those of other diseases.

Removal of the tumor, with the surrounding kidney tissue (nephrectomy), is required, but metastases may occur a dozen years after all signs of the tumor were removed in a successful operation.

Embryoma of the kidney, also called Wilms' tumor, is a malignancy that appears in children under age six, and especially in those under three. (*See* WILMS' TUMOR.) The chance of a cure by nephrectomy is much higher if the embryoma is found and surgery initiated before the tumor starts its expected rapid growth and metastasis. It may metastasize to the lungs, liver, and brain. Chemotherapy with actinomycin or nitrogen mustard as well as irradiation are used to supplement surgical tumor removal.

CANCER OF THE URINARY BLADDER. Hematuria (blood in the urine), and painful and frequent urination are the first signs of cancer of the bladder. Later there may be pain, anemia, and complications caused by the blocking of the urinary passages, including hydronephrosis (distention of parts of the kidney) and sepsis (infection with poisonous by-products). Carcinoma, the most common malignancy of the urinary bladder, is removed by surgery (transurethral resection). Most of the problems occur in expansion of the cancer to nearby tissue, rather than by metastases.

Papillomas, small growths from the sides of the urinary passages, are sometimes classed as malignant. They may be destroyed by electrocautery, which utilizes electricity to "burn off" the growths.

When cancer of the bladder is so extensive as to require removal of the entire bladder and surrounding tissues, the ureters (urinary passages to the kidneys) may be diverted to open into the colon or through the skin (a cutaneous ureterostomy).

CANCER OF THE SKIN. More persons get skin cancer than any other malignancies. But fortunately, most skin cancers are curable, and they are seldom fatal. Furthermore, they are easily prevented. Of all cases of cancer in men, about one in five is confined to the skin; among women, the ratio is about one in ten. The high cure rate is partly due to the fact that precancerous lesions and cancer are easily identified on the skin surface.

Most skin cancer is basal cell carcinoma and is often found on the nose, eyelids, or elsewhere on the face. Like other skin cancers, it seems to be caused, or at least aggravated, by exposure to the sun for long periods. People who do most of their work, or most of their playing, outdoors have the highest rate of basal cell carcinoma. It occurs more readily among blond, blue-eyed individuals.

Basal cell carcinoma of the skin grows slowly, starting as a small, rounded lump or swelling with a waxy appearance. Later, if not removed, it ulcerates in the center and a scab grows over it. Finally, if still untreated, it may invade adjacent tissue or destroy eye or nose tissue. It seldom metastasizes to remote parts of the body.

Squamous cell carcinoma of the skin usually grows faster. It may resemble the basal cell variety somewhat, but the lump is often red and cone-shaped. It tends to metastasize to lymph nodes more often than the basal cell type.

The carcinoma may be preceded by benign dermatoses (skin blemishes or lesions). Some of these precancerous growths may be senile keratosis (deterioration of an aged person's skin), radiodermatitis (caused by radiation exposure), and xeroderma pigmentosum (a rare childhood disease with changes in skin color). (*See* KERATOSIS.)

Almost all basal and squamous cell skin carcinomas can be quite effectively eliminated by surgical removal. If the cancer has started to spread, nearby lymph nodes also will be removed. Irradiation treatment may be used separately or as an adjunct to surgery.

MELANOMAS. The ordinary mole, or nevus, may turn malignant, particularly if irritated again and again by rubbing. Thus moles on the feet, palms of the hands, or genital areas (near the sex organs) should be removed while still benign. When they become malignant they are called melanomas or melanocarcinoma. About seven of ten melanomas occur in women—usually not until puberty and most commonly in women over forty-five. (*See* MELANOMA; MOLES.)

When a mole starts to become cancerous, it may change in color, shape, or general appearance. Itching, bleeding, and pain at the site also may signal the conversion of a benign mole to a melanoma.

Melanomas occur in the eye and may result in the loss of sight. Many melanomas will metastasize to the liver, bones, lungs, lymph nodes, and other parts of the body. A form called malignant melanoma spreads rapidly through lymph nodes and may metastasize through the bloodstream. Surgical removal is the best treatment for melanomas, although some that are widespread may respond to regional perfusion chemotherapy. Irradiation has only limited use for melanomas.

CANCER OF THE LYMPH NODES. Any malignancy originating in the lymph nodes is called a lymphoma. The most common type, lymphosarcoma, originates in the reticuloendothelial system. This is the system of tissue cells and white blood cells (leukocytes) which removes damaged cells and foreign matter that may have penetrated the tissues. Its functions are vital and may be greatly impaired by cancer growth.

The first signs of lymphosarcoma are enlarged lymph nodes near the surface of the body, although the malignancy often begins in the lymph nodes of the abdominal region, the liver, or spleen. Some lymphosarcomas may start in the bone.

In follicular lymphoma, much less common than lymphosarcoma, the structure of the lymph nodes is replaced by follicles—saclike cell masses.

Granulomatous lymphoma, or Hodgkin's disease, starts with a painless enlargement of the lymph nodes, followed by fever, weight loss, and other systemic symptoms. (*See* HODGKIN'S DISEASE.)

Since extensive removal of lymph glands is usually impractical, lymphomas are generally treated with irradiation and with chemotherapy agents such as nitrogen mustard, triethylene melamine (TEM), and steroids.

Although lymphomas may never be completely cured, modern chemotherapy has kept many cases in remission for many years past the five-year period rated as indicating a cancer cure.

Lymphomas are much more common among men. Hodgkin's disease is most common among adults from about twenty-five to forty-five years of age, while other lymphomas are more common among those over forty-five or fifty.

LEUKEMIA. Leukemia is a disease characterized by malignancy of the tissues which produce white blood cells. It has some similarities to lymphoma. Acute leukemia is a disease of children under ten years, while the chronic myeloid and lymphatic types are more common among the aged. For a detailed discussion of the disease, see LEUKEMIA.

CANCER OF THE BONE. Cancer originating in the bone is rare except among children and young adults, but it often is a site of secondary cancer which has metastasized from elsewhere in the body.

Primary cancers of the bone are sarcomas, since they all involve connective tissue. The most common type is osteogenic sarcoma, which usually starts in bone-forming cells of the leg. It is most often found among males between the ages of ten and twenty-five.

Ewing's sarcoma appears among males of the same age range as osteogenic sarcoma. It is typified by "onion-layer" formation of new bone under the periosteum, the fibrous sheath which surrounds bones, and it invades the trunk or long bones of the leg.

Chondrosarcoma has its start in cartilage tissue, often in the femur or pelvic areas. It is one bone cancer which is more common among adults, usually occurring in men and women aged thirty to fifty.

Myelomas are tumors that originate in the marrow of bones. In multiple myeloma there is cancerous growth of certain blood cells. (*See* MYELOMA, MULTIPLE.)

Symptoms of cancer of the bone include aching in the affected bones, especially at night. Thus, children's so-called growing pains should not be dismissed casually. If a pain lasts for several days, the child should be examined by a physician. Sometimes, however, there may be no pain at first, and the clue to bone cancer may be an accidental detection of the hard growth on a bone.

Bone cancer often metastasizes to other bones or the lungs. Removal of the cancerous bone, or complete amputation of a limb, may be necessary. Chemotherapy and radiation may also be used.

CANCER OF THE BRAIN. Malignant or nonmalignant tumors of the brain may produce identical or similar symptoms. One symptom is intracranial (within the skull) pressure, much like concussion, which results in headache, nausea, vomiting, problems of eyesight, and dizziness. The pressure may damage nerve tissue, sometimes permanently. Other damage can occur if the cancer directly alters the brain cells. Thus, there is an urgency if brain tumors are suspected.

Sometimes the first clue to a possible brain tumor is a change in the individual's personality. A gentle, easygoing person may suddenly show signs of hostility or irritation. He may do strange things. Or he may get epilepsy—a nervous system disorder characterized by seizures and loss of consciousness. The pattern of symptoms depends upon which part of the brain is affected.

The tumor may be detected by one or more varied techniques: examination of brain wave patterns (electroencephalography); analysis of spinal fluid obtained by lumbar puncture; general X rays; cerebral angiography (use of contrast media to outline brain blood vessels during X ray); or pneumoencephalography (an X ray after using air to displace fluid in areas of the brain for contrast). Another technique is brain scanning, with devices that note how certain injected radioactive substances pass through the brain. Still another is ultrasonography, in which ultrasound (beyond the wavelength heard by the ear) is used to detect distortions of the brain structure. (*See* SCANNING; ULTRASONOGRAPHY.)

There is something about disorders of the brain that frightens people. However, many tumors, both malignant and benign, have been removed successfully by neurosurgery with few, if any, after effects.

The brain is a common site of tumors among children. One of them is an astrocytoma, a cancer of star-shaped cells of the cerebellum, which is often cured by surgery. Another malignant tumor of all ages is a glioma (or glioblastoma). This is cancer of the neuroglia, the supporting structure of the brain and central nervous system.

Radiation and chemotherapy are used for treating some brain cancers when surgical removal is not possible. (*See* BRAIN TUMORS.)

CANCER OF THE SPINAL CORD. Cancer of the spinal cord may cause changes in parts of the body served by the central nervous system. It may result in a diminished ability to use certain muscles, particularly those of the legs. The patient may have trouble walking or standing. He may have back pain, particularly at night. His ability to feel and sense may be altered or lost.

Both brain and spinal cord tumors may be the result of metastasis from a primary cancer of the lung, breast, or another part of the body. Sometimes tumors along the spine are removed by surgery. Radiotherapy and chemotherapy are also used.

ORAL CANCER. Oral cancer, or cancer of the mouth, is often preceded by leukoplakia, a whitish area on the mucous membrane (lining) of the mouth. (*See* LEUKOPLAKIA.) Other sores or ulcers also may be precancerous. Some of them may be caused —or at least irritated so that they become cancerous—by pipe or cigar smoking. Excessive use of alcoholic beverages, failure to keep the mouth clean, and venereal disease also have been linked to oral cancer. Ill-fitting dentures, which irritate mouth linings, have been blamed for oral cancer in some patients. None of these ideas are well documented.

The most common site of oral carcinoma is on the tongue, and the second is on the lip. Other sites may be the roof or side of the mouth, the soft palate, and the gingiva and buccal mucosa—tissues close to the teeth.

Smear tests can often give clues to early oral cancer even if there are no lesions or blemishes in the mouth. Some dentists take these smears routinely.

Closely related to cancer of the mouth itself are malignancies of the larynx, pharynx, salivary glands, and nasal passages. Treatment by surgery or irradiation is most successful if these cancers can be detected early, for they may metastasize along lymph nodes.

Hoarseness or difficulty in swallowing may be the first sign of cancer in the throat area.

CANCER OF THE THYROID. Most goiters (enlargements of the thyroid) are nonmalignant. They occur most frequently among women, but when men get goiters, the growths are more likely to be cancerous.

Thyroid carcinoma usually develops very slowly. Sometimes the patient neglects to report the lump in his neck until several years after noticing it. In other cases, the individual does not even detect any thyroid enlargement. He may first notice a swelling in his neck lymph nodes, or a bone pain— the result of metastases from a "silent" cancer of the thyroid gland. It may also metastasize to the lungs and elsewhere.

The cancer may involve both of the two lobes of the thyroid gland and require a thyroidectomy (removal of the gland). If the tumor is only in one lobe, then a hemithyroidectomy (removal of one lobe) may be performed.

Irradiation may be used for some thyroid tumors, either from an outside source of radiation or through radioactive iodine (I-131). The latter is taken up only by certain types of thyroid tumors, so it is not used in all cases.

Thyroid carcinoma may occur at any age, including childhood, but it is most common among adults, especially those over age forty-five.

GLANDULAR CANCERS. Tumors of hormone-producing parts of the body (endocrine glands), such as the adrenal glands, may have a feminizing or masculinizing effect, depending on which hormones are increased or decreased as the result of the tumor. There may be, for example, abnormal growth of body hair in a woman or a deepening of her voice. There may be an enlargement of the breasts in a man.

Other changes, such as an increase in blood pressure, may result from tumors which alter those hormones affecting circulation. Adrenal tumors, whether benign or malignant, are usually removed. When the function of a hormone-producing gland is impaired by such corrective surgery, it may be necessary for the patient to receive supplementary cortisone or hormone products for the rest of his life.

OTHER CANCERS. One class of malignancies are cancers of the soft tissues. There are many types, named for the cells from which

Estimated Cancer Deaths for All Sites, Plus Major Sites, by State—1972

State	All Sites Number of Deaths	Death Rate per 100,000 Pop.	Breast	Colon-Rec-tum	Lung	Oral	Skin	Uterus	Pros-tate	Stomach	Leu-kemia
Alabama	5,200	141	425	500	1,100	100	125	275	325	200	200
Alaska	200	67	15	15	50	5	10	10	10	10	10
Arizona	2,400	124	200	250	600	50	50	100	150	90	125
Arkansas	3,300	161	225	375	850	60	60	125	250	125	200
California	32,000	147	3,100	4,000	6,700	700	475	1,100	1,400	1,500	1,400
Colorado	2,800	130	250	375	475	40	40	90	175	100	150
Connecticut	5,200	165	500	850	900	150	70	150	250	275	250
Delaware	900	159	70	125	200	25	20	25	30	30	30
Dist. of Columbia	1,600	186	175	200	325	70	10	70	80	60	40
Florida	13,900	201	1,100	1,800	3,200	325	200	400	800	600	500
Georgia	6,200	130	550	650	1,400	175	100	300	375	275	275
Hawaii	900	118	50	80	150	30	30	20	30	100	50
Idaho	1,000	139	90	125	175	20	10	25	80	40	70
Illinois	19,600	176	1,900	2,800	3,900	425	250	700	1,000	900	900
Indiana	8,500	166	800	1,300	1,700	175	150	325	450	275	350
Iowa	5,100	188	475	800	750	90	80	150	350	200	275
Kansas	3,900	170	375	550	650	90	70	125	275	100	200
Kentucky	5,200	160	400	700	1,100	150	100	225	300	150	275
Louisiana	5,700	148	450	600	1,300	150	100	225	325	275	250
Maine	2,000	202	175	300	400	30	20	70	125	90	80
Maryland	6,300	158	600	800	1,400	175	80	225	300	200	200
Massachusetts	11,100	200	1,200	1,700	2,000	250	125	300	475	550	400
Michigan	14,200	163	1,300	1,800	2,900	275	175	450	750	550	550
Minnesota	6,300	171	550	950	950	125	80	150	450	325	275
Mississippi	3,500	146	275	375	650	60	70	175	250	175	200
Missouri	8,600	186	800	1,200	2,000	200	125	300	550	300	400
Montana	1,200	166	100	150	175	20	15	40	70	50	60
Nebraska	2,700	183	225	425	450	50	40	70	175	125	150
Nevada	700	124	60	70	125	15	10	20	25	10	30
New Hampshire	1,500	202	150	250	300	30	20	50	80	40	70
New Jersey	13,700	182	1,400	2,200	2,800	275	150	425	550	650	500
New Mexico	1,200	108	100	125	200	20	20	40	50	50	50
New York	37,000	192	3,900	5,800	6,900	750	425	1,100	1,500	1,900	1,400
North Carolina	6,600	126	600	650	1,300	150	100	325	375	250	350
North Dakota	1,100	169	90	150	175	15	15	25	70	60	50
Ohio	18,900	175	1,800	2,700	3,800	400	225	700	900	750	750
Oklahoma	4,300	170	350	500	850	80	90	150	300	175	200
Oregon	3,500	167	300	475	800	70	60	125	200	150	200
Pennsylvania	23,000	197	2,200	3,600	4,200	500	275	800	1,100	1,000	950
Rhode Island	1,900	207	200	350	350	60	30	50	80	100	60
South Carolina	3,300	123	300	325	750	70	60	175	200	125	150
South Dakota	1,200	177	70	175	175	15	20	40	100	50	80
Tennessee	6,100	149	550	750	1,300	150	125	250	375	225	275
Texas	16,400	142	1,300	1,700	3,700	325	350	600	800	700	900
Utah	1,100	99	90	150	150	15	25	40	80	50	60
Vermont	800	191	60	125	150	20	15	30	50	30	40
Virginia	6,600	136	600	750	1,400	150	100	275	375	250	275
Washington	5,300	170	500	700	1,100	150	70	175	300	225	275
West Virginia	3,200	185	225	400	750	70	50	150	200	150	125
Wisconsin	7,600	177	750	1,200	1,200	150	70	225	450	375	325
Wyoming	500	149	30	60	75	5	15	10	40	15	20
United States	345,000	166	32,000	47,000	69,000	7,500	5,000	12,000	18,000	15,000	15,000

American Cancer Society

they originate, such as fibrosarcoma, liposarcoma, angiosarcoma, etc. They may take root in the flesh of many parts of the body. Often they are retroperitoneal—that is, they grow in the tissues behind the peritoneum, the membrane which lines the abdomen. The choice of treatment depends upon their nature and location.

Cancer does not often originate in the mediastinum, the chest area that encloses the lungs and other organs, but it may be the site of metastases from lung and other cancer.

CANCER IN CHILDREN. Cancer so often affects the aged that we sometimes fail to watch for signs of it among children. The fact is that cancer is the second leading cause of death among children under the age of fourteen. (Trauma—or physical injury—is the first.)

Among the most common cancers of children under ten years of age are leukemia; kidney malignancies, including Wilms' tumor; retinoblastoma; brain and nervous tissue tumors (medulloblastoma and neuroblastoma); and sarcoma. Hodgkin's disease is more common in children over about five years. Ewing's sarcoma, osteogenic sarcoma of the bone, and lymphosarcoma are common cancers in children over the age of ten. As in the case of most cancers, the causes of many childhood malignancies are unknown. Some apparently may be traced to inherited or genetic factors or to influences on the infant's body in the prenatal (before birth) state.

Cancer Chemotherapy.
Various human cancers can be satisfactorily retarded and sometimes eliminated by using newly developed chemical compounds. This form of cancer treatment is called chemotherapy. (*See* CHEMOTHERAPY.)

Cancer Detection.
At present, since early surgical removal is the best available weapon against cancer, early detection of a cancerous growth is the most important step toward cure. Cancer as a cause of death is on the rise and now ranks third behind heart disease and kidney disease.

Physicians have many facilities at hand to help them detect a cancer, but the real key to conquering this disease is self-examination by the individual. Each person must be aware of his body and aware of changes that occur in it. Following are major bodily changes which one should watch for.

1. Any persistent skin growth which enlarges or changes color or consistency *may* be cancerous and should have a biopsy. (*See* BIOPSY.) Skin cancer is the most common type of malignant disease but has a 90 percent cure rate when attended to properly.

2. The presence of a lump in the female breast, whether painless or painful, can indicate cancer. Every woman should without fail examine her breasts once a month. Approximately one-quarter of all female cancers arise in the breast. Bleeding from the nipple, changes in the contour of the nipple, and small dimples in the skin of the breast should also be looked for.

3. Bleeding is an important sign. In the female, unexplained vaginal bleeding or vaginal bleeding after sexual activity can be a sign of carcinoma of the cervix of the uterus. (*See* UTERUS.) Pelvic pain, leakage of urine or fecal matter from the vagina, and any foul-smelling discharge from the vagina are possible signs of cancer.

Bleeding is also an important sign of cancer involving the bowel. Red blood or tarry black material passed during a bowel movement may indicate a tumor within the bowel. Likewise, a change in bowel habits, such as diarrhea or constipation, may point toward an internal cancer.

Blood in the urine (hematuria) should also be noted and attended to by a physician. Hematuria is the most common early finding in cancer of the kidney and bladder.

4. Persistent cough, chest pain, coughing up blood, and shortness of breath are all significant complaints. They should be heeded because an underlying lung tumor may be the cause. Lung cancer is a lethal disease: only 5 percent of patients live five

years after the diagnosis is made. Early detection is critical.

5. The appearance of a lump (lymph node) in the neck, above the clavicle (collarbone), in the armpit, or in the groin should be reported to a physician. Many diseases can cause such a lump, but cancer is one of these.

6. Many generalized sensations may be due to a cancerous growth. Among these are unexplained weight loss, excessive fatigue, changes in personality, headache, and leg pains. (*See* THROMBOPHLEBITIS.)

Due to advanced technology and recent advances in laboratory testing, the physician has many ways to approach cancer detection. In spite of these advances, the patient's history and a physical examination still rank first in importance. They form the starting point of the doctor's search. After completing them, the physician may use any of the following special diagnostic tools.

Direct visualization of a diseased body organ may be helpful in making the diagnosis. A pelvic examination in women by insertion of a speculum can be easily done and, in combination with a Pap smear, can be very useful. (*See* PELVIC EXAMINATION.) Tumors in the esophagus and stomach can be seen by inserting a special flexible tube with a light in the end. These are called esophagoscopes or gastroscopes respectively. Tumors of the lower bowel can be seen after inserting a lighted metal tube called a proctoscope into the rectum. A similar but smaller tube (cystoscope) can be inserted into the bladder through the urethra and a search made for a bladder tumor.

X-ray examination is an important and much used tool. Simple X rays of the chest, abdomen and pelvis, skull, and various bones can often detect a cancer in those regions. Special X-ray exams, using fluids which show up on the X ray and therefore outline body cavities and passages, are often employed. These fluids (contrast media) can be injected into arteries, thereby show-

ing an artery displaced by a nearby tumor. This is called angiography. The contrast medium can be injected into veins and picked up by the kidneys to show any abnormal growth there. This is termed an intravenous pyelogram (IVP). Similar fluids can be placed in the esophagus, stomach, small intestine, large intestine, gallbladder, and urinary bladder, thereby defining any neoplastic growth within them.

Similar to a simple X ray but using a slightly different technique is the mammogram, or breast X ray. This test can often detect a possible cancer in a breast that may feel normal. It is often used in women as a screening test or on "high-risk" women (single women over thirty years old, women who have had cancer of one breast, or women with a family history of breast cancer).

Radioactive scans of various organs are now being used more and more. Certain harmless radioactive elements are known to collect in specific organs after they are injected into an arm vein. Their distribution within that organ can be determined by a sensing device much like a Geiger counter. A picture similar to an X ray is then produced, and from this any abnormality is detected. Scans can be performed on the brain, thyroid gland, lung, liver, kidney, and bones.

The biopsy, which allows direct microscopic examination of diseased tissue, is unequaled in reliability and must be performed before treatment is initiated. (*See* BIOPSY.) A biopsy can take many forms but one in particular is the key to actual cancer detection and deserves emphasis. This is the Papanicolaou smear or cytology smear. Every adult female should, without fail, have a yearly pelvic examination and Pap smear. This simple and painless test has the potential to virtually eliminate carcinoma of the uterine cervix as a cause of death. Any specialist trained in obstetrics-gynecology and most other physicians can perform the test, which involves scraping a few cells off the cervix and placing them on a microscope slide. This slide is then stained and viewed under the microscope. Using this method, the physician can detect changes in the cervix which appear before actual cancer starts growing. At this very early stage of the disease a simple operation can cure the patient.

Cancer of the Skin. The most common form of cancer in man is cancer of the skin. Fortunately, 95 percent of all skin cancers can be cured with medically approved treatments. Most cancers of the skin can be treated successfully because of the skin's accessibility. Precancerous or cancerous tumors can be recognized visually by a trained physician and can often be felt by the fingers while they are still very small. The location of the tumor on or under the skin eases the task of total removal.

CAUSES OF SKIN CANCER. The prevalence of skin cancer is understandable when one considers that the skin is one of the largest organs of the body. Its external locations and its role as a protector of the body against outside forces play a definite part in making the skin more susceptible to cancer. To a greater degree than other organs, the skin is liable to environmental attacks that can be cancer causing.

Today, doctors agree that continued and frequent exposure to sunlight, specifically ultraviolet light, is the leading cause of skin cancer. This is supported by the fact that more than 90 percent of all skin cancers appear on skin areas exposed to ultraviolet light rather than areas normally protected by clothing. Continued, excessive exposure to certain chemicals, such as coal tar, pitch, arsenic compounds, and paraffin oil, and to radium and X ray, may produce precancerous skin changes. Certain scarring processes, such as those resulting from burns and a few scarring diseases of the skin, appear to make the development of cancer more likely.

Most skin cancers appear in the middle

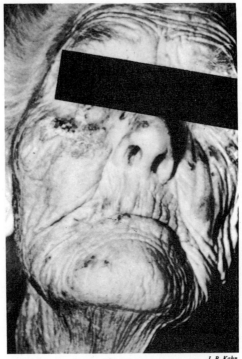

J. B. Kahn

Dark patches on the face of a very old woman are skin cancer lesions which resulted from excessive exposure to the sun.

and later decades of life. They also occur most often on exposed areas of people who have fair, ruddy, or sandy complexions and those who are exposed to great amounts of sun, such as farmers, sailors, and outdoor sportsmen. Geographical location also plays a role. Since the sun is the primary cause of skin cancer, there is a much higher incidence in areas with the greatest number of hours of sunlight per year, including the southwestern United States, southern California, and southern Florida.

While some cancers develop from normal, healthy skin tissue, most of them develop from areas where abnormal changes or conditions have been apparent for a long time. In addition to the precancerous conditions already cited, actinic keratoses, moles, and leukoplakia are considered to be precancerous lesions.

Actinic keratoses are the most common of the precancerous conditions. A keratosis is a dry, scaly patch or clump of patches, usually darker than the surrounding skin, which appears on exposed areas of the body. A certain percentage of all actinic keratoses become cancerous. (*See* KERATOSES.)

Moles themselves are harmless, benign growths, but sometimes skin cancers may look like moles or develop at the same sites as moles. Thus moles must be carefully observed for suspicious changes in color, growth, bleeding, or irritation. (*See* MOLES.)

Leukoplakia is a white, scaly thickening of the lip or membranes of the mouth which may predispose to cancer. (*See* LEUKOPLAKIA.)

TYPES OF SKIN CANCER. Cancer of the skin may be one of three types: basal cell cancer, epidermoid cancer, and malignant melanoma.

Basal Cell Cancer. This is the most common type of skin cancer. It very rarely, if ever, spreads to distant parts of the body. In the simplest and most common form it appears as a small, firm, translucent, gray nodule or bump on the skin, usually on the forehead, cheeks, nose, or other exposed areas, such as the backs of the hands. Since it is painless and rarely bleeds, this form is often unnoticed until it begins to grow more rapidly.

Another form of basal cell skin cancer appears as a raised, scaly patch of keratosis, which is noticed because it bleeds easily when rubbed or scratched. A fully developed basal cell cancer is easily recognized. It has a central area of ulceration circled by a raised, grey, pearly edge. It is a painless, slow-growing ulcer which does not heal.

Epidermoid Cancer. Epidermoid cancer is another common form of skin cancer which may appear like basal cell cancer but which spreads more rapidly. The epidermoid type of skin cancer usually starts in the form of a warty, crusty keratotic area

or several such areas on the cheek, ear, neck, or back of the hand. This form often becomes infected and may be tender. The ulcerating form of epidermoid skin cancer is usually a shallow, nonhealing ulcer which spreads over the surface of the skin, sometimes including a wide area, but rarely grows down far into the deeper tissues. On unexposed areas of the body, epidermoid skin cancers may arise in old scars of burns or infections, appearing as a nontender, raised, firm, pinkish, flesh-colored small area on the normal skin. The fact that epidermoid skin cancers grow more rapidly than basal cell cancers may attract attention to them.

Malignant Melanoma. The most dangerous—and fortunately rarest—type of skin cancer is the malignant melanoma. This type spreads very early to other parts of the body. A malignant melanoma may arise from what appears to be a mole, because these malignant growths usually look like bluish-black moles that are raised above the surface. One of the most definite signs of danger in a mole is the appearance of a dull, diffuse, brownish zone spreading from it. If a mole is irritated and becomes larger, blacker, or bleeds, it should be seen at once by a doctor, as it may be a malignant melanoma instead of a mole. In fact, any increase in size, change in shape, deepening of color, bleeding, or ulceration of a painless sore or mole that does not heal may be cancerous unless proved otherwise.

DIAGNOSIS AND TREATMENT. Diagnosis of the common kinds of skin cancer is comparatively simple. Unlike many cancers, it is readily accessible so that a piece of suspected tissue can be removed in a doctor's office for pathologic examination with little or no pain or trouble. This procedure, known as a biopsy, helps to establish definitely whether or not cancer is present.

Cancer can be treated by surgery, X ray, radium, or drugs. All are used in treating cancer of the skin and all of them can effect cures. The particular form of treatment depends on the type of cancer and the state of the disease. (*See* CANCER.)

Cancer Prevention. Until the exact cause of cancer is known, it will be difficult to indicate how best to prevent this illness. A vast accumulation of clinical and laboratory data has led to many theories regarding the cause of cancer. Some theories involve chromosomal abnormalities and chemical alterations. Some investigators view cancer as a disease of tissues rather than of isolated cells and are studying the cells with regard to renewal of tissue masses. They also work with the blood supply and growth characteristics of malignant tissues. (*See* MALIGNANT.) Still other investigators see cancer as a disease of a whole organism. They study immunity problems nutritional factors, and the total environment of the cancer. (*See* IMMUNIZATION.)

In spite of all the questions that remain unanswered, there are certain scientifically based actions which the average person can take to help prevent cancer. The following discussion will point out some of these actions.

Certain agents in our environment are known or strongly believed to cause various kinds of cancer. These agents are called carcinogens. (*See* CARCINOGENS.) It is reasonable to assume that if contact with these carcinogens is kept to a minimum, certain cancers can be prevented. The most important such agent in our society today is the cigarette. Lung cancer is a deadly disease and its incidence continues to increase. When carefully examined, the information linking carcinoma of the lung with cigarette smoking is irrefutable.

The power of radiant energy to cause cancer (particularly leukemia) is well known. (*See* CARCINOGENS.) Each year, more and more atomic energy is being used in our country. More and more atomic-energy plants are being constructed close to large population centers. In the event of an atomic disaster at one of these plants, many citizens would die, many of these from cancers. Strict safety regulations and constant evaluation of industrial methods are essential. A little forethought can prevent thousands of needless deaths.

Some cancers are in a sense prevented when so-called precancerous changes are detected and the affected organ is removed or partially removed. The best example of this involves the Pap or cyto smear for carcinoma of the cervix. Using this simple test, early signs of impending cancer can be detected and appropriate surgery performed. (*See* CANCER DETECTION; CERVIX.) Every adult female should have an annual Pap smear without fail.

Cancroid. Growths of tissue with characteristics of cancer, but which are not necessarily malignant, are termed cancroid. Literally the word means cancerlike. It can also refer to skin cancer that shows varying degrees of malignancy. Thus an abnormal proliferation of cells resulting in a tumor which is not a cancer is cancroid. (*See* MALIGNANCY; SKIN.)

Candida. This is a fungus of the yeast family which is normally present in many body tissues, but which occasionally is the cause of fungal infection. There are many species of *Candida,* each having specific areas of disease conditions. In normal persons *Candida* usually are present in the mouth, vagina, sputum, and stools. Thus they are also to be found in the gastrointestinal tract. It is when these fungi gain the upper hand that infection occurs.

Candidiasis is a disease mainly involving the skin, which also extends to the kidneys, heart, and brain. Initial symptoms of this and most other candida infections include itching and burning; later fever may develop when the infection spreads internally.

Treatment in any affected area begins with washes to flush the fungi out, and drugs used internally and externally to destroy them. (*See* CANDIDIASIS; CERVICITIS; VAGINITIS.)

In many cases, candida infection can be prevented by proper hygiene—particularly of the mouth and vagina. Total elimination is practically impossible, but the amount of the fungus present can be controlled. Reinfection after recovery is often a problem if hygienic measures are not followed.

Candidiasis. The yeastlike fungus called *Candida* (or *Monilia*) *albicans* causes a number of variations of the disease candidiasis. It may attack the skin, the mucous membranes of the mouth and vagina, the fingernails, the folds of the fingers, the intestinal tract, and infrequently internal organs such as the liver or kidneys. The skin lesions generally are whitish and soggy, with reddening of the surrounding skin. The patches often resemble curdled milk. If they are scraped, the skin underneath looks raw and may bleed. In some cases of vaginitis, itching may be the only obvious sign of candida infection. (*See* VAGINITIS.)

The candida fungus may be present on the normal skin or mucous membrane and cause no symptoms until something triggers it into activity. Candidiasis often appears along with problems of malnutrition, imbalance of the endocrine system, or blood disorders. It occurs more often among infants and the elderly than among persons of other ages. It often flares up in vaginitis during pregnancy and may be passed on to the newborn during birth—by unclean hands of the mother or nurse, or by nursing from a bottle or the mother's breast.

So-called diaper rash is often a candida infection. Infants as well as adults may become infected with "thrush," or candidiasis of the mouth membranes. The tongue may also be involved. The infection apparently may pass from the mouth to the intestines, then to the anal area via excrement. Cleanliness is an obvious aid in prevention.

Candida infections in folds along the side of the mouth result in the condition called perlèche. (*See* PERLÈCHE.)

The housewife who does lots of scrubbing around the home, professional cleaning women, and other workers whose hands are wet for long periods are susceptible to candidiasis between the fingers. It is most likely to occur in persons whose hands are fat or shaped so that there is poor ventilation between the fingers. Painful cracks with infection may appear in the folds where the fingers join the palm. The disease may also involve the skin covering the base of the nail, and the nail itself. Fingernails may become ridged and discolored.

Candidiasis is treated by diagnosing and remedying any accompanying conditions of malnutrition or systemic disease, and by the use of anti-fungal therapy. Nystatin is a useful anti-mycotic (fungus-destroying) agent used in mouth rinses for thrush, in suppository tablets for candida-caused vaginitis, and in solution for soaking other parts of the body. Aqueous gentian violet may be prescribed for daubing on the lesions. Corticosteroid creams are often of value.

Like other fungal infections, candidiasis may be associated with diverse skin infections, such as intertrigo or ringworm. (*See* FUNGAL DISEASES.)

Canker Sores. The shallow ulcers that appear under the tongue, on the inside of the lip, or elsewhere in the mouth are commonly called canker sores. This is a popular synonym for aphthous ulcers or ulcerative stomatitis, the technical names. A slight blister usually appears first. This rubs off and forms a raw, painful ulcer in the center of a reddened area. The sores may appear singly or in groups, and may have a glossy covering or "false membrane."

The cause of these ulcers has not been found. (Another common eruption of the mouth, the fever blister or herpes simplex, is caused by a virus. *See* HERPES SIMPLEX.)

Irritants seem to be to blame for canker sores, as they are often associated with loose teeth, ill-fitting dentures, or dental decay, and clear up when these conditions are remedied. Some patients find that the ulcers flare up when they eat certain types of foods, such as citrus fruits, nuts, and rich chocolate. By trial and error, some persons are able to find the particular item causing the irritation, and eliminate it.

Diluted hydrogen peroxide and other mouthwashes give relief in many cases. Ointments containing antibiotics also aid healing, but often the canker sores do not respond well and run a course of several days to a few weeks before they disappear. They tend to recur from time to time. If the ulcers do not disappear or are widespread, it makes good sense to see your physician. He will determine whether the lesions are really canker sores or another type of problem.

A canker sore should not be confused with a chancre (pronounced shan-kur), an ulcer-type lesion found at the point where such diseases as syphilis, tularemia, or sporotricosis enter the body. (*See* SYPHILIS; TULAREMIA.)

Cannabis. A close relative to the hops and fig plants, *Cannabis sativa* is the plant commonly known as marijuana, kif, maconha, hashish, bhang, charas, or dagga. Although named by Linnaeus in 1753, the cannabis plant has been known to man since 2500 B.C., when it was listed in a Chinese book of pharmacology. (*See* MARIJUANA.)

Cannabis has been used in times past for treatment of arthritis, malaria, headaches, stomach ailments, and constipation. Around 1100 B.C., the "Giver of Delight" and "Liberator of Sin" began to assume a new use—in religious rites. Cannabis was called holy or sacred grass in Hindu culture, and as it spread in use throughout Asia, Africa, and South America, its reputation spread. Its euphoria-producing properties are well known throughout the world today.

Cannula. A tube designed for insertion into a body vessel, duct, or organ is called a cannula. Frequently a cannula is made of a plastic material and has a needle or trocar (sharp, pointed rod) inside to facilitate its insertion. It can be placed into a vein so that intravenous fluids can be given. An artery can also receive a cannula so that arterial samples can be easily collected or arterial blood pressures recorded. The trachea (windpipe) is frequently cannulated so that oxygen and anesthetic gas may be administered during surgery. (*See* ANESTHETIC.) A cannula can also be placed in the abdomen, bladder, or any other body cavity for a variety of tests and treatments.

Cantharides. Also known as Spanish fly, cantharides is a preparation of powdered blister beetles used medicinally as a diuretic, skin irritant, and aphrodisiac. The active principle in the drug is called cantharidin. It is marketed as cantharidin plaster, blistering fluid, cantharidin ointment, and tincture of cantharidin. (*See* APHRODISIAC.)

The drug is sold, under a doctor's prescription, with many warnings. It is intensely irritating and should not enter the mouth, eyes, or other sensitive areas. It cannot be used before the patient's kidneys have been checked, as it is absorbed through the skin. It causes blistering, due to heat and perspiration, if applied to a part of the body on which the patient lies.

Cantharidin poisoning is accompanied by intense pain in the stomach, kidneys, urinary organs, and alimentary canal. Diarrhea and vomiting occur, and the individual has a desire to urinate constantly. In some cases the pulse is weak, and the patient may collapse.

Capillaries. The smallest of the blood vessels, the capillaries, are in a sense the most important. All segments of the circulatory system, of course, are critically necessary. But it is in and around the capillaries that the life processes made possible by blood are carried out. Here the body tissues are nourished, stimulated to growth, repaired, and cleaned of waste products—here the body lives.

Capillaries are sometimes thought of as being at the outer ends of the circulatory system. But they also can be pictured in an intermediate position. They are the connecting link between the outer reaches of the arterial system, the arterioles, and the outermost link in the venous system, the venules. Throughout nearly every part of the body, capillaries form a network. (*See* BLOOD CIRCULATION.)

Capillaries are microscopic vessels with walls only one cell thick and a cross-section large enough to pass only one red blood cell at a time. Blood moves steadily here, not spurting as in the arteries but smoothly, at about one inch a minute.

The walls are a type of tissue called semipermeable membrane, so thin that it allows materials such as oxygen, sugar, amino acids, and fluids to pass through it from the bloodstream into the tissue fluids (where any excesses eventually move into the lymph system). In the other direction, the thin wall passes carbon dioxide, lactic acid, and by-products of metabolism back into the bloodstream for disposal.

In the lungs, for example, the capillary semipermeable walls are the gateway through which oxygen moves into the bloodstream. Oxygen molecules in the 700 million tiny air sacs of the lungs, the alveoli, move through this semipermeable membrane by a process called diffusion. In this process, molecules of a given material move from a greater concentration of the material to a lesser concentration. Oxygen molecules, then, diffuse through the lung and capillary walls from the air on the lung side to the blood on the capillary side. And the oxygen-laden blood moves from the capillaries to venules and back to the heart.

The reverse process takes place when blood molecules unload their carbon dioxide, which diffuses from the greater concentration in the red cell hemoglobin to the lower carbon dioxide concentration in the lungs. (*See* HEMOGLOBIN.)

Capsule. An enclosure formed by a number of tissues around other tissues or organs is called a capsule. The capsule surrounding the kidney is fibrous, while the capsule enclosing the ducts and arteries of the liver is composed of connective tissue. The word is also used to describe the membrane limiting and protecting bacterial cells.

Carbohydrates. Most of the energy in the food we eat comes from substances called carbohydrates. They contain sugars or materials that our bodies can convert to sugar—and then to energy.

The name carbohydrates was derived from the composition of the substance: carbon, hydrogen, and oxygen. When digested, all carbohydrates which serve as food are broken down into simple sugars. These are then changed, through a series of chemical reactions, into carbon dioxide and water, yielding energy for work.

A sufficient supply of carbohydrates in the diet is necessary for the proper utilization of fat. When fat is used as a source of energy without enough carbohydrates, a condition known as acidosis may develop. One type of acidosis occurs in diabetics if they do not use insulin. (*See* DIABETES MELLITUS.)

Each gram of carbohydrate utilized in the body as a source of energy yields approximately four calories, or units of energy. (*See* CALORIES.) When one eats more carbohydrates than the body needs, the material is stored as glycogen in the liver and as fat. Sugar eaten in amounts too great to be utilized by the body or in too-concentrated form dulls the appetite for more essential foods. It may also ferment in the digestive tract, irritating the membranes as well as causing discomfort.

Important sources of carbohydrates are breads and cereals, potatoes, lima beans, corn, dried beans and peas, and fruits—fresh, dried, or sweetened. Considerable amounts of carbohydrates are furnished by sugar, syrup, jelly, jam, and honey.

The terms starch and carbohydrate are not synonymous. Starches are carbohydrates, but not all carbohydrates are starches. Carbohydrate is a general term used to identify one class of food components. Proteins, fats, vitamins, and minerals are other such general terms.

Carbohydrates themselves can be divided into classes. One class is simple sugars, such as grape sugar and common table sugar. Another class is starch.

In plants, starch is called the "storage" form of sugar. The sweetness of fruits depends upon the kinds and amounts of simple sugars produced when starch is broken down by the ripening process or by cooking.

In humans, the energy from starch can be utilized only after it is broken down to simple sugar by digestive enzymes. The most important enzyme that functions in the digestion of starch is found in saliva. While saliva is thoroughly mixed with food in the mouth by chewing, the major part of starch digestion is carried out by the salivary enzyme after the food reaches the stomach. Food, especially starchy food, must be chewed well to allow time for adequate secretion and the mixing of saliva. (*See* NUTRITION.)

Carbolic Acid.   An obsolete name for phenol is carbolic acid. It is obtained from coal tar or prepared synthetically. In solution, carbolic acid, or phenol, cauterizes the skin and mucous membranes. It is used as an antiseptic, germicide, disinfectant, and local anesthetic. (*See* ANESTHETIC; DISINFECTANTS AND ANTISEPTICS; TETANUS.)

Carbon.   The element carbon is a nonmetal that occurs free in nature—in pure crystalline form as diamonds. Graphite is also carbon, but in a different crystalline form. Coal, charcoal, lampblack, and soot are also mainly carbon, but in noncrystalline form.

The naturally occurring carbon is a mixture of two stable isotopes, mainly carbon 12 with some carbon 13. There are also four radioactive isotopes. Of these, carbon 14 has the longest half-life (6360 years). (*See* HALF-LIFE.) It has been especially useful in biomedical research because it can be incorporated as a tracer into various foods and drugs taken into the animal body, and can then be followed as these substances are transported, stored, and eventually excreted.

Chemical compounds of carbon, especially the carbohydrates, fats, and proteins, are absolutely essential in the structure of all living things. Such compounds are called *organic* to distinguish them from chemical substances of purely mineral origin, which are called *inorganic.* The distinction is hard to maintain consistently, however. Many minerals, like limestone and coral, are really the products of living things, while chemists have been able to make artificially many carbon compounds, like urea, that are normally formed by and found in living organisms. In general, the chemistry of carbon compounds is called organic chemistry.

Because carbon atoms have the ability to hang together in chains and rings and also to combine with atoms of hydrogen, oxygen, and nitrogen in so many different configurations, organic chemistry is exceedingly complex, but its applications in medicine are exceedingly important. (*See* CARBOHYDRATES; CARBON DIOXIDE; CARBON MONOXIDE; FATS; PROTEINS.)

Carbonated Drinks.   It was once believed that the carbon dioxide dissolved in the water of certain springs made it useful in treating disease. To increase the supply of supposedly medicinal water, the first processes for artificial carbonation were developed about two hundred years ago.

Carbonated drinks, more commonly called "soda pop," are bottled under pressure. Some of the carbon dioxide combines with water to form carbonic acid, which gives the characteristic sharp taste. When the bottle is opened, much of the dissolved gas bubbles away into the air or into the drinker's digestive tract. (*See* CARBON DIOXIDE.)

Most people can drink reasonable amounts of carbonated drinks without discomfort, except for an occasional burp. But people with ulcers and other digestive problems have more than enough gas and acid as it is. Diets prescribed for them usually exclude carbonated drinks.

Carbon Dioxide. This colorless, odorless gas passes out of the lungs when we exhale. It is one of the body's end products of metabolism. Plants absorb carbon dioxide and water to synthesize certain carbohydrates, and then release oxygen into the air.

Some environmentalists are concerned that man's activities are generating increasing amounts of carbon dioxide that may be effecting changes in global weather patterns. (*See* CLIMATE.) It has been known for many decades that carbon dioxide in the atmosphere produces a "greenhouse effect" —heat is trapped in the lower atmosphere, possibly increasing the temperature at the earth's surface. This has led some to predict that if man continues to increase the atmospheric content of carbon dioxide by, for example, burning fossil fuels, the earth's surface temperature will rise sufficiently to melt the ice caps and thus inundate many of the world's major cities. Others dismiss this prediction by pointing out that other components of air pollution, such as particulate matter, have a cooling effect on earth temperature as they absorb and scatter the sun's radiation. (*See* AIR PÒLLUTION.)

Carbon Disulfide. Carbon and sulfur form a compound (CS_2) called carbon disulfide, a volatile, colorless liquid that is exceedingly useful in industry but also highly flammable and poisonous. It has been used on a large scale in the manufacture of other chemicals, especially certain plastics, and in the processing of rubber.

The odor of carbon disulfide is not especially strong or unpleasant, but inhalation of the vapor causes acute poisoning like that by chloroform, with the possibility of sudden collapse and death. Workers can tolerate twenty to fifty parts per million in an industrial atmosphere for perhaps thirty minutes under emergency conditions. For prolonged exposure the maximum acceptable concentration is given variously as three to twenty parts per million. Exceeding these limits results in a chronic poisoning that is slow to appear, with headache, vertigo, excitement, loss of weight, paralyses and seizures, degenerative changes in the nervous system and other important organs, and toxic blindness.

The treatment is generally supportive, not specific. Prevention has been made possible by the development of a technology that permits the handling of large quantities of the liquid without allowing it to escape into the air.

Carbon Monoxide. One of the main examples of gaseous pollutants, produced by the incomplete burning of carbon in fuels, is carbon monoxide (CO). It is colorless, odorless, and slightly lighter than air. Carbon monoxide emissions can be prevented by supplying enough air to insure complete combustion. When this occurs, carbon dioxide, a natural constituent of the atmosphere, is produced instead of carbon monoxide. Almost two-thirds of the carbon monoxide emitted comes from internal-combustion engines, and the overwhelming bulk of that comes from gasoline-powered motor vehicles.

When carbon monoxide is inhaled, it displaces oxygen in the blood and reduces the amount carried to the body tissues. Death by asphyxiation occurs when too much is inhaled—a risk taken by persons who stay in closed garages while an automobile engine remains running. At levels found in city air, it can slow the reactions of even the healthiest persons, making them more prone to accidents. Moreover, it is believed to impose an extra burden on those who already suffer from anemia, diseases of the heart and blood vessels, chronic lung disease, overactive thyroid, or even simple fever. Cigarette smokers, who are already inhaling significant amounts of carbon monoxide in tobacco smoke, take on an additional CO burden from polluted air.

Studies have shown that exposure to 10 parts per million of CO for approximately eight hours may dull mental performance. Such levels of carbon monoxide are commonly found in cities throughout the world. In heavy traffic situations, levels of 70, 80, or 100 parts per million (or higher) may be common for short periods. (*See* AIR POLLUTION; AUTO SAFETY; SMOKING.)

Carbon Tetrachloride. The volatile, nonflammable, colorless liquid with the formula CCl_4 is carbon tetrachloride. In the past, its pleasant smell, its effectiveness as a solvent, and the fact that it is nonflammable recommended it for many industrial uses. It became popular for removing stains, extinguishing fires, and carrying on many manufacturing processes. It also had anesthetic properties. (*See* ANESTHETIC.)

Unfortunately, it was found that the use of carbon tetrachloride also had serious drawbacks. Animals anesthetized with it, though they might recover for a time, would die hours later with severe symptoms of irremediable damage to liver and kidneys. In industry, its incautious use caused chronic poisoning. Fatalities were reported after its use in homes as a spot-remover. Its usefulness in putting out fires was offset by the fact that heat decomposed it into exceedingly noxious gases like chlorine, phosgene, and hydrogen chloride, which were especially lethal in confined spaces.

A housewife trying out a new solvent for cleaning in the home should make it a general policy to work only in a well-ventilated place away from any possible source of flames or sparks. Actually, carbon tetrachloride should not be used in the home at all, and when it is necessary in industry, steps must be taken to protect the workers. (*See* VENTILATION OF THE HOME.)

Carbuncles. A boil that has more than one core of infection and pus is called a carbuncle. Like a boil, a carbuncle is caused by the bacteria staphylococci invading hair follicles. The infection may be accompanied by sickness throughout the body. There may be fever and changes in the composition of the blood, particularly an increase in the number of leukocytes (leukocytosis). Carbuncles are extremely painful and disabling, and require professional medical attention. Treatment is similar to that for boils. (*See* BOILS.)

Carcinogens. Although we still do not know the cause or causes of cancer, certain agents in our environment have been shown to cause cancer. These agents are called carcinogens. Carcinogenic (cancer-causing) materials can be grouped into four major categories: (1) chemical, (2) viral, (3) physical, and (4) hormonal.

CHEMICAL. One of the first controversies regarding cancer etiology (causes) was focused on a chemical: chimney soot. During the 1700's in England, doctors noticed that chimney sweeps had a high incidence of cancer of the scrotum, due to direct contact with coal soot for long periods of time. Experiments in 1915 showed that skin cancer could be caused by applying liquid coal tar to the ears of rabbits. Shortly after this, coal tar was purified and the carcinogen isolated as a group of chemical compounds known as polycyclic hydrocarbons. There are more than one thousand such chemicals which have been shown to produce various kinds of cancer in animals after application to the skin, injection into body organs, or oral feedings. A chemical (2-'b-naphthylamine) used in the aniline dye industry is known to cause bladder cancer in man.

Other kinds of chemicals, including chromium, cobalt, arsenic, iron dextran, nitrogen mustard (a nerve gas), and several plastics, have the potential to produce tumors in many animals. Plastics are used to make artificial vessels in man, but there has never been a report of these plastics causing cancer.

The chemical carcinogens which affect man most widely are the hydrocarbons inhaled with cigarette smoke. The body of evidence for this conclusion is now overwhelming and cannot be ignored. Some statistical studies show that the death rate from bronchogenic carcinoma (lung cancer) in those persons smoking a pack or more of cigarettes per day is fifty times that of the nonsmoker. Clinical and experimental evidence for this correlation is growing daily.

VIRAL. It has been proven that viral agents can induce cancer in experimental animals. (*See* VIRUSES.) There are four large groups of viruses which are known to be carcinogenic in animals: papovirus, adenovirus, poxvirus, and myxovirus-like. The virus is believed to alter the reproduction apparatus of normal cells in some way which turns them into neoplastic (tumor-producing) cells.

Even though there can be no doubt that viral agents cause various cancers in animals, no conclusive evidence has been presented which shows this is true in man. Viral particles have been isolated from solid tumors in man, but this alone does not prove the virus caused the cancer. Similarly, viruslike particles have been seen by electron microscopy inside human malignant tumor cells. The best data so far available on this topic concern a lymphoma present in Africa known as "epidemic lymphoma," or Burkitt's lymphoma. (*See* LYMPHOMA.) There is much statistical evidence which supports the theory that this cancer is virus induced. In addition, viruses have been seen in the tumor cells of patients with Burkitt's lymphoma. Research in this field actively continues and will probably soon yield valuable findings.

PHYSICAL AGENTS. Among the forms of physical energy which can cause cancer are the so-called ionizing radiations produced by such agents as X ray and atomic energy. The early experimenters in the field of X ray learned quite vividly how X rays can induce cancer. Many of these men developed skin cancer on their hands and arms after long exposure to their new ray. A high rate of leukemia among radiologists also points up the danger of X-ray overexposure. Miners in the radium and uranium mines developed a great deal of lung cancer from inhaling these radioactive ores. Those Japanese who survived Nagasaki and Hiroshima show a ten- to fifty-fold increase in the incidence of leukemia. Routine X-ray examinations release very little ionizing radiation and cause no damage to the average citizen.

Exposure to sunlight and other sources of ultraviolet light may also induce the formation of certain skin cancers. People whose jobs require them to be in direct sunlight for long periods of time, such as farmers and sailors, have notably higher incidence of such cancers.

The mechanism by which radiant energy induces cancer remains unclear. Most investigators think that the energy alters the reproductive mechanisms within the cells, thus changing them to cancerous cells. Others believe the radiant energy in combination with a virus brings about this cellular change.

Other forms of physical injury are thought to induce cancers. Many cases have been reported which tell of a skin cancer developing over an area previously burned. Many claims have been made that an injury (particularly an automobile injury) caused a cancer to form. There is, however, no good evidence that a single blow can induce neoplastic growth. Repeated trauma to a part of the body is somewhat different. Cancers of the mouth have occurred after irritation to that region by poor-fitting dentures or by warm clay tobacco pipes. There is also an increased incidence of cervical cancer among women who have borne many children, thus lacerating the uterine cervix.

HORMONES. Certain animal tumors can be induced by the administration of hormones, particularly estrogens. (*See* ESTROGENS.) Some experimenters feel that the hormones act directly on the cells, thus transforming them to neoplastic cells. Others believe the hormones merely change the cell's chemical environment, thus enabling another agent (virus or chemical) to enter and alter the cell. With the considerable research being done in this field, more information will soon be available.

Carcinoma. Those specialized cells which cover the internal and external surface of the body, including the linings of vessels and body cavities, are called epithelial cells. Malignant cancers which arise from these epithelial cells are termed carcinomas. Since there are many varieties of epithelial cells, there are several types of carcinomas. (*See* CANCER.)

Cardiac Arrest. Most familiar of all depictions of the "heart attack" in fiction and drama is the victim who falls gasping to the floor, or the surgical patient who suddenly expires on the operating table. Such an event is actually "cardiac arrest," a sudden end to circulation caused by a stoppage of effective heart action.

It is cardiac arrest that most frequently kills persons with heart disease, particularly coronary diseases. Cardiac arrest is the worst effect of abnormal heart conditions, and all heart care and heart disease treatment is aimed ultimately at preventing it.

Death is the certain result of a cardiac arrest unless the heartbeat is started again within no more than four minutes. Beyond this time, oxygen starvation irreparably damages the brain to the point that it no longer can sustain life processes in the body.

When the victim gasps and falls, or begins to fail during surgery, immediate aggressive steps must be taken to restore normal heart action or, if the patient is already unconscious, to resuscitate him. Not a sec-

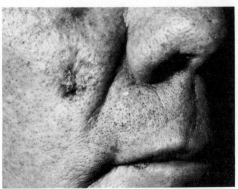

Armed Forces Institute of Pathology

Carcinoma on the cheek. This is a type of cancer composed of connective tissue and epithelial (skin) cells.

ond can be lost in the work to save his life.

If the heartbeat is erratic, a normal rhythm must be restored; if it is missing, a regular beat must be induced. The goal of immediate cardiac treatment is to keep the victim alive long enough to get his strength back while, at the same time, resting and restoring the regular pumping action of the heart. Emergency treatment to restore the heartbeat and breathing action include the use of bottled oxygen and mechanical resuscitators, and massage and electric shock treatment direct to the heart muscle. (*See* FIBRILLATION.)

A number of conditions can cause cardiac arrest. Drug poisoning is one, and if patients show any signs of toxic reactions to medications, the possible danger of an arrest should be prepared for. Patients with coronary conditions, as noted, should be suspect as liable to cardiac arrest. If necessary, any person suspected of developing an arrest condition should be watched scrupulously and monitored for heart action.

Two kinds or degrees of abnormal heartbeat (arrythmias) may change pumping action enough to adversely affect circulation: atrial *flutter*—partial irregularity of heart action; and atrial or ventricular *fibrillation*—completely uncontrolled, disorganized heartbeat.

Flutter or fibrillation in the action of the

upper chambers (the two atria) of the heart may affect circulation or they may not. But when these arrythmias are in the lower chambers, the ventricles, they can stop the pumping of blood to the brain and the rest of the body and cause immediate death unless resuscitation is started instantly. This emergency treatment must be maintained until the heart is beating effectively again.

Cardiogram. The record on paper which shows the force and form of the movements of the heart is called an electrocardiogram. (*See* ECG; ELECTROCARDIOGRAPHY.)

Cardiologist. Within the specialized field of medical practice called internal medicine, physicians active in the subspecialty of cardiovascular disease—disease of the heart and circulatory system—are called cardiologists (*See* CARDIOLOGY).

Physicians practicing in this field must not only know intimately the abnormalities of the heart and blood vessels, and be highly skilled in their treatment; they must also be thoroughly educated in the function of the heart and vascular system (physiology), in the detection and recording of sickness and symptoms of sickness involving the cardiovascular system or related to it (diagnosis), and in corrective steps whether they involve drugs, diet, surgery, a special regimen of living, or other methods (treatment).

Physicians are approved, for the practice of cardiology, by the Subspecialty Board of Cardiovascular Disease of the American Board of Internal Medicine.

Cardiology. In medicine, the scientific study of the heart, its functions, and diseases is known as cardiology, from the Greek *kardia*: heart, *logos*: word or reason. The practice of cardiology is a subspecialty of the specialized field of internal medicine. (*See* CARDIOLOGIST; HEART.)

The history of cardiology is interwoven with the entire history of science in both the Eastern and Western worlds. For an understanding of the heart, blood, and circulation ranks equally with an understanding of the substances of life on earth and an understanding of the bodies in the heavens as a prime goal of thinkers since the records of man have been written and preserved.

The names in this history are the names of scientific history: Hippocrates, Aristotle, Leonardo da Vinci, Paracelsus, Emperor Hwang-ti, Erasistratus, Galen, Andreas Caesalpinus, Michael Servetus, William Harvey, René Laennec, and Paul Dudley White.

Before the diseases of the heart, blood vessels, and blood could be understood, the heart, vessels, and blood themselves had to be understood. Cardiology was for many hundreds of years a long history of physiology, before it was joined to the medical treatment of the circulatory system.

EARLY CARDIOLOGICAL THEORIES. An early name in this record is Claudius Galenus or Galen of Pergamon, a Greek anatomist, physiologist, physician, and, at one time, team doctor to the Roman gladiators. He is thought to have lived from about 130 to 201 A.D. He was a determined, singleminded, and authoritarian physician and teacher who demanded—and widely received—the acceptance of his theories about the human body and its functioning, including the circulation of blood. His theories about circulation later were proved wrong.

According to Galen, the liver produced the blood, which did not circulate but ran here and there among the organs as needed. Yet Galen did discover correctly that the arteries carry blood, which was an advance over the earlier theory of such scholars as Erasistratus that the arteries carried "pneuma" or air. Still, Erasistratus, who lived four centuries earlier (born ca. 300–310 B.C.) in Alexandria, learned through dissection of bodies that the heart works like a pump and that there are tiny blood vessels--capillaries—connecting the arteries to the veins.

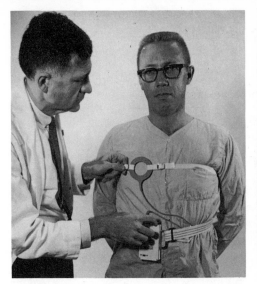 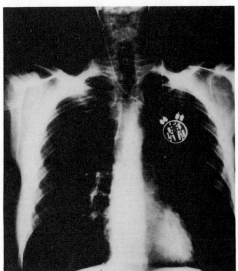

National Institutes of Health

The medical specialty of cardiology has produced many benefits for the patient with a heart problem. Here a cardiologist (heart specialist) at the National Heart Institute adjusts a battery-operated coil which sends impulses to a radio receiver implanted in the chest, as shown in the X ray. Wire electrodes from the implanted unit are attached to the carotid sinus nerves of the neck. The device stimulates the nerves that control the muscles of the heart responsible for the timing of the heartbeat.

TWO "FIRSTS," MANY HELPERS. Credit for the first discovery and description of how the parts of the human circulatory system are related and operate is disputed. There are many claimants, but among others Andreas Caesalpinus, or Cesalpino, of Italy and William Harvey of England both have solid bases for their claims. But much prior and contemporary work by others in explaining the heart and circulation must be seen as part of our total understanding of cardiology today. Among these were the following:

Leonardo da Vinci, 1452–1519, was the Italian genius who made excellent anatomical drawings, brilliantly anticipating the anatomies prepared from much later physiological studies.

Michael Servetus, 1509–1553, a Spanish theologian and physician, disproved Galen's ideas about circulation and showed accurately how the pulmonary circuit operates.

Andreas Vesalius, 1514–1564, a Flemish physician and surgeon, is called the father of modern anatomy. His anatomical studies resulted in drawings that, for the first time, correctly showed the details of the circulatory system. The anatomical methods he developed are still used today.

Marcello Malpighi, 1628–1694, an Italian physiologist and entomologist, founded microscopic anatomy and was the first to describe the complete circuit of blood in the human body.

Rev. Dr. Stephen Hales, 1677–1761, was an apparently adequate English theologian but also an innovative scientist who invented the manometer, the device still used to take the blood pressure. He used his first manometer in about 1708 to take the blood pressure of a dog, and subsequently took the pressures of other animals. For at least one pressure experiment on a horse he used a 1/6-inch brass tubing, inserted in the femoral artery (large artery in the groin that supplies the leg), and glass tubing of about the same diameter and nine feet high. This glass tube indicated the pressure in inches of height.

William Withering, 1741–1799, an English physician, was led to his famous writing on digitalis by his avocational interest in botany. He heard of a woman who cured dropsy with her tea made of twenty or so herbs, analyzed it, and found that its active ingredient was foxglove. His book on the medicinal plant, *An Account of the Foxglove*, was the first scientific discussion of the subject.

René Laennec, 1781–1826, a French physician, was forced into the invention of the stethoscope by the plumpness of a patient and the proprieties of his day. A rather heavy young woman, apparently suffering from a heart ailment, had come to him for examination of her symptoms. He was frustrated, though, in his attempts to examine her, first by the fat layer over her chest and, second, by his fear of the impropriety of the types of examination then used for heart sounds. The usual choice was either palpation (feeling with the hands) or percussion (thumping). He believed her bosom was no proper place for these methods, nor even for the only method of auscultation then used (listening with the ear pressed against the body). And so he rolled a sheet of paper into a cylinder, placed it against her chest, and heard what he needed to hear. Using the same principles he later went on to make a wooden version of his stethoscope. (*See* AUSCULTATION.)

Probably equal credit must be given to Andreas Caesalpinus and William Harvey as being the first to discover human circulation of blood. Still, there is some distinction between the work of the two.

Caesalpinus, 1519–1603, was an Italian botanist, mineralogist, physiologist, and physician. He knew well, apparently, how the circulatory system worked. He accurately described the capillaries and how they functioned in circulation.

William Harvey, 1578–1657, an English physician and anatomist who studied in Italy, undoubtedly knew about the extensive investigation and writing of the older Caesalpinus. After his innovative description of the circulatory system, Harvey went on to give mathematical proof of its functioning.

Other important individuals and events in the development of cardiology include:

• The modification of the mercury manometer for use in taking human blood pressure. This was the work of an Italian physiologist, Scipione Riva-Rocci, in 1906.

• The invention, by Sir James MacKenzie in 1908, of the polygraph for making chart recordings of the pulse. MacKenzie, a Scot, was a practicing physician.

• The invention of the electrocardiograph in 1906 by William Einthoven, a Dutch physiologist who won the Nobel prize for this achievement.

New developments during this period, however, were not limited to instruments. For example, Dr. James Herrick, a U.S. physician, stated in 1912 that the cause of a long-lasting severe chest pain was a kind of heart attack resulting from blockage in the coronary artery—a coronary occlusion.

PHYSIOLOGY AND MEDICINE WORK TOGETHER. A recurrent theme in these stories of the innovators of cardiology is the joining of the skills of the anatomist and the physiologist to those of the physician. As late as 1900 the medical and physiological aspects of the field now called cardiology were still separate. Medicine dealt with sickness, with abnormality; physiology concentrated on normal structure and conditions. In the twentieth century the two have finally merged.

In the four decades before World War II, cardiovascular medicine was developed as a successful means of treating heart and vascular diseases. The heart specialist, called a "cardiologist," became skilled in the technicalities of cardiac and vascular physiology as well as the technologies of a new battery of instruments—X rays, fluoroscopes, and electrocardiographs. Medications that successfully controlled or eased the effects of heart conditions came into general use, such as digitalis for failing heartbeat, nitroglycerine for severe heart pain, and quinidine for irregular heartbeat.

Since World War II, intensive research has made cardiology a highly developed medical specialty. The advances have come in all the major phases of the specialty, including physiology, biochemistry, surgery, pharmacology, and roentgenology.

Greater chemical control of heart and vascular disease is possible with the antibiotics to fight infections, such as those caused by the streptococci, and tranquilizers and relaxants to control blood pressure and ease serious hypertension. Better understanding of food chemistry and metabolism has led to radical changes in ideas about human diet—the prohibition or severe limiting of saturated fats and of carbohydrates. American society has moved a long way toward "outlawing" fatness as an inevitable and even allowably comfortable condition of life.

Another comparatively recent change has come in examining techniques. No longer must the cardiologist remain in the dark about the patient's exact condition. He can see the heart on X-ray film by means of angiocardiography, and the vessels by means of angiography. And cardiac catheterization allows him to examine the heart directly.

Today, continuing progress in cardiology, including surgery, makes possible the curing of more and more patients who would have been incapacitated or lost only a few years ago. Organ transplants, vascular transplants, and mechanical hearts have all been tried with some successes, some failures. Attempts to cure cardiac and vascular disease continue.

Cardiospasm. A spasm of the muscle fibers around the opening of the esophagus into the stomach is called a cardiospasm. (*See* STOMACH.) Cardiospasm should not be confused with achalasia of the esophagus. (*See* ESOPHAGUS; GASTROINTESTINAL SYSTEM.)

Carditis. An inflammatory condition of the heart is called carditis, from the Greek words *kardia* (heart) and *itis* (inflammation). (*See* HEART.) More specifically, this term usually is used to refer to an inflammatory heart condition that is one result of rheumatic fever. Since carditis affects all three heart layers—the inner layer, or endocardium; the heart muscle, or myocardium; and the outer layer, or pericardium—it is sometimes called *pan*carditis.

Rheumatic fever is a complex condition, often difficult to recognize, to diagnose, to treat, and to assess once it is over. It affects the patient in stages, to varying degrees and for varying lengths of time, and it may flare up again repeatedly.

There is an infectious organism involved in rheumatic fever, *Hemolytic streptococci,* but as far as medical researchers know now, it is involved only indirectly. The sickness that is called by the general term "rheumatic fever" may come two to four weeks after a streptococcus infection. It apparently is an extreme sensitivity to the organism itself, the strep germ. This is different from a sickness caused by the infectious processes of the germ.

The heart often is affected by rheumatic fever carditis in two stages, a first active stage and an inactive or later stage. The active stage of carditis may last long after the other signs of rheumatic fever are gone. Or there may be a serious effect on the heart although all other symptoms of the rheumatic condition seemed quite mild, if they were noticed at all. After the active stage has passed, the later condition of the heart may seem to bear no relation at all to the severity of the active stage.

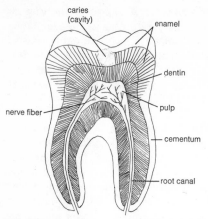

caries
(cavity)

enamel

dentin

nerve fiber

pulp

cementum

root canal

The arrow points to recurrent decay under an old filling. If such decay is not discovered, the pulp may become exposed. Infections and toothaches frequently result if the tooth is not treated.

Often rheumatic fever inflammation affects the outer layer of the heart, the pericardium, but this is the least serious type of carditis. The most immediately serious, because it causes the most deaths, is myocarditis, when the inflammation penetrates to the heart muscle itself. Yet this type does heal, and in most cases it leaves no permanent damage.

It is rheumatic endocarditis, inflammation of the heart lining, that ultimately is the greatest problem. Here the disease forms small nodules on the lining and heart valves. These heal but form scar tissue on which later infection can gain a foothold and cause serious, chronic heart trouble.

To treat rheumatic carditis conditions, the physician prescribes bed rest to guard against straining the heart during the active disease; penicillin to fight any live streptococci germs (although none may be present by then); aspirin-type drugs to reduce inflammation; and as many electrocardiograms, X rays, and blood tests as he feels necessary to keep a close watch on the condition of the patient's heart. Since the patient may have become even more sensitive than before to hemolytic strep, the doctor

may also prescribe a continuing course of penicillin to combat invading germs.

Caries. At least 98 percent of Americans suffer from caries—the scientific name for tooth decay or cavities at sometime during their lives. Tooth decay is almost as common as the common cold. (*See* TEETH.)

Decay starts in enamel, the hard, protective, outer covering of the tooth. Unless checked by dental treatment, decay spreads into the dentin, a softer, ivorylike substance forming the body of the tooth, and finally into the pulp, or tooth nerve. If decay is neglected too long, the tooth will be lost.

Overwhelming scientific evidence suggests that decay results primarily from the action of certain bacteria, always present in the mouth, on fermentable carbohydrates, especially sugar. The bacteria produce acids that can dissolve tooth structure. Whether the acids destroy the enamel depends partly on the strength of the acids and the length of time they are in contact with the tooth. There is some indication that the most damage is done in the first fifteen minutes after sweet foods are eaten.

Many other causes for tooth decay have been suggested—including malnutrition and emotional problems. But there is little scientific evidence to support any of these theories.

Teeth, like other organs of the human body, are intended to last a lifetime. With proper care they will. Sound care includes brushing teeth immediately after eating. To be effective, brushing must result in the cleaning of all accessible tooth surfaces. One suggested method is to brush your teeth the way they grow: down on the upper teeth, and up on the lower teeth. The chewing surfaces should be brushed with a scrubbing motion. Most people can clean their teeth adequately with a handbrush. Electric toothbrushes may make brushing easier. Your dentist can recommend the best brush for you.

In preventing tooth decay, what you do

eat is perhaps less significant than what you *don't* eat. A diet proper for general health is equally suitable for good dental health. While no way has been found to remove bacteria permanently from the mouth—although brushing will temporarily decrease the number of bacteria—sugar in the diet can be eliminated or at least greatly reduced. No harm to nutrition will come from cutting down on candies, jams, sweetened drinks, cakes, and cookies.

Routine dental checkups are also important if decay is to be controlled. Decay may start as soon as a child has teeth and may increase rapidly. Children should have their first dental examination between the ages of two and three years. After that, checkups should be made as often as the dentist recommends.

Early treatment is important for both the primary (baby) and the permanent teeth. The first teeth should remain in place—and not be lost due to neglected decay—until the permanent teeth are ready to come in.

Once a cavity has formed, the teeth can be restored only by removing the decayed part of the tooth and replacing it with a filling. A decayed tooth cannot repair itself. When tooth decay is treated early, restoring the tooth causes little or no discomfort. Less of the tooth will have to be removed than if a person waits for the danger sign of a toothache before going to the dentist. (*See* TOOTHACHE.)

The fluoridation of water supplies is now recognized as the most effective, practical, and economical method for reducing the high rate of tooth decay in entire communi-

Caries, or tooth decay, is one of the most common medical problems. Children as well as adults should have regular dental examinations. If caries is found, it should be treated immediately to avoid loss of teeth or other complications.

American Dental Association

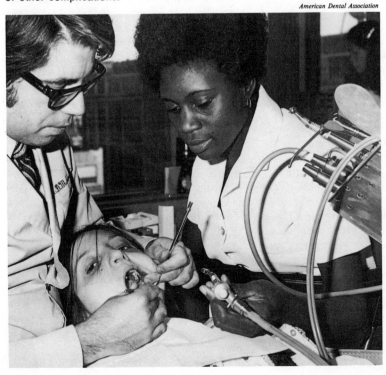

ties. Though the protective effect of fluoride is built into the teeth during childhood, the benefits last for a lifetime. Reductions of up to 65 percent in new tooth decay have been reported in communities in which ten-year studies on fluoridation have been conducted. Fluoridation of a community's water supply is the best way of helping to develop decay-resistant teeth. But children living in areas that do not have fluoridation can still obtain many of the benefits of fluoride by having a dentist or a dental hygienist apply topical fluoride solutions to their teeth.

Dental scientists are currently studying the possibility of developing a vaccine or some other immunization method against tooth decay. Animal experiments have shown some promising results, but scientists caution that it is much too early to predict just when such methods may become available for the treatment of humans.

Carotene. This is a yellow or red pigment found in foods, which the body chemically converts to vitamin A. Carotene is abundant in carrots, from which it derives its name. It is also present in high concentrations in sweet potatoes, milk, egg yolk, and certain green, leafy vegetables. In some foods, the color of the chlorophyll masks the yellow of the carotene.

In vegetables such as corn, there is more carotene and more potential vitamin A in yellow varieties than in white. (*See* VITAMINS.)

When a large quantity of carotene is present in the blood, the patient may show a pigmentation of the skin resembling jaundice. This condition is called carotenemia. (*See* CAROTENEMIA.)

Carotenemia. If you eat too much food containing the pigment carotene, you can get a yellowish tint to the skin, or carotenemia. The term literally means "carotene in the blood." (*See* CAROTENE.)

Carotene is found in carrots, oranges, egg yolk, squash, sweet potatoes, spinach, and other fruits and vegetables. The discoloration of carotenemia is due to secretion of the carotene through pores of the skin.

Carotenemia is harmless and will disappear if you cut down consumption of the food involved. But this condition may be confused with jaundice, a yellowing of the skin which may be due to serious blocking of the bile ducts or to liver damage. When in doubt, check promptly with your physician. Carotenemia is mistaken for jaundice so frequently that it is sometimes called pseudo-jaundice (false jaundice). (*See* JAUNDICE.)

The word carotenosis also is used to refer to the yellowing of the skin in carotenemia.

Carrier. A carrier is an apparently healthy person who is infected with some pathogenic organism, but who is at the same time immune to its effects, who accidentally transfers the organism to another person, who in turn becomes ill. (*See* CONTAGIOUS DISEASES.) A genetic carrier is a person whose chromosomes contain a pathologic mutant gene which may be transmitted to his or her children. In some conditions, a genetic carrier may be detected by an appropriate laboratory test or physical sign. (*See* GENETICS.)

Carsickness. Many children and adults experience nausea, dizziness, or vomiting as a result of riding in a car. This is known as carsickness, or motion sickness. The same symptoms may occur while riding in elevators or airplanes. (*See* MOTION SICKNESS.)

Cartilage. Another term for cartilage is gristle. It is a tough and flexible substance that is usually found in conjunction with the rigid tissue called bone. There are three general classifications of cartilage: hyaline, fibrous, and elastic.

"Hyaline" means glassy or transparent.

Hyaline cartilage is most commonly found covering the ends of bones at the joints. In this case it is also called articular (joint) cartilage. It is one of the parts of the joint that deteriorate in osteoarthritis. A type of hyaline cartilage is also embryonal—it is found in the unborn fetus and in the child and is a base for the later formation of bone. The ends of the ribs, which must yield in the breathing process, are composed of hyaline cartilage, as are parts of the nose, larynx, trachea, bronchi, and bronchial tubes.

"Fibrocartilage," as the name implies, is more fibrous than hyaline tissue. It joins certain bones together. It is the cushioning material of which the disks between the vertebrae of the spine are composed.

"Elastic" cartilage, like that of the external ear, springs back into position if it is moved. It also is found in the ear canal (auditory tube) and parts of the larynx and epiglottis.

Usually cartilage has a bluish cast, but as a person ages it may turn cloudy and become less transparent. Calcification, if it occurs in disease or in aging, tends to make cartilage harder and less flexible.

Unlike bones, cartilage contains no nerves, and seldom any blood vessels. (*See* BONES; JOINT.)

Cast.   A fractured (broken) bone is often immobilized in a plaster of Paris cast. The plaster in the cast is composed of calcium sulfate, produced by heating gypsum to 248° to 266° F. After the fracture is lined up, a tube of cotton stockinette is slipped on the extremity. This is well padded, then wrapped with strips of plaster dipped in water until the cast is thick enough to provide support. The plaster is then smoothed. The thickness required depends on the part of the body—an arm requires a much lighter cast than does a leg. A walking cast is made by putting a small rubber disk on the heel of a leg cast.

Casts should be kept dry because of the padding inside. If the skin under a cast be-

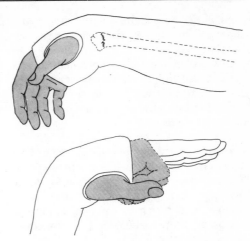

A cast for a broken wrist sometimes is extended above the elbow to prevent movement of the healing bones. Wrist casts permit movement of the fingers at all three joints.

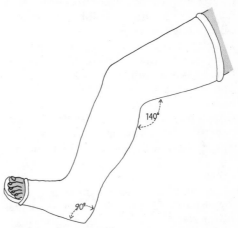

Casts must be properly placed so that fractures will heal correctly. When, for example, the bones of the lower leg (the tibia and fibula) are broken, the cast is extended above the knee and down over the foot. This prevents movement of the knee and ankle, which could strain or separate the healing bones. The knee and ankle are flexed (bent) at angles which best maintain good circulation.

gins to itch, the doctor may permit the patient to shake some powder inside the cast. The outside of a cast can be kept clean by wiping it with a damp cloth. It can be made even whiter by polishing with white liquid shoe polish diluted with water. An old, flesh-colored, nylon stocking slipped over a cast will make it less conspicuous and easier to put clothes on. It may be necessary when wearing a leg cast to slit the inner seam of trousers and replace it with a zipper or Velcro fastener.

Castor Oil. A popular cathartic, or laxative, is an oil obtained from the seed of *Ricinus communis,* and is known as castor oil. It is often given in combination with orange juice, which makes swallowing the castor oil more palatable. (*See* CATHARTICS; LAXATIVES.)

Castration. Loss of the testes at any time, with subsequent loss of some or all male sexual characteristics, is called castration. If the loss occurs before puberty it is called eunuchism. Results of castration depend upon the time of life in which the testes are removed. The condition is one form of hypogonadism. (*See* HYPOGONADISM, MALE; MALE HORMONES; TESTES.)

Catalepsy. When people are hypnotized, they often lapse into a state of "catalepsy." They will hold their body in any position in which it is placed, as will a jointed doll. (*See* HYPNOSIS.)

The condition also occurs among some persons with schizophrenia or other mental disorders.

The treatment of catalepsy depends on what has caused it. If the cataleptic person has been hypnotized, he will be released from the state as part of the hypnotic technique. If a mentally disordered patient lapses into catalepsy, the method of treatment will be determined by the nature of his disorder.

The word should not be confused with "cataplexy." (*See* CATAPLEXY.)

Cataplexy. Almost everyone has had the experience of receiving shocking news which makes him stop rigid in his tracks or drop his jaw momentarily. An extreme reaction of this type is called cataplexy.

The cataplectic person may be so shocked by a simple emotional experience (such as laughter) that his muscles go limp and he is unable to move for some minutes. He may just stare, or drop and lie motionless on the ground.

Some persons first have signs of cataplexy, then drop off to sleep (narcolepsy). The reasons for both conditions are unknown, but may be related to the control centers of that part of the brain called the hypothalamus. (*See* NARCOLEPSY.)

The word cataplexy should not be confused with catalepsy, a quite different condition. (*See* CATALEPSY.)

Cataracts. When the lens, a normally transparent portion of the eye, becomes opaque (nontransparent) the condition is known as a cataract.

The opacity may be very slight and stop the passage of only a small portion of light. Often, however, the clouding of the lens grows steadily worse, with progressive blurring of vision. If vision is entirely blocked by the opacity, the cataract is said to be mature.

There are various types of cataracts. One of the most common is the senile cataract, which seems to be a result of aging. Most people over the age of sixty have some degree of opacity of the lens, although it presents a critical problem only for a few of them.

Congenital cataracts are those present at the time of birth. They may be the result of a poisonous condition in the embryo. Some cataracts at birth are the result of the mother's illness with German measles (rubella) during the first three months of her pregnancy. (*See* GERMAN MEASLES.)

In the normal eye, protein fibers in the lens are transparent. In the formation of cataracts, the protein becomes chemically changed, or denatured, and gradually coagulates in spots which become opaque. Finally, the coagulated proteins receive deposits of calcium, and a further loss of transparency results.

DIABETIC AND SUGAR CATARACTS. Cataracts are a common complication of diabetes mellitus, a disorder of the body's utilization of sugar. The exact cause of the opacity is unknown.

In addition to the typical diabetic cataract, there are two other types of sugar cataracts. One is caused by high intake of galactose and the other by that of xylose, both types of sugar. (*See* DIABETES MELLITUS.)

The development of sugar cataracts seems to be more related to improper use of sugar by the body and the lens than to the amount of sugar consumed. High levels of certain sugars have been known to induce cataracts in laboratory rats, but there is no evidence that this same cause-and-effect relationship exists in a normal human.

However, we do know that a healthy lens must be properly nourished. So it follows that a well-balanced diet will help you keep the lens and the rest of your eye in its best condition.

OTHER CAUSES. Cataracts may also be caused by physical damage to the eye, by overexposure to X rays, by high doses of drugs such as steroids, and by consumption of poisonous chemicals. If you are taking medication, be particularly alert for changes in your eyes.

Although eyestrain is not good for the eyes, lots of reading, close work such as sewing, and watching motion pictures are not known causes of cataracts. Watching television is not a cause, either, unless you happen to sit too close to a defective color set which emits harmful radiation.

Heat, developed from infrared or microwave radiation, has been known to cause cataract. The intense heat of the infrared rays endured in some occupations has resulted in cataracts known as "glassblower's cataract." High-voltage electricity passing through the eye is another cause.

Cataracts sometimes occur in individuals with hormonal imbalances and thyroid disturbances, but a cause-and-effect relationship is hard to determine. Advanced and untreated glaucoma—an increase in fluid pressure within the forward part of the eye—may result in cataracts, but otherwise there is no connection between the two disorders. (*See* GLAUCOMA.)

SYMPTOMS OF CATARACT. Cataracts are usually bilateral. That is, they usually occur in both eyes at the same time. The individual with opacity will notice that he does not see as well as before and will experience varied blurring of images, but he will not have any pain and the eye will be without obvious signs such as redness or discoloration.

The opacities may easily be detected, however, by the ophthalmologist (eye specialist) through an instrument called an ophthalmoscope, which enables him to look inside the eye. Or he may use illumination by a slit lamp to see the signs of the cataract.

EXAMINATION AND TREATMENT. If opacities are detected the doctor will first try to correct any underlying disease or improper nutrition and halt the use of suspect drugs or chemicals. If the opacities are not too far advanced, he may simply ask the patient to return periodically to determine if the cataract is getting worse or remains unchanged.

The doctor may put eye drops into the eye when examining for cataract. These are mydriatic, which means that they dilate (widen) the pupil, the opening which controls the entry of light. The dilation makes it easier for the doctor to look inside.

The patient should understand that these drops are not treatment. Cataracts are not cured by eye drops.

Some people fail to have their eyes examined for cataracts or other possible problems because they have read an eye chart and found that their vision has an excellent 20/20 rating. These figures, however, show only the ability of the eye to see letters in focus at various distances; they give no clue to the blurring common to cataracts.

The treatment for an advanced or mature cataract is its removal. Whether a cataract not severe enough to cause blindness should be removed will depend in part upon the health and occupation of the patient.

One surgical method is to remove the lens with forceps. A newer technique, which often has fewer complications, is to use cryoextraction. This consists of making a surgical opening and inserting a metal instrument cooled to far below freezing. The lens freezes to the instrument and is gently pulled out. Another way to take out the lens is with suction, using an instrument called an erysiphake. An enzyme, alpha-chymotrypsin, is sometimes used to weaken the ligaments holding the lens in place and thus ease removal.

After cataract removal, eyeglasses are used to do the refracting (light bending) formerly done by the lens. These glasses have thick lenses, as considerable refraction is necessary. Contact lenses, which fit directly over the cornea, often are better. (*See* CONTACT LENSES; EYEGLASSES.)

Further suggestions on how to avoid cataracts are given in the article EYE CARE. For details on the relationship of the lens to other parts of the eye, and the way it focuses, see the articles EYE and EYESIGHT.

Catarrh. Inflammation of the mucous membrane with a free discharge of secretions, especially in the air passages of the nose and throat, is sometimes called catarrh. The term comes from a Greek word meaning "to flow down." The word is now rarely used as a scientific term. A physician will usually describe an inflammation in a specific place, such as the larynx (voice box) or pharynx (throat), as laryngitis or pharyngitis. When the inflammation is spread throughout the membrane lining of the upper air passages, it is called upper respiratory disease. (*See* NOSE; THROAT.)

Catatonic. When a person has a form of schizophrenia (a common mental illness) in which he exhibits phases of stupor and excitement, bizarre body postures, or periods of staring into space for hours listening to voices, he is said to be catatonic. (*See* SCHIZOPHRENIA.)

Cat Bites. When a child or adult is bitten by a cat, the wound should be treated immediately. (*See* ANIMAL BITES; CAT-SCRATCH FEVER; FIRST AID.)

Caterpillar Bites. There are many species of caterpillars throughout the world which, when touched, cause such a violent reaction that the victim believes he has been bitten. The resulting skin disease appears as a result of contact with the fine, bristly hairs covering the insect's body: each hair contains a toxic substance.

Aside from the inflammatory skin reaction and, in some cases, a true allergy reaction, the caterpillar hairs can cause other problems. When removed from the insect's body by a strong wind, these hairs float about in the air. If imbedded in the eye, they can cause conjunctivitis; if inhaled, they produce irritation and pain of the respiratory tract.

The most common example of the poisonous caterpillar found in the United States is the puss caterpillar. Located primarily in the Southern states, puss caterpillars become so numerous at certain times of the year that dermatitis epidemics result.

After contact with the caterpillar, symptoms of intense pain and itching develop. Red blotches followed by raised rashes then develop. The itching rash may last from a few hours to several days, depending upon the degree of exposure and the allergic reaction of the victim.

An old-fashioned remedy, ammonia, may help alleviate these symptoms, but if the reaction is severe, consult a physician.

When exposure has been heavy, the victim may have nausea, vomiting, fever, and swelling of the affected area. In many cases,

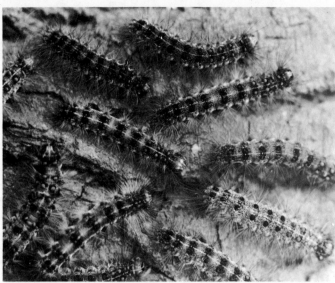

Furry or long-haired caterpillars are often the causes of a skin rash due to the toxic substances they secrete.

U.S. Department of Agriculture

if the exposed area is about the head and neck, the victim may develop temporary paralysis. These symptoms occur because of the system's rapid absorption of the powerful toxin secreted by the caterpillar.

Cathartics. Laxatives, especially those that act by irritating the bowels, are sometimes called cathartics. Habitual use of cathartics aggravates constipation. They should never be taken for abdominal pain.

Castor oil, Epsom salts, and cascara are among the most familiar cathartics, but phenolphthalein, the active ingredient in many trademarked candy and chewing-gum laxatives, is probably the drug most widely used today. One disadvantage of phenolphthalein is that it may cause skin eruptions.

Many people still think that a cathartic is good treatment for a cold, or for the common feverish illnesses of children. The fact is that the action of cathartic drugs tends to deprive the body of food and water that it badly needs, making the sufferer feel worse instead of better. Much more dangerous is the use of a cathartic when there is

abdominal pain. The pain may be due to appendicitis, and there is always the possibility that the appendix may burst, causing peritonitis, a dangerous and sometimes fatal infection.

Habitual users of cathartics often complain that they must take something in order to have a bowel movement. This is because the overstimulated bowel eventually loses tone and no longer responds naturally to the presence of waste material. (*See* CONSTIPATION; LAXATIVES.)

Catheter. Any tubular instrument that is used to drain fluid from a body cavity is referred to as a catheter. These tubes are usually made of rubber or plastic. The most common type of catheter is a urinary catheter (an indwelling type is a "Foley catheter"), which is passed through the urethra and into the bladder. (*See* BLADDER; URETHRA.) This catheter is then connected to a plastic bag which collects the urine drained from the bladder. The catheter must be sterile and must be inserted using sterile technique so that infectious bacteria will not be introduced into the bladder.

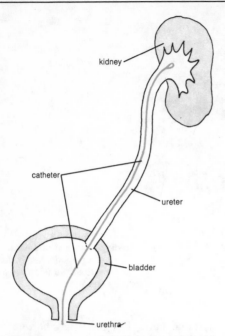

kidney

catheter

ureter

bladder

urethra

A catheter is a flexible tube that is inserted into the body for various purposes, such as to permit drainage or obtain a sample of a fluid. Here we see how a catheter is inserted through the urethra and bladder and upward through a ureter to a kidney.

Here is a catheter used to check blood and internal pressure within the heart chamber and its vessels. The catheter is inserted into the arm and pushed up through a vein to the heart.

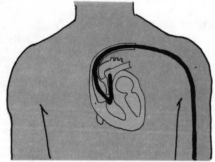

Cat-Scratch Fever. One animal-transmitted disease of which little is known is called cat-scratch fever. Caused by the scratch or bite of domestic cats, it is par-

ticularly dangerous because the cat does not appear to be sick.

Following introduction of the virus into the victim's body, symptoms appear in eight to twelve days. In most cases of cat-scratch fever, the disease is not attributed to the initial scratch or injury because of the long time between attack and illness.

When symptoms set in, the patient (usually a child) has a mild fever, swelling and pain of the lymph glands around the wound, aches and pains, and mild prostration. Redness and swelling appear at the site of the healed scratch or bite. This sign should be noted when describing the illness to a physician.

Treatment consists of bed rest during the most severe symptoms, and treatment with antibiotics. In mild cases, the disease runs its course in one to three months; in severe cases, deaths have been reported. (*See* ANIMAL BITES; RABIES; WOUNDS.)

Caul. The portion of the amniotic sac covering a child's head at the time of delivery is sometimes referred to as the caul. Most generally this sac breaks during labor, before the child is delivered. (*See* BAG OF WATERS.) If the bag does not break, the child is born surrounded by it.

Superstition once had it that a child born with a caul would never die by drowning.

Cauliflower Ear. Professional boxers and wrestlers sometimes have ugly malformations of the auricle, or outer part of the ear. Sometimes it looks more like a piece of cauliflower than an ear, hence the name. (*See* EAR.)

The cauliflower ear develops in this way: First an injury results in blood being drawn out of the blood vessels and collecting between the cartilage of the ear and the layer of tissue called the perichondrium.

The blood clot (hematoma) may continue to form for as long as a week if not treated. Then fibrosis, the growth of abnormal tissue, begins. New cartilage grows, making a permanent deformity.

The ear will follow this cycle every time it is injured, if treatment is neglected or inadequate.

Ice packs should be used as a first-aid measure for several hours after the injury to the auricle. This will not always prevent a hematoma from developing, but should limit its size.

Within a few days after the injury, the physician should draw out the blood from the hematoma with a hypodermic-like hollow needle. In some cases he may make an incision to permit drainage.

The ear should then be bandaged firmly with gauze. The pressure of the bandage prevents the area formerly occupied by the hematoma from again filling with blood or other fluid. Injections of antibiotics may also be given.

Removal of blood or fluid from the auricle should be performed only by a physician, as there is danger of infection. If the perichondrium is infected a serious, stubborn problem called perichondritis may develop. (*See* PERICHONDRITIS.) Any cuts or openings into the auricle, whether resulting from the injury or made by a surgical instrument, must be carefully disinfected.

Correction of a cauliflower ear, once it has developed, is a problem for a plastic surgeon.

In athletics, excellent helmets and other protective coverings are available to protect the ears. These can prevent injuries which might result in cauliflower ear. Unfortunately, children and athletes often neglect protecting their ears and ignore injuries, under the mistaken notion that the ear structure is not easily damaged.

Causalgia. Some weeks after even a minor injury to a nerve in a hand or foot, a sharp and persistent pain may appear in the area of the injury. This is called causalgia and may include reddening of the skin and local cold sweating. Sometimes the skin may become smooth, filled with watery fluid, and may lose its hair. Once in a while the skin may be warm, dry, and scaly.

The area also becomes very sensitive to touch, and the individual may become quite nervous in his effort to avoid such pain producers as movement, pressure of clothing, or even a breeze. In some cases the pain can be relieved with analgesic drugs until it disappears with time. But sometimes it will not go away unless the nerves to the painful area are cut surgically.

Causalgia and variations of the problem are sometimes called by other names, such as trophic edema, reflex dystrophy, or sympathetic dystrophy.

Cautery. The professional medical procedure called cautery (or cauterization) consists of burning off waste or defective tissue by means of actual heat or by electrical or chemical agents.

It is used to remove diseased matter from the skin or from the skinlike mucous membranes which line openings into the body. Growths called polyps, for example, may be removed from the passages of the nose or from the female cervix or uterus by cautery.

Cancerous growths are more often removed by surgery or radiation, or by drug administration, but in some cases cautery may be used.

Cauterization also has been used by doctors to stop hemorrhaging or severe bleeding from open wounds.

Cautery with electrical methods is termed electrocautery. When chemical means are used it is called chemicocautery, and techniques using heat are named thermocautery.

Cecum. The pouchlike structure at the junction of the small and large intestines is called the cecum, or blind gut, from a Latin word meaning blind. The appendix is an extension of the cecum. (*See* APPENDIX; INTESTINES.)

Celiac Disease. This disease should be distinguished from a complex known as the "celiac syndrome," which appears in varying degrees by signs and symptoms of malnutrition—foul, greasy feces, a distended abdomen, and secondary vitamin deficiencies. "Celiac disease," on the other hand, is a gluten-induced disease which affects the intestines. It is not known whether the basic defect exists in the body's enzyme activity or in an inborn error of metabolism, which accentuates or precipitates the disease when wheat or rye products are ingested, leading to difficulty in absorbing intestinal fat.

Celiac disease can be triggered by a variety of mechanisms. This includes ingestion of wheat or rye gluten, dietary deficiencies, chronic infections, and sometimes psychologic trauma. The disease is sometimes categorized as "starch intolerance," and expresses itself differently in different age groups. At the present time it is rare in the United States and Western Europe, probably because of improved nutrition and the low incidence of chronic infections. But the disease has been observed in caucasoid children of almost all national origins, though rarely in negroids and mongoloids. Both sexes have been equally affected, most patients being between the ages of six and eighteen months (though some symptoms may appear earlier). The disease rarely occurs after two years of age.

The symptoms of the disease include chronic or recurrent diarrhea, progressive malnutrition, and, in prolonged cases, whatever effects secondary deficiencies may cause. The feces are characteristically foul-smelling, bulky, and greasy.

An excellent treatment is the exclusion of wheat and rye gluten from the diet, and limiting the intake of fat. Patients then gain weight rapidly, and the nature of the feces improves. Relapses may sometimes occur during upper-respiratory-tract infections, or when dietary instructions are not followed.

It must be remembered that there are many other causes for malabsorption. (*See* MALABSORPTION SYNDROME.)

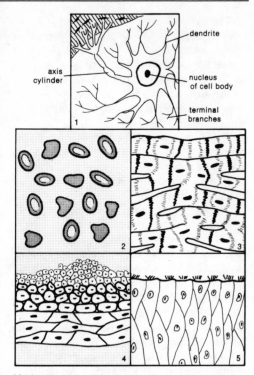

Various types of human cells are illustrated here. 1 is a typical neuron, or nerve cell, with its components. 2 shows some blood cells. 3 shows cells of heart muscle tissue. 4 is an example of epithelial tissue such as is found on the surface of the body.
5 is epithelial tissue from the intestinal lining, showing waving hairy projections called cilia which help sweep along the intestinal contents.

Cell. The basic unit of living creatures from which all tissues and organs are built is the cell. While all cells have certain characteristics in common, there are great degrees of diversity. Cells thus are specialized to form bone, blood, muscle, nerves, or skin. All cells are kept intact and protected by a membrane. Within the cell, fluids contain nutrients, reproductive capabilities, and all basic systems necessary for life.

Cells of the body reproduce by mitosis, whereby each cell splits in two. This is the process by which the original fertilized egg grows in size in geometric progression. Differentiation into the various systems of the body is controlled by chromosomal directions inherited from the two parents.

Cells together form tissues, and tissues in turn form organs. The study of cells is cytology. (*See* CYTOLOGY; ORGANS; TISSUES.)

Cellulitis. The skin infection known as cellulitis is similar to erysipelas, except that cellulitis is more severe and invades deeper tissues of the body.

Both diseases involve red, hot blemishes on the skin. Cellulitis may penetrate the lymph vessels. Treatment is similar to that for erysipelas. Antibiotics are used to fight the micro-organisms which cause the diseases. (*See* ERYSIPELAS.)

Orbital cellulitis is an infective problem of the eyelids, with redness and inflammation. It may be a complication of a sinus infection. The swelling may cause an outward bulging of the eye. In most cases the cellulitis promptly responds to treatment with antibiotics.

Cellulitis may occur in the mouth below the tongue, and the inflammation may spread and obstruct breathing passages. In serious cases the tissues must be opened up surgically for drainage, and emergency measures taken to keep air passages open. Antibiotics are used to destroy the infecting organisms.

Centrifuge. In medical practice and research it sometimes is desirable to break down a substance into its components so that these can be viewed under the microscope, measured, tested chemically, and observed in various ways. Imposing centrifugal force is an excellent way to break down or separate substances, such as the liquids and semiliquids common in medicine. A device for creating this force is called a centrifuge.

A common type of centrifuge for use in a physician's office or medical laboratory consists of a mount for whirling test tubes horizontally, powered by a hand crank or electric motor.

To analyze the blood sample taken in a doctor's office, for instance, a test tube containing the patient's blood is fastened into the mount and spun. (*See* BLOOD.) The centrifugal force throws the formed elements, that is, the white and red cells and platelets, down against the bottom of the tube. When the tube is taken out, the bottom will be filled with a dark red, sedimentlike substance, the compressed corpuscles and platelets. The upper part of the tube will be filled with a pale yellow liquid, the blood plasma.

Centrifuges also are used in medicine to separate other materials to be analyzed, such as urine.

Cerebellum. The part of the brain that is responsible for the coordination of body movements is called the cerebellum. (*See* BRAIN; NERVOUS SYSTEM.)

Cerebral. This is a descriptive word referring to the cerebrum, or upper brain. It is also used to refer to the brain in general. The cerebral cortex, for example, is the wrinkled outer layer of the cerebrum—the "gray matter" which enables us to talk, to think, to create. The term cerebral palsy, on the other hand, means a defect in muscle coordination resulting from damage to the brain, but the damage may be in the cerebrum, the cerebellum (lower brain), or elsewhere. (*See* BRAIN; CEREBRAL PALSY; CEREBRUM.)

Cerebral Palsy. The word "palsy" means a lack of muscle control. Cerebral refers to the brain. Thus a person with cerebral palsy has muscular coordination problems related to the brain.

Nearly all cases of cerebral palsy have their beginning before or during birth. The brain cells of the developing infant may be

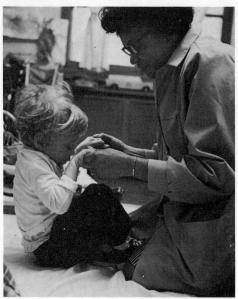

United Cerebral Palsy Association of Greater Chicago

A cerebral-palsied child receives the painstaking care needed to prepare these severely handicapped youngsters for happy, productive living.

damaged in various ways. Insufficient oxygen reaching the brain is one. It can occur during birth, such as when labor is prolonged, if there is pressure squeezing off the umbilical cord's supply of blood, or if any other difficulty occurs.

Such brain damage also may appear among children born of a mother who had German measles (rubella) during her pregnancy. (New German measles vaccines may reduce brain damage from this cause to a minimum.) Other virus diseases acquired by the mother before giving birth may also result in a child's having cerebral palsy.

Another cause is a blood incompatibility between mother and father, also called the Rh factor disease. Transfusions and other new methods have been used to reduce Rh factor problems and may make possible a reduction in the number of cases of cerebral palsy resulting from this cause.

Most of the cases of cerebral palsy are of the spastic type. This means that the brain damage results in tight, drawn muscles which make walking difficult and impair the use of arms and hands.

In the athetoid type, the patient's muscles jerk or move him involuntarily in various ways when he wants to hold still. In some patients these movements occur constantly.

Another is a rigid type of cerebral palsy in which the patient has muscles that do not respond with normal speed. Children having this condition move very slowly.

Ataxic cerebral palsy is characterized by a poor sense of balance. The patient falls easily and often. Tremors may be the only sign in some of these patients, but may be combined with other symptoms of cerebral palsy.

Along with these prominent symptoms may be an assortment of other difficulties such as speech problems, an awkward grin, and disturbances of hearing and seeing.

While there is no cure for cerebral palsy, early recognition of the disease will help many children train themselves to compensate for their handicaps. Special teachers, who understand the problems of the child with cerebral palsy, are employed by many school systems. They help the child train new muscles to do the jobs which the muscles under improper brain control cannot do.

Corrective exercises, braces, and surgery also help improve the child's ability to grow and adjust himself to the world about him. Eyeglasses and hearing aids also are a boon to those with cerebral palsy. Care must be taken by parents and friends not to complicate the physical problems of the disease by creating emotional ones. Cerebral palsied persons need to feel as wanted yet as independent as possible.

Drugs have been found to reduce some of the effects of cerebral palsy, such as muscle spasms and convulsions, but they cannot cure the disease. Research is being conducted to determine whether surgery on the brain itself may help. Experiments indicate that drugs may help the unborn or newborn baby use available oxygen more effectively, thus reducing oxygen deficiency brain damage.

At least a half-million persons, many of them still children, are afflicted with cerebral palsy. If you are planning a family, you can help reduce the chances of cerebral palsy and other complications by seeking good medical care and by reading the articles in this book on PREGNANCY and PRENATAL CARE.

Cerebrospinal Fluid. A protective cushion around the brain and spinal cord is the cerebrospinal fluid, sometimes called spinal fluid. It is a clear, colorless liquid derived from plasma—the fluid portion of the blood—and similar to it chemically.

The spinal fluid comes from two clumps of blood vessels called the choroid plexuses in open passages (ventricles) in the center of the brain, and from other vessels along one of the membranes lining the space around the brain and spinal cord. The fluid flows through the inner passageways around the brain and spinal cord, in the space between the membrane layers, and eventually is absorbed again into the circulating blood.

If the flow is blocked, so that the fluid cannot drain away, it produces a condition called hydrocephalus, in which there is dangerous pressure on the brain. (*See* HYDROCEPHALUS.)

Physicians use spinal fluid to help diagnose a number of diseases. They may measure the pressure of the fluid, withdraw a sample to test for infection or other abnormalities, or inject a dye or other substance into the fluid to aid in X-ray diagnosis of such problems as tumors and spinal injuries.

They may also inject a drug, such as procaine, into the fluid for spinal anesthesia. (*See* ANESTHESIA; BRAIN; SPINE.)

Cerebrum. The largest part of the human brain is the cerebrum. Its wrinkled gray outer layer—the cerebral cortex—makes up 80 percent of the volume of the brain. The complicated folds and wrinkles of the cortex permit a maximum surface inside a small space. If it were stretched out, the cortex would be about three feet long and two feet wide.

Down the midline, a curtainlike membrane divides the cerebrum into two halves—the cerebral hemispheres. Each hemisphere controls the opposite side of the body. In a right-handed person, the left side of the cerebrum is dominant, and some areas on this side are more developed. In a left-handed person, the right side is usually dominant.

The frontal lobes of the cerebrum, directly behind the forehead, are the most sophisticated part of the brain and the most recent in man's evolutionary development. This is the part of the brain with which we learn, remember, plan, reason, and make moral judgments. In the center is the motor area, which regulates muscles and movement. At the back is the sensory area, where sensations such as touch, pain, sound, and temperature are received and interpreted. (*See* BRAIN.)

Cerumen. The waxlike secretion found within the outer ear is known as cerumen, or earwax. (*See* EAR; EAR CARE; EARWAX.)

Cervicitis. Inflammation or infection of the cervix (the opening from the uterus to the vagina) is given the medical name cervicitis. (*See* CERVIX OF THE UTERUS.)

One of the most common problems of the female sex organs, cervicitis may occur to three women out of every four at some time during their adult years, or three of every five who have children.

One of the first noticeable symptoms of cervicitis may be the presence of blood in the vaginal discharge (*See* LEUKORRHEA), or some other change in its color, consistency, quantity, or odor. There may be pain in the lower back or middle abdominal region, as well as pain during menstruation, urination, or sexual intercourse. There also may be frequency and urgency of urination, or uterine hemorrhage (similar to heavy menstruation).

On examination, the family doctor or gynecologist will find ulceration and abnormal growth of cervical tissues, and odorous, thick, or blood-streaked cervical mucus. Tests also will show that the mucus has acidity and is injurious to sperm, often causing infertility.

Recurrent (chronic) cervicitis can be a major factor in spontaneous abortion (miscarriage) or infections after childbirth. It also can cause pain in the cervix during childbirth.

Chronic cervicitis also sometimes is a symptom of venereal disease (syphilis or gonorrhea) or tuberculosis of the uterine cervix. These possibilities must be checked carefully by the physician and treated if found. If you are more than twenty-five years old, he probably will take a smear test to check for signs of cervical cancer. (*See* PAP SMEAR TEST.)

Antibiotics usually are prescribed to treat sudden or severe cervicitis. This should be brought under control before the menstrual period begins, if possible, or the infection can spread upward through the uterus. If the menstrual period begins before the infection is brought under control, local surface treatment of cervical tissues is usually withheld until after it has ended.

If the uterus of a woman with chronic cervicitis becomes tipped backward, this helps cause repeated attacks and aggravates the condition by blocking normal circulation. Replacing and holding the uterus in its proper position usually can be achieved with a special instrument called a pessary in the vagina. This is a relatively painless, simple procedure that helps lessen the abnormal congestion of blood in tissues of the cervix and adjoining organs.

Warm douches of water-soluble vaginal creams or acetic acid (vinegar) may be prescribed. Be careful not to use any product that has not been specified by your doctor, or you might make the condition worse.

In mild cases, the cervical area may be cauterized (damaged tissues burned off and bleeding coagulated) with mild silver nitrate or sodium hydroxide solution at a time halfway between menstrual periods. Deeper infections may require surgical cauterization by a hot galvanic wire instrument or diathermy treatment.

Sulfa or hormone medications also may be given orally beginning just before the menstrual period. In extreme cases, surgical repairs or removal of part of the tissue may be needed. As a last resort, hysterectomy (removal of the uterus) may be performed. (*See* HYSTERECTOMY.)

Cervix. The word cervix originates from the Latin and means constricted or narrowed portion or neck. This is applied to a number of parts of the body and its organs.

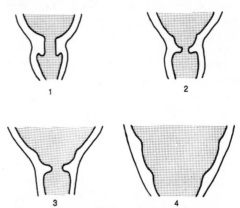

Stages in the stretching of uterine cervix during childbirth are shown above. (1) Cervical canal stretches open; mucous plug has already passed out of canal. (2) and (3) Thick walls of cervix begin to stretch thinner as baby's head pushes down from top. (4) Fully dilated, the cervical canal is ready for baby's birth.

When used alone, the term cervix usually refers to the lower outlet of the uterus (womb). This is the cylindrical section which normally is very small; it stretches large enough to permit the birth of a child at the end of each pregnancy, then shrinks again. (*See* CERVIX OF THE UTERUS.)

Less often, the word "cervix" is applied to the narrow outlet or neck of the bottom of the bladder, called the cervix vesicae. (*See* BLADDER.)

"Cervical vertebrae" are those spinal bones which are narrower and fit inside the neck of the body. There are seven of these. (*See* SPINAL CORD; SPINE.)

Cervix of the Uterus. The narrowed, cylindrical portion at the bottom of the uterus (womb) is called the cervix (neck) of the uterus, or often simply the cervix.

The cervix surrounds the opening at the bottom of the uterus. It projects into the top of the vagina through the front wall above the bladder. (*See* UTERUS.)

The supravaginal portion is located above and outside the vagina, between the rectum and the bladder. The vaginal portion is located inside the walls of the vagina.

The opening of the cervix has two lips, the front (anterior) and rear (posterior).

CERVICAL ANATOMY. The tissue of the cervix is not as thick as that of the rest of the uterus, but is highly flexible. The cervix normally resembles a small cylinder with the bottom opening almost completely closed.

Yet this small cervical opening stretches wide enough to deliver a baby's head at the close of pregnancy. Then soon afterward it tightens nearly shut again.

In the woman who has never borne a child, the opening in the cervix is a small slit, so small it barely permits passage of a probe (slender, flexible rod used for medical examinations). The lips are smooth and rounded, much like a small doughnut.

The cervical canal is about one inch long, running from its internal opening into the cavity of the uterus to its external opening into the vagina. It is narrower at the ends than in the middle of the cervical cavity.

Folds run lengthwise from top to bottom of the mucous lining inside the canal. Extra folds radiate from these, making the canal resemble a tree with branches. These folds and curves fit into each other so that the canal remains nearly closed.

After the first pregnancy, the radiating folds tend to disappear. The cervical canal and its outlet become wider. The lips are irregular and wrinkled in appearance, often with diagonal scars from tears during childbirth.

The lining of the cervix is a continuation from the endometrium inside the uterus, and is similar in composition. Called the endocervix, it is a mucous tissue which contains many compound racemose glands (resembling bunches of grapes). These secrete a clear mucus which fills the spaces remaining in the cervical canal and helps block out infection.

CHILDHOOD DISORDERS. A female child is occasionally born with an improperly formed cervix. For example, there may be a double cervix when the uterus is partially or completely duplicated.

In other rare cases the uterus (or a duplicate) may lack a cervix. If there is no uterine outlet into the vagina, the menstrual discharge, if any, accumulates inside the uterus and cannot be released.

Such failure to menstruate is more often due to a hymen completely closed over the vagina, whereas it normally has some opening. (*See* MENSTRUATION; VAGINA.)

Teen-age girls and women who have not been married or are virgins are subject to the same cervical problems as married women. Most infections of the female genital tract are rare among younger children and infants, however. Cancer of the cervix also is rare among little girls.

Gonorrhea in children also is different from that in adults and rarely affects their cervix. But children can acquire it from contaminated materials as well as directly from an infected person, such as during birth. (*See* GONORRHEA.)

INFECTIONS AND INFLAMMATIONS. Infections and inflammations of the cervix are called cervicitis. It usually is noticed because of a creamy discharge which is emitted through the vagina. But there may be spotting or bleeding after accidents or injuries. (*See* CERVICITIS.)

Spontaneous bleeding at other times usually is for different reasons. There should be laboratory tests of the secretions and tissues, as well as a physical examination to pinpoint the cause.

Bleeding between menstrual periods, after intercourse, or repeated hemorrhages commonly are due to cervical polyps. Other causes could be uterine, metabolic, or hormonal problems. Cancer of the cervix is less common than these. (*See* CANCER.)

CERVICAL POLYPS. Polyps may develop on the mucous membrane anywhere in the body. They resemble long or rounded lumps of tissue hanging from a narrow attached strip.

Cervical polyps are benign (noncancerous). Occasionally, however, certain types of cervical cancer may resemble a polyp, so the tissue must be studied carefully.

Polyps of the cervix are small and have red, smooth surfaces. There frequently are many of them at one time. They usually are found in a cervix where infection is chronic, but they also may be found when no infection is present.

Filled with many blood vessels, polyps tend to bleed from the tip. They are attached to the endocervix inside the cervical canal, but often are long enough to hang down outside the opening into the vagina.

Polyps may cause no noticeable symptoms at all, or there may be irregular bleeding, usually spotting, more noticeable just a few days before menstruation begins. There may also be leukorrhea, a creamy discharge. This can be worsened in such cases by intercourse or douching.

Sometimes the polyps are completely hidden and too small to be found easily. Even if they are found, examination must be thorough because other problems may be present at the same time. The polyps must be removed surgically.

Cesarean Section. The delivery of an infant through incisions in the abdominal

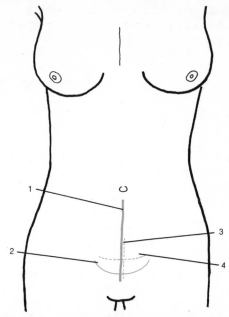

Classical cesarean section, which is used less often now, involves only one vertical incision as shown in the diagram. This goes directly through all layers of tissue from the abdominal skin on into the wall of the uterus itself.

In other cases there may be a series of separate incisions through the various layers of tissue involved. In the two-flap, or low cervical, cesarean section, three incisions are used: abdominal (1), peritoneal (2), and either a uterine longitudinal (3) or transverse (4).

In an extraperitoneal cesarean section, the incision through the peritoneal cavity is avoided by going below it through the tissues around the bladder. Thus there is only the abdominal incision (1) and a low transverse uterine opening (4).

and uterine walls is known as a cesarean section. Although cesarean section is not without hazard to both mother and child, it is used commonly in those cases where the child is too large (or the mother's pelvis too small) to permit normal vaginal delivery. On other occasions, illness in the mother or fetal distress makes delivery by cesarean section advisable.

Once a woman has had one child delivered by this method, subsequent children are usually born this way, thus not risking a rupture of her previous scar. However, normal vaginal deliveries are possible even though a woman has had cesarean deliveries.

Cesarean section can help prevent injuries to an infant during birth and thus improve his chances for survival. Often an obstetrician will wait until a woman has gone into labor before operating, rather than risk delivering a premature infant. (*See* CHILDBIRTH; LABOR; PREMATURE BIRTHS.)

Although the origin of the term is obscure, legend once had it that Julius Caesar was born in this way.

Chafing. When two delicate skin surfaces persistently rub against each other, or when a foreign substance rubs against the skin, it becomes irritated and "chafing" results. The skin is red, raw, moist, and painful. Secondary infections with bacteria and fungi may easily occur. (*See* FUNGUS INFECTIONS.)

Excess weight, tight-fitting or rough clothing, improperly fitted shoes, and irritating substances in contact with the skin are common causes of chafing. Babies may develop chafed skin from diapers; overweight women often experience chafing under the breasts and on the inner surfaces of the thighs. Other common sites of chafing are under the arms, in the groin, and between the fingers and toes.

Keeping the skin clean and dry is important in the management of simple chafing. The skin should be thoroughly dried after bathing, paying particular attention to chafed areas. Dusting powder and simple creams and ointments such as cold cream and zinc ointment will help to relieve chafing. More severe cases may require more active treatment with various medications. Antibiotics may be required if there is secondary infection.

To prevent recurrences of chafing, the underlying cause of irritation must be removed. For obese people this may mean losing weight. In other cases properly fitted shoes or a larger, looser garment may solve the problem. (*See* SKIN; SKIN CARE.)

Chancre. The first visible sign or symptom of syphilis is a sore known as a chancre, or hard chancre. It usually develops about three weeks after exposure at the site of syphilis infection. Since syphilis is most often contracted through sexual contact, the chancre is usually located on the genital organs. But it may be located anywhere on the skin or mucous membranes.

A typical chancre is a solitary, firm, elastic, painless nodule. Its borders are well defined when pressure is applied. The diameter is usually about one-fourth to one-half inch. The surface erodes and an ulcer develops. This primary lesion of syphilis slowly heals, but other symptoms of the infection, such as fever, persist. (*See* SYPHILIS.)

Another type of chancre, known as a soft chancre, develops on the genital area from infection with a pathogen different from the one responsible for syphilis. This infection, known as chancroid, is also contracted by sexual contact. Syphilis and chancroid infections are often contracted simultaneously. The soft chancre appears a day or two after the sexual contact. The sores are usually multiple, small, oval, soft, yellow-grayish pustules with slightly undermined edges and a reddened periphery. This bacterial infection responds quickly to antibiotic treatment. (*See* CHANCROID.)

Chancroid. A relatively uncommon venereal disease characterized by small skin lesions, ulcers, and inflammation of lymph glands, is called chancroid. It usually is spread by sexual intercourse. For a more detailed description, *see* VENEREAL DISEASE.

Chapping. When the skin becomes excessively dry, reddened, rough, and cracked, the condition is called chapping.

The primary cause of chapping is dehydration, or loss of moisture from the outer layer of the skin (the epidermis). Dehydration causes loss of flexibility and considerable brittleness, which leads to cracks—the condition commonly referred to as chapped skin.

This problem usually occurs when there is a sudden drop of humidity, as in cold weather, because in a cold, dry atmosphere the outer layer of skin loses water to the air.

Frequent contact with water, incomplete drying of the skin, as well as excessive use of soaps, detergents, and other chemicals may alter the outer layer so that its water-holding capacity decreases, and chapping results. Inflammation of the skin may follow chapping when these conditions are not corrected promptly.

Some people, especially the elderly, are particularly susceptible to chapping because their oil glands and sweat glands are not as active as they used to be.

Chapping can be counteracted by restricting the frequency of washing, exercising special care to dry the skin after bathing, and limiting the use of soaps and detergents. Women should wear protective rubber gloves for household tasks requiring the hands to be in water.

The liberal use of lubricating (emollient) creams and lotions which hinder evaporation of water from the skin is very helpful.

Lips are especially vulnerable to chapping because their sensitive surface is frequently moistened. They should be protected with a coating of lipstick, chapstick, cold cream, or petrolatum before going out in the cold.

Proper humidity control in the home helps to counteract the excessively dry air which contributes to chapping.

If chapping does occur, the affected area should be protected from infection. Cracks in the skin may be treated with a mild ointment such as cold cream or petrolatum. If the irritation is prolonged, a doctor should be consulted. (*See* DRY SKIN; SKIN; SKIN CARE.)

Charley Horse. When the major muscle (the gastrocnemius) forming the back or calf of the leg is torn, a condition known as a "charley horse" develops. If the strain involves a tear in the back of the heel or in the Achilles tendon, the condition is called "tennis leg" or "golfer's leg."

Many leg cramps occur during the night and are quite painful. Most victims of nocturnal "charley horse" cramps are women. The most common causes of night cramps are improper shoes, pregnancy, osteoarthritis, and a disease known as Moenckeberg's sclerosis. This form of sclerosis develops calcium deposits on the artery walls, thus slowing down the flow of blood.

Immediate treatment begins with gentle massage above and below the sore area. Ice packs on the affected muscles will help eliminate swelling and reduce pain. As this is a sprain, it should be treated like one. (*See* SPRAINS.) If severe pain persists, see your physician.

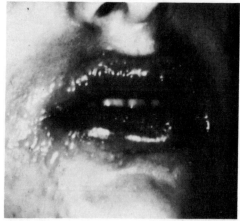

J. B. Kahn

Cheilosis is a condition in which the lips and sides of the mouth are marked by fissures (cracks) and dry scaling. Vitamin B deficiency, a habit of repeatedly licking the lips, or a fungus infection can be a cause.

Cheilosis. A condition marked by dry scaling and fissuring of the lips and corners of the mouth is called cheilosis or cheilitis. The corners of the mouth first become inflamed. Then cracks and fissures, which usually become infected and bleed, occur in this area. The lips themselves may become similarly affected. Cheilosis occurs in several, disorders, but is most commonly associated with deficiency of riboflavin (vitamin B₂). (*See* VITAMINS.)

Chemical Burns. Burns produced by contact with chemicals resemble those produced from boiling water and fire. They may range from mild first-degree burns, with irritation, redness, inflammation, and swelling, to severe third-degree burns, with permanent destruction of tissue and even death. The severity depends on the chemical producing the burn and the length of time it remains in contact with the skin.

Strong acids and alkalies are most often responsible for chemical burns. Some examples are ammonia, sulfuric acid, hydrochloric acid, phenol, sodium hydroxide, and potassium hydroxide. These chemicals are widely used in industry and are found in many household products. Some are incorporated into cosmetics, especially hair treatment preparations. Doctors use solutions of certain acids to remove skin growths such as warts and keratoses.

Chemical burns are a particular hazard in industries where caustic chemicals are utilized; employees should be careful to follow the posted safety procedures for handling such chemicals.

Many products found in the household, especially corrosive cleaners such as oven cleaners and drain cleaners, lye, and similar products, contain caustic chemicals capable of producing chemical burns. It is advisable to check the labels of all household products for cautionary statements regarding potential dangers and proper use. Such products should absolutely be kept out of the reach of children. A child may pour the product on his skin and suffer a severe skin burn; worse yet, he may drink the product, severely burning the mouth, esophagus, and stomach lining.

Certain hair preparations, while safe under normal conditions of use when directions are followed, may produce chemical burns if allowed to remain on the skin (or scalp) for too long, or if not properly diluted before use. These products include certain hair straighteners, hair bleaches, and chemical depilatories. Any product that changes or destroys hair is also capable of destroying skin, as both are composed of the same material, keratin. When such products are used, the directions should be carefully followed as to proper dilution, length of application, and other precautions the manufacturer may recommend.

If a chemical burn does occur, the skin should be rinsed at once with copious amounts of running water. If the eyes are affected by a chemical, they should be thoroughly rinsed by spraying or pouring water into them; this may require assistance, as the individual may not be able to hold his eyes open because of pain. First aid for chemical burns is the same as for other burns. A doctor should always be consulted as soon as possible. (*See* BURNS; FIRST AID.)

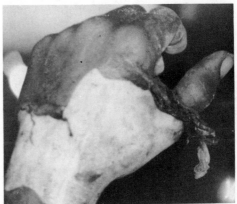

Walter Reed Army Institute of Research

Gasoline burns.

Chemical Warfare. Although chemistry has long been used in military science, in the twentieth century chemical action has been combined with the physical energy of bullets and explosives. The chemical agents used in this specific type of warfare are called war gases, smokes, and fire producers (incendiaries).

Each chemical weapon is classified according to its primary physiological effect on the human body—that is, the immediate result, not secondary complications or after effects. The severity of injury is proportional to strength of dosage (concentration of chemicals) and length of exposure.

There are many types of chemical agents used to make gases, smokes, and incendiaries:

1. Choking gases are lung irritants which affect the respiratory system and often cause death. They cause inflammation of the bronchi, trachea, and lungs. Examples of choking gas agents are chlorine, phosgene, and diphosgene. The effect on the body lasts from several minutes to three hours; the gas remains effective in the air for less than ten minutes.

2. Blister gases are known as vesicants because they cause the skin to blister. These gases cause injury to any part of the body that comes in contact with the liquid or vapor. Inflammation, burns, and tissue damage follow external or internal contact with no immediate pain or effect on the body. (See MUSTARD GAS.)

3. Sneeze gases, often called irritant smokes, are released into the air in particles which cause sneezing, respiratory pain, and mental depression when inhaled. Although the effects are severe (twelve hours) there have been no deaths reported from their use. Mechanical filters used in a gas mask canister offer protection.

4. Blood gases, or systemic poisons, are chemical agents which act on the heart or nerve reflexes or interfere with the absorption and taking in of oxygen. Carbon monoxide, hydrocyanic acid, and cyanogen chloride have not been effectively used for war purposes because the chemical agents are too light to remain in the air long enough to be effective. (See NERVE GAS; TEAR GAS.)

Chemotherapy. The use of chemical compounds in the treatment of disease, especially cancer, is called chemotherapy. (See CANCER.) It would seem that this type

of therapy ought to be the best weapon against tumor cells, since chemicals seek out these cells wherever they are in the body. Unfortunately, this is not the case. The search for chemical agents that will concentrate themselves only in tumor masses and destroy the cancerous cells is intense. Several good drugs are in use today. In general, however, chemotherapy is disappointing and often merely resorted to as a last effort after surgery and radiotherapy have failed. (See RADIOTHERAPY.) Very good results have been reported in certain cancers when surgery, radiation, and chemotherapy all are used.

There are several different categories of chemotherapeutic agents. Each type has a different effect on the cells. Generally, however, these agents are effective because they interfere with the internal mechanisms and reproductive processes of the cell. But they also influence normal cells and tissues. Particularly sensitive to these drugs are the cells of the bloodstream and bone marrow (blood platelets and white blood cells).

An important difference exists between tumor cells and most normal body cells, which makes the tumor cells more liable to be damaged. Tumor cells divide (multiply, reproduce) almost constantly. That is, a large fraction of the cells in a tumor will be dividing at any given time. Normal cells, in contrast, have quite long periods of time during which they rest. Most of the chemicals used affect the cells during the time of their reproduction process. Therefore, tumor cells are more vulnerable to the effects of chemotherapeutic drugs than are normal cells. The problem is that it is difficult to eradicate every single tumor cell because at the time the drug is given some, even a few, of the tumor cells will be resting and therefore not vulnerable.

There are basically five groups of anti-tumor drugs now in use: (1) alkylating agents, (2) anti-metabolites, (3) hormones, (4) antibiotics, and (5) miscellaneous drugs. The following discussion will outline these groups, their characteristics, and provide a few examples of each group.

ALKYLATING AGENTS. These drugs act upon cellular compounds which are necessary for the life of the cell. Cellular enzymes and DNA are especially damaged. (*See* DNA.) Normal cells usually damaged are those of the bone marrow, the lining of the intestine, and the hair follicles (hair roots). Among these drugs are nitrogen mustard, cyclophosphamide (Cytoxan), and phenylalanine mustard (Alkeran).

ANTI-METABOLITES. The action of these drugs is primarily dependent on interference with the production of DNA, by blocking the action of an enzyme on one of the essential constituents. The anti-metabolite chemically resembles the normal constituent, and displaces it in combination with the enzyme. Thus the essential reaction is not completed. Commonly used drugs in this category are methotrexate, 6-mercaptopurine, 5-fluorouracil, and cytosine arabinoside.

HORMONES. These agents have been used for many years for treating carcinoma of the breast and prostate. Usually they are prescribed after surgery has failed or in cases where the tumor is too advanced to be surgically removed. The exact effect of hormones on cancer cells is unknown, but hormones are most effective against tumors that have arisen from organs normally influenced by hormones. Included in this group are estrogens (diethylstilbestrol), androgens (testosterone compounds), progestins (progesterone derivatives), and various steroids (e.g., Prednisone).

ANTIBIOTICS. Several of these anti-bacterial drugs have been used to treat cancer. The results have generally been poor. A few of these drugs, however, have been useful against specific tumors. Actinomycin D interferes with cell reproduction. It has been used effectively against choriocarcinoma and Wilms' tumors in children. Mitomycin C is the only chemical agent discovered so far which has good activity against stomach cancer. Mithramycin has been shown to be highly effective against one form of cancer of the testis. Daunomycin is sometimes used to treat acute leukemia. Bleomycin is a drug first developed in Japan, but now being used in this country against a variety of cancers.

MISCELLANEOUS DRUGS. Procarbazine is a chemical useful against Hodgkin's disease, ovarian cancer, and one type of cancer of the lung. Vincristine may be useful in arresting acute leukemia, lymphoma, some breast cancers, and Wilms' tumor. Vinblastine, similar to vincristine, has been used against lymphoma, choriocarcinoma, and breast cancer. A chemical agent abbreviated DTIC is the only drug known to be effective against melanoma. One of the acute leukemias has been shown to respond to an enzyme called L-asparaginase.

The use of chemotherapy alone has been generally ineffective in curing people of their cancers. Usually the physician resorts to this form of therapy after surgery and radiotherapy have failed. There are, however, a few kinds of tumors in which chemotherapy has sometimes rendered a complete cure. Among these, choriocarcinoma is a prominent example. Great progress has been made recently in the treatment of this tumor using methotrexate, actinomycin D, and vinblastine. By administering actinomycin D in combination with radiation or vincristine, several investigators have cured cases of Wilms' tumor. Burkitt's lymphoma has also been cured using cyclophosphamide. An occasional cure of acute lymphocytic leukemia has been reported using prednisone and methotrexate.

(For complete descriptions of these cancers, see CANCER and the specific tumor in question.)

Chemotherapy, much like radiotherapy, has some serious side-effects. (*See* RADIOTHERAPY.) Most of these are a result of drug damage to normal cells of the body. Among the side-effects is a decrease in the number of white blood cells and blood platelets. White blood cells normally act to ward off bacterial invaders, thus various infections can occur in people treated with these drugs. Blood platelets are part of the normal blood-clotting mechanism. Patients treated with some of these drugs may therefore bleed or bruise easily. The hair follicles of the body are easily damaged by many of these agents, thereby causing hair loss (alopecia). Fever is a general response brought on by many of these chemicals. Nausea, vomiting, and diarrhea are frequent side-effects. The nervous system can also sometimes be damaged, causing blindness, brain disorders, and nerve palsies.

In summary, some complete cures are possible using chemotherapeutic agents. More often, patient benefit results from an increase in survival time and from decreased discomfort. Chemical agents can also sometimes diminish the severity of disorders which affect the body's biochemistry, and which result from chemicals produced by the tumor (paraneoplastic syndromes). (*See* CANCER.) New chemotherapeutic drugs are now being sought. Perhaps one of them will furnish the long-sought cure for cancer.

Chest. The section of the body from the neck down to the bottom of the rib cage, containing the heart and lungs, is the thorax or chest. The skeleton of the chest is comprised of the thoracic vertebrae at the back, the ribs, and the sternum, or breastbone. This skeleton provides rigidity for the body's upright position, offers protection to the internal organs, and aids in the breathing process. (*See* BREATHING.)

The chest is lined by the parietal pleura, which aids movement of the lungs. This membrane also lines the lungs and the heart. (*See* PLEURA.)

The heart is comprised of four chambers, with two auricles and two muscular ventricles. (*See* HEART.) The major blood vessels enclosed within the chest are the aorta, the pulmonary arteries, the pulmonary veins, the precava, and the postcava.

Most of the respiratory system lies within the chest. The tough trachea brings air into the chest and continues on until it splits into two bronchi. The bronchi then enter the lungs and end in bronchioles. The bronchioles in turn end in the alveoli, the individual units of the lungs where air is taken up by capillaries and carried throughout the body. (*See* LUNGS; RESPIRATORY SYSTEM.)

The only organ in the chest that is outside the circulatory and respiratory systems is the esophagus, which transmits food to the stomach.

The chest proper ends with a muscular, tough membrane called the diaphragm, which separates the thorax from the abdomen and aids in breathing.

Cheyne-Stokes Breathing. Periods of loud, difficult breathing interrupted with periods of breathlessness are known as Cheyne-Stoke breathing or respiration. It is often seen in patients with cerebral arteriosclerosis, senility, heart disease, and other conditions. (*See* LUNGS; RESPIRATION.)

Chickenpox. Varicella is another name for chickenpox, one of the most common diseases of children. It is caused by a virus and transmitted from one child to another by nasal droplets or by the moist crusts that fall off the skin eruptions.

Shingles is a closely related disease. This usually infects adults rather than children, and is also caused by the varicella virus or one very much like it. (*See* SHINGLES.)

The typical rash of chickenpox appears on the child's skin within two or three weeks after exposure to the virus. Reddish areas appear, smaller than a dime, each with a blister in the center. They are usually seen on the trunk, face, and scalp, but sometimes elsewhere on the body, such as the eyelids or the membranes lining the openings to the nose and throat.

The skin outcroppings may be preceded by a day or two of fever, poor appetite, headaches, and restlessness. Special care should be given to older children in poor physical condition and to babies who contract chickenpox.

Chickenpox nearly always is mild and complications are rare. But heed this warning: if your child has been given corticosteroid treatments for any reason, call your physician at once when any signs of chickenpox appear. The disease can have severe complications in children who have been taking this type of medication.

The tiny chickenpox blisters itch, and hardly any child can resist scratching them thus spreading the infection. A pair of mitts (be sure they are clean and sterile!) over the hands of small children or infants will help keep eager fingernails from tearing away at the skin lesions. Cutting the fingernails short also is effective.

Calamine lotion or other salves or powders may be suggested by your physician to soothe the itching. If the eruptions are complicated by bacteria, other medications may be advised.

As the blister is scratched off or falls off from rubbing, it leaves a small open sore, which soon dries into a crust. New eruptions appear in groups while the earlier spots are drying and flaking off.

Permanent scarring from chickenpox seldom occurs unless other infections take hold in the open sores. You can reduce this risk by keeping the child's hands and body clean with mild soap and water. This precaution also will help reduce the chances of spreading the disease to others. Adults may break out with shingles on exposure to a child with chickenpox.

The contagious period for chickenpox lasts about ten days, starting about one day before the first spots are noticeable, and continuing until new ones stop appearing. The skin sheddings no longer can transmit the virus when the sores cease being moist and are dry and flaky.

When your child has chickenpox he should be kept isolated until the spots dry out. As long as he has a temperature, he should be kept quiet and in bed. He may

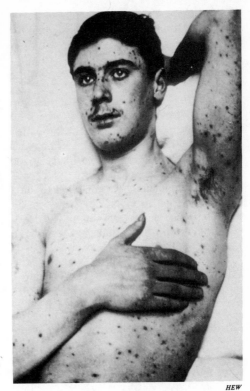

HEW

A severe case of chickenpox.

be given showers or tub baths, but should be guarded against chills.

Chickenpox is what doctors call a self-limiting disease. It runs its course within a week or two. Rarely, there may be serious complications such as pneumonia or encephalitis.

Chigger Bites. The larva of a tiny mite causes the red itching rash called chigger bites. The mites belong to a group of tiny insects which inhabit grass and other plants. Identical or similar insects are called harvest or grain mites.

The mite larvae may attach themselves to the parts of the body they reach first, such as ankles, legs, and bare arms, or they may move unnoticed to moist areas, such as between the thighs or the pubic region.

They inject an enzyme into the skin which has a digestive action to convert tissue and blood to a form acceptable to the chigger's special appetite. After feeding for up to four days or so, the chigger will drop off. The enzymes produce an itch. In allergic persons, the red eruptions can be quite severe.

Prevention is the best remedy, for there is little that can be done to stop the mite feeding cycle once it has begun. So-called repellents should be applied to clothing and to the skin whenever one is likely to be exposed to chiggers. The commercial products available usually do not repel the larvae, but poison them. Some of them contain benzyl benzoate, diethyltoluamide (deet), ethyl hexanediol, and dimethyl phthalate, most of which also repel mosquitoes.

Calamine lotion will soothe the itching skin. In severe cases with many chigger bites, ACTH, steroids, or antihistamines may be used. (*See* CALAMINE LOTION.)

Chilblains. Sometimes red, itchy eruptions occur on the skin from exposure to the cold, but without actual freezing of the tissues. This is known as chilblains, or pernio.

There may be blistering of the skin, edema (a collection of fluid in the area of swelling), and ulcers. Most chilblains yield to simple measures and go away, but if the same area is repeatedly exposed to cold, there may be permanent damage to the skin.

Chilblains occur mostly on the hands, feet, arms, or legs. The affected extremity should be elevated slightly and permitted to warm up slowly at room temperature.

Never massage chilblains or apply heat or cold packs. Irritation may lead to infection. If you are subject to chilblains, keep the vulnerable parts well protected when outside in the cold, and go inside occasionally to warm up. (*See* FROSTBITE.)

Child Behavior. If a child's emotional as well as physical needs are being met, he will be happy, healthy, and reasonably well behaved regardless of his age or the size of the family. If the child has a need that is not being met, he will (unintentionally) resort to whatever techniques he hits upon that come closest to fulfilling that need. (*See* FAMILY PROBLEMS.)

Physically, a child should have a well-balanced diet which is adequate to meet, but not to exceed, his personal physical requirements. (*See* NUTRITION.) He needs enough sleep, relaxation, and exercise to suit his needs and limitations. He should have periodic physical, dental, eye, and ear examinations, and corrective treatment when needed. (*See* CHILD HEALTH.)

Intellectually, a child needs the opportunity to express himself in a great variety of ways. Then he can find the one that best suits his own unique talents and interests. Emotionally, a child needs love and affection expressed openly by himself, by both parents, and by other children toward him and each other. He needs positive reassurance that he is still loved even when he is being punished. He should know at all times that you trust him and expect good behavior. Research shows a child will live up to the best or the worst that his parents (or teachers) expect of him.

Parents should discuss and agree on basic rules and bounds for behavior. This will help the child, and will help them too by

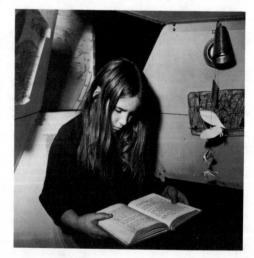

clarifying their own roles in guiding him. These rules should be enforced firmly and consistently, with punishment suitable to the nature of each problem. Don't threaten punishment and fail or forget to make good on it. Rules are meaningless if nothing happens when they are broken. Both parents should cooperate in this discipline as partners bearing equal responsibility. But they should be fair to the child and willing to discuss a problem honestly and reasonably.

Do not overreact to a situation, or punish severely for normal childish forgetfulness. And do not expect too much of a child. Do not ask a child to do something that one of his parents could not normally do (unless the parent has a physical handicap). Remember, he will form habits like his parents', no matter how severely you lecture or punish him. If one parent has temper tantrums or fits of anger or hostility—expressed or deliberately withheld—the child will also have these reactions. You cannot keep them secret; he will "feel" and react to the emotional tension.

If you do not express your approval of his good behavior, the child will never know you approve. If you tell him only what is wrong with everything he does, he will think everything he does is wrong, and

become discouraged and despondent. Always be honest and sincere, and point out to your child those ways in which he has improved. If you always express your approval first, he will not mind a few gentle suggestions for further improvement.

Give him the freedom and experience of gradually doing new things on his own, and don't constantly pick at him about details. Don't assume he knows what you mean, because he won't!

Emotionally, a handshake or pat on the back is good, but it is not always enough. There is nothing wrong with a father or mother giving a warm hug or kiss to a child, or to each other while the child is watching. If you have difficulty expressing affection, start practicing now or while your child is small—and don't stop when they grow older.

If this kind of normal family affection is always forbidden or confined to secrecy or the bedroom, your child may grow up mistakenly thinking that sex is the only means of achieving emotional satisfaction. When that child needs emotional reassurance during normal adolescent development, he or she is likely to make the mistake of seeking sexual gratification instead. (*See* TEEN-AGER.)

Brian Cara, Avery Coonley School, Downers Grove, Illinois

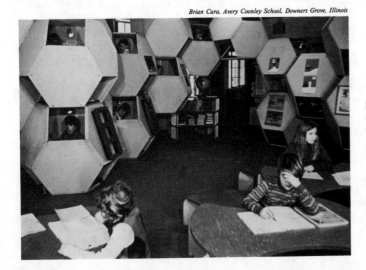

New learning spaces called polyhedrons, designed for this Illinois private school, allow a child to learn at his own pace. Results of this experimental classroom setup showed that students studied harder, their attention spans lengthened, and their work became more original.

Typical Behavior of Children Up to Age Six

Average Age	Question	Average Behavior
3–6 months	What does he do when you talk to him?	He awakens or quiets to the sound of his mother's voice.
	Does he react to your voice even when he cannot see you?	He typically turns eyes and head in the direction of the source of sound.
7–10 months	When he can't *see* what is happening, what does he do when he hears familiar footsteps . . . the dog barking . . . the telephone ringing . . . candy paper rattling . . . someone's voice . . . his own name?	He turns his head and shoulders toward familiar sounds, even when he cannot see what is happening. Such sounds do not have to be loud to cause him to respond.
11–15 months	Can he point to or find familiar objects or people, when he is asked to? ("Where is Jimmy?" "Find the ball.")	He shows his understanding of some words by appropriate behavior; for example, he points to or looks at familiar objects or people, on request.
	Does he respond differently to different sounds?	He jabbers in response to a human voice, is apt to cry when there is thunder, or may frown when he is scolded.
	Does he enjoy listening to some sounds and imitating them?	Imitation indicates that he can hear the sounds and match them with his own sound production.
1½ years	Can he point to parts of his body when you ask him to? ("Show me your eyes." "Show me your nose.")	Some children begin to identify parts of the body. He should be able to show his nose or eyes.
	How many understandable words does he use—words you are sure *really* mean something?	He should be using a few single words. They are not complete or pronounced perfectly but are clearly meaningful.
2 years	Can he follow simple verbal commands when you are careful not to give him any help, such as looking at the object or pointing in the right direction? ("Johnny, get your hat and give it to Daddy." "Debby, bring me your ball.")	He should be able to follow a few simple commands without visual clues.
	Does he enjoy being read to? Does he point out pictures of familiar objects in a book when asked to? ("Show me the baby." "Where's the rabbit?")	Most two-year-olds enjoy being "read to" and shown simple pictures in a book or magazine, and will point out pictures when you ask them to.
	Does he use the names of familiar people and things such as *Mommy, milk, ball,* and *hat*?	He should be using a variety of everyday words heard in his home and neighborhood.
	What does he call himself?	He refers to himself by name.
	Is he beginning to show interest in the sound of TV or radio commercials?	Many two-year-olds do show such interest, by word or action.
	Is he putting a few words together to make little "sentences"? ("Go bye-bye car." "Milk all gone.")	These "sentences" are not usually complete or grammatically correct.

Average Age	Question	Average Behavior
2½ years	Does he know a few rhymes or songs? Does he enjoy hearing them?	Many children can say or sing short rhymes or songs and enjoy listening to records or to Mother singing.
	What does he do when the ice-cream man's bell rings, out of his sight, or when a car door or house door closes at a time when someone in the family usually comes home?	If a child has good hearing, and these are events that bring him pleasure, he usually reacts to the sound by running to look or telling someone what he hears.
3 years	Can he show that he understands the meaning of some words besides the names of things? ("Make the car go." "Give me your ball." "Put the block in your pocket." "Find the big doll.")	He should be able to understand and use some simple verbs, pronouns, prepositions, and adjectives, such as *go*, *me*, *in*, and *big*.
	Can he find you when you call him from another room?	He should be able to locate the source of a sound.
	Does he sometimes use complete sentences?	He should be using complete sentences some of the time.
4 years	Can he tell about events that have happened recently?	He should be able to give a connected account of some recent experiences.
	Can he carry out two directions, one after the other? ("Bobby, find Susie and tell her dinner's ready.")	He should be able to carry out a sequence of two simple directions.
5 years	Do neighbors and others outside the family understand most of what he says?	His speech should be intelligible, although some sounds may still be mispronounced.
	Can he carry on a conversation with other children or familiar grownups?	Most children of this age can carry on a conversation if the vocabulary is within their experience.
	Does he begin a sentence with "I" instead of "me," "he" instead of "him"?	He should use some pronouns correctly.
	Is his grammar almost as good as his parents'?	Most of the time, his speech should match the patterns of grammar used by the adults of his family and neighborhood.

U.S. Dept. of Health, Education and Welfare

Research has shown that babies and older children who do not receive open affection and warm approval from their parents, brothers, sisters, and others will grow up unable to express their feelings in normal ways. The results may be disastrous later to their own lives, their marriages, and their children unless positive steps are taken to overcome problems as soon as they are noticed.

Childbirth. The birth of a child is always an awesome event. The exact time when a child will be born cannot be calculated with precision, though a child is born approximately 280 days after the wo-

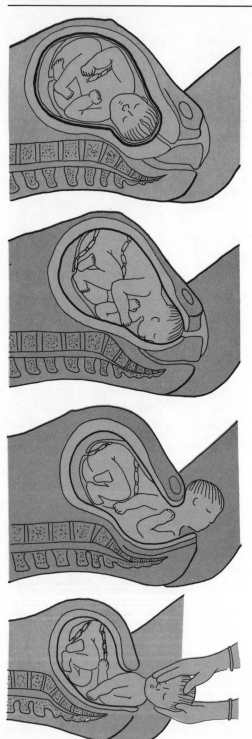

Four stages in the birth of a baby are illustrated from top to bottom. Top, infant in
uterus when labor begins. Next, baby and
uterus press downward as labor progresses,
with baby's head passing through cervix and
pelvic region. Third, head has emerged but
shoulders are still inside. Last, shoulders
usually must turn in order to pass through
birth canal.

Emergency First Aid Procedures for Delivering a Baby

Sometimes a baby is born before the doctor arrives, or before the mother can leave home to get to the hospital. This emergency is unusual, and is not as likely with a first baby as it is with later babies.

If you are a prospective mother faced with this problem, try not to feel frightened. When a baby is born so quickly that you cannot reach the doctor or get to the hospital in time, it nearly always means the birth is normal. You would probably have had time to get the doctor, or go to the hospital, if the birth was going to be difficult.

Certain things can be done which will make it easier for both you and the baby. You cannot do these things yourself. So get someone to stay with you until the doctor comes, and give your helper these instructions:

1. Be sure the doctor or an ambulance has been called.
2. See that the mother is lying down comfortably.
3. Wash your hands thoroughly.
4. Do not touch the area around the vaginal entrance.
5. Place a clean towel under the mother's hips for the baby to come onto. If you have time, protect the bed with newspapers.
6. Let the baby come naturally.
7. If the bag of water has not broken, and the baby is born still inside the sac, puncture the sac with a pin or tip of scissors. Wipe the sac and fluid away from his face and head with the inside of a clean handkerchief.
8. As soon as he is born, wipe the baby's mouth, nose, and face with the inside of a clean handkerchief. Do not use cotton or paper tissues.
9. Move him carefully to a clean spot between the mother's legs, with his head elevated a little and away from

any fluid or secretions. Do not stretch the cord. Let it remain a little slack.
10. If the doctor has been called and is on his way, you do not need to tie the baby's cord. Leave it attached. Leave the baby in a clean spot between the mother's legs, but cover his body with a blanket or towel to prevent chilling. Leave his head uncovered so he can breathe.
11. If you have not been able to reach the doctor, or if he cannot get there within an hour, the cord should be tied.
    - Tie the cord tightly in two places about 2 inches apart with clean pieces of tape or strong twine. The tie nearest the baby should be about 6 inches from his navel.
    - Cut the cord between the two ties with a clean pair of scissors.
    - Wrap the baby in a clean flannel square or blanket, with his face uncovered, and lay him on his side in a warm place.
12. Let the afterbirth come by itself. *Do not pull on the cord to make it come out.* Save the afterbirth in a basin or newspaper for the doctor to examine.
13. As soon as the afterbirth has passed out, place your hands over the mother's uterus (a firm lump just below her navel).
14. Cup your hands around the mother's uterus and massage the uterus several times to keep it firm. If it does not stay firm, hold your hands around it until it does.
15. Clean the mother's buttocks and lower thighs, but do not touch the area around the vaginal entrance.
16. Make the mother comfortable and see that the baby is warm and breathing. Give the mother a hot drink, such as tea, if she wishes.
17. Do not leave the mother until the doctor comes.

man's last regular menstrual period. (*See* PREGNANCY.)

Regular uterine contractions signal the beginning of labor. Coordinated muscular action begins at the small of the back and proceeds wavelike to the front of the abdomen. These contractions are painful, rhythmic, and involuntary. (*See* LABOR.) If the woman has been under a doctor's care for the course of her pregnancy, she will follow her doctor's instructions, allowing enough time to get safely to the hospital. (*See* PRENATAL CARE.)

Once she has arrived at the hospital she will be taken to the labor and delivery rooms. There she is checked for the frequency, intensity, and duration of her contractions, the amount of bloody "show" (the mucous plug from the cervix), and the status of the membranes. Her temperature, pulse, blood pressure, and breathing rate are recorded. The fetal heart tones and movements are also observed. A urine specimen is taken to be analyzed, and a blood sample drawn.

If delivery is not imminent, the vulva and perineum are usually shaved or "prepped." Sometimes an enema is given to facilitate labor.

The woman continues to labor until the cervix is fully open or dilated to approximately four to six inches. During this time both she and the infant are examined regularly. The bag of waters usually breaks sometime during labor, but this is not always the case. (*See* BAG OF WATERS; CAUL.) Sometimes the physician will rupture the membranes in an effort to speed labor. Drugs, too, can be given to stimulate uterine contractions.

When the infant's head reaches the vagina (a condition known as crowning), the woman is ready for normal delivery. She is then draped with sterile garments and adjusted into position. Usually she lies on her back with her legs spread and elevated.

Depending on the preferences of both the woman and her physician, she is anesthetized to minimize pain during this stage. Anesthesia can range from total anesthesia (usually involving a gas) to such techniques as pudendal, caudal, or paracervical blocks which numb various nerves in the lower part of the body. These usually involve shots. In the absence of these, a local anesthetic is sometimes given for the episiotomy. (*See* EPISIOTOMY.)

Normal vaginal delivery is accomplished without the use of instruments. The size and positioning of the infant sometimes make instruments necessary, however. (*See* CHILDBIRTH COMPLICATIONS.) In other cases an infant may have to be delivered through an abdominal incision, a procedure known as cesarean section.

If the woman is conscious during vaginal delivery she is coached to bear down and push to help in delivering the child.

Once the child is completely out of the birth canal, the umbilical cord is clamped and cut. The child is then checked to make sure it can breathe on its own and that no obvious difficulties exist. It is then properly identified and sent to the hospital nursery where it is cleaned and kept warm.

After delivery of the placenta, the woman's episiotomy is repaired and she is cleaned and sent to a recovery room. There she is observed closely until any anesthesia has worn off and the uterus is firm. She is then moved to a hospital room.

The woman remains hospitalized for at least three days or more, though she is usually encouraged to be out of bed as much as she can. (*See* POSTNATAL CARE.) Her body typically returns to normal prepregnant condition within six weeks.

Childbirth Complications. Any conditions which make labor and delivery more difficult can be considered childbirth complications. These can range from those conditions present even before pregnancy to those which develop (sometimes quite suddenly) during its final stages.

If the woman has been under the supervision of a competent obstetrician throughout her pregnancy, she will rarely have cause for concern. When complications develop during childbirth, the obstetrician's special skills will help to minimize them.

Any type of difficult labor is referred to as dystocia. Labor becomes unduly long as a result of abnormalities in the mechanics involved—for example, uterine contractions insufficient to move the child through the birth canal; faulty positioning or abnormal development of the fetus; or malformation or disproportion of the birth canal. An unusually small pelvis or large child, or an obstruction in the birth canal, can complicate childbirth and even preclude normal vaginal delivery.

The use of too much anesthesia or analgesia can become a complication if it interferes with necessary uterine contractions. Excessive anesthesia or other drugs administered during labor can also lead to respiratory difficulty, a slow heartbeat, and diminished oxygen in the infant.

Excessively strong uterine contractions, on the other hand, can bring on so-called precipitate labor. In other instances, labor of less than three hours results from lack of resistance from the soft parts of the pelvis. The rapid transit through the birth canal sometimes has serious consequences for the infant. Uterine contractions close together can deprive the infant of sufficient oxygen. Rapid labor also risks delivery of the infant before the mother can reach the hospital.

The position of the child in the uterus during labor can sometimes lead to complications. Normally the child lies with its head down into the pelvis. Delivery is made with the back of the head toward the front of the pelvis. Variations from this normal position range from rotations of the head to feet-first deliveries.

If the head is somewhat molded or squeezed, the large fontanelle (the soft spot) of the infant's skull may appear first. This condition is known as "bregma delivery." At times the brow or even the entire face can appear first. The appearance of an arm, shoulder, or leg as the so-called presenting part can also complicate delivery.

At the thirtieth week of pregnancy, about 25 to 35 percent of all babies are resting head up in the womb. This position is known as "breech presentation." By the time the child reaches full term at thirty-eight weeks, however, it has generally turned to head-down position. Breech deliveries at term appear in only 3 to 4 percent of all cases. If the child's bottom appears first, with the feet up by the head, the delivery is called a "frank breech." A "complete breech" occurs when the legs are flexed across the child's middle.

If the child is resting crossways in the uterus, the position is known as "transverse lie." Cesarean section is sometimes necessary for such children, since normal vaginal delivery can prove difficult and hazardous.

The cause of malpositioning of the infant within the uterus cannot always be determined. At times it is due to an unusually large or small fetus, multiple pregnancy, weak uterine muscles, or small pelvis.

Forceps are sometimes used to speed delivery. Their use occurs particularly when the mother has become exhausted or should not risk heavy labor, or if the fetus has appeared in an abnormal position or is having difficulty which would make speedy delivery desirable.

Use of forceps can be classified as outlet forceps or midforceps depending on the location of the infant's head when forceps are attached. An episiotomy may sometimes be enlarged to allow more room for these and other types of difficult deliveries. (*See* EPISIOTOMY.)

The birth canal can become obstructed if the placenta is attached overlapping the cervix. This condition is known as "placenta previa." Other placental difficulties include "abruptio placentae," in which the placenta becomes detached from the uterine wall far in advance of the delivery. Both these conditions can lead to maternal hemorrhage and can endanger the lives of both mother and child.

Such childbirth complications as placenta previa, malpresentation, abruptio placentae, fetal distress, unproductive labor, or disproportion of the child's head with respect to the mother's pelvis can generally be handled by cesarean section delivery.

Other conditions sometimes requiring cesarean section include toxemia, maternal diabetes, previous pelvic surgery, cervical cancer, erythroblastosis, or previous cesarean section. (*See* CESAREAN SECTION.)

After the membranes have ruptured, there is a chance that the umbilical cord may slip through the cervix, a condition known as "prolapsed cord." If the cord becomes squeezed, the infant may be deprived of blood and oxygen. The woman is usually confined to bed once the bag of waters has broken.

Rupture of the membranes usually leads to labor. Infection can result with subsequent danger to the child if labor does not take place within several hours after the bag of waters has broken. Premature rupture of the membranes is probably one of the most frequent causes of premature births.

Premature labor accounts for 50 percent of infant mortality associated with birth. The cause of at least 60 percent of such labors is not known. (*See* PREMATURE BIRTHS.)

Delivery of a multiple pregnancy can be more complicated, particularly since the infants will sometimes assume a variety of positions for delivery. Prematurity is also a frequent problem. At times the infants will become hooked together and have to be untangled for delivery. Delivery of so-called Siamese twins which are physically joined together provides even more challenge. A number of these births do not survive, however.

Other deformities of the fetus, such as hydrocephalus, can make labor more difficult since the infant's head is sometimes too large to fit through the pelvis.

Excessive fluid in the bag of waters, a condition known as polyhydramnios, is usually associated with defects in the infant or the placenta. Such conditions as abruptio placentae, uterine dysfunction, and postpartum hemorrhage can develop in association with polyhydramnios. An abnormally low volume of amniotic fluid, on the other hand, can cause pressure injuries (such as

clubfoot) to the infant since he is unprotected by cushioning fluid. (*See* BIRTH DEFECTS.)

If a woman has had six or more pregnancies, she is usually classified as a "grand multipara." The maternal death rate for such women, according to some studies, is four times greater than normal. Since the woman's uterus has been stretched repeatedly in previous pregnancies, the child is more able to assume an unusual position. In fact, the incidence of malpresentations is increased by at least 100 percent. The women also show more incidence of ruptured uterus, postpartum hemorrhage, and placenta previa and abruptio placentae. High blood pressure, heart disease, diabetes, and anemia are also more common among such women.

Bleeding during labor or in the twenty-four hours following delivery can be serious if left untreated. Low blood volume can cause a woman to go into shock.

Tears in or lacerations of the birth canal can occur if the infant passes through it too quickly and the skin does not stretch. At times some of these tears become fistulas. (*See* VAGINAL FISTULAS.) If an episiotomy has not been made large enough, further tearing can result.

Rupture of the uterus is a serious complication of childbirth which can lead to hemorrhage and death if not treated quickly. Occasionally, abdominal surgery must be performed and the damaged uterus removed. Rupture can occur spontaneously or as a drug-induced complication when uterine contractions become unusually strong. Both mother and child are endangered by so-called tumultuous uterine contractions.

If the uterus turns inside out following delivery, the condition is called "uterine inversion." The cause of this rare condition cannot always be pinpointed. Sometimes the condition can occur if the umbilical cord is pulled before the placenta has separated from the uterine wall.

If fragments of the placenta remain

within the uterus after delivery, bleeding and sometimes infection can develop. More commonly, postpartum bleeding results from relaxation of the uterine walls. Only occasionally do vaginal and cervical lacerations account for hemorrhage.

An oral temperature of more than 100.4° F. for any two days within the ten days following delivery can indicate so-called "puerperal infection." Attention to cleanliness and sterile techniques during delivery have greatly decreased the occurrence of such infection. In earlier days, infection and "childbed fever" were common causes of maternal mortality.

Although the United States still has a relatively high maternal mortality rate, improved obstetric technique continues to minimize childbirth complications.

Child Care. Good child care practices are different in our time than earlier in the century. Then, physicians made a great many home visits to care for acute infectious diseases. In the last twenty years alone, tremendous progress has been made in the prevention of illness and the methods of treatment of infants and children. With the virtual disappearance of many infectious diseases due to immunizations and antibiotics, there is now an emphasis on the psychological and social aspects of child care. The goal of pediatric medicine is to help the child reach adulthood in the best state of physical, emotional, and social development that is possible for him to achieve.

At birth, the interruption of circulation from the placenta forces the infant to make a series of anatomic and physiologic changes in order that it may survive and thrive as an independent being from its mother. The most important of these alterations are the adaptation of the respiratory, circulatory, digestive, and urinary tracts, some of which must be made immediately if the baby is to live, while others take place during the first four to six weeks of life. During this newborn period, the child re-

quires special care and observation by the mother and physician. Since the infant is usually born in the hospital, the care of the newborn for the first few days is provided by the hospital staff. As soon as the infant leaves the hospital, the care and nurturing become the responsibility of the mother, or mother-substitute.

The newborn, in order to flourish, must be provided with a continuous, warm, interacting relationship with his mother. He needs not only food but gentle stimulation, to be held and fondled and to hear someone talk to him. He reacts to the adequacy of care and thus becomes emotionally secure for his level of development. Through these daily predictable experiences and nurturing, he develops a confidence in the goodness of the world and, through that, an attitude of trust.

The time of the child's first feeding will vary according to the physician's instructions—usually between eight and twenty-four hours after birth, and will consist of sugar and water. The American Academy of Pediatrics recommends breast feeding thereafter as the method of choice; but if the mother does not wish to breast feed, there is no scientific reason why she should. The bottle is not harmful and can provide adequate nutritional intake for the infant. (*See* FORMULA.) After that, the child's diet should be carefully adjusted to his age and physiological stage of development.

The regulation of feeding goes beyond dietary needs and includes observation of a variety of behavioral signs and symptoms which are related to the rhythm of appetite and sleep, capacity to take solids, self-selection of foods, play activities, emotional reactions, and so forth. (*See* INFANT CARE.)

The newborn does not have clearly differentiated waking and sleeping periods; his waking is usually a response to the pain of hunger, or the discomfort of being wet and cold. By the end of the first month, however, a more definite pattern develops, and waking periods are more clearly separated from sleep, though the infant may continue to wake and cry because of hunger. Crying will usually stop when he is given food or when he is changed. At three or four months he shows more consistency and establishes a schedule that is more or less stable thereafter.

From birth to one month, the infant's crying is hardly ever accompanied by tears, but between one and two months, tears appear and from then on will accompany crying. By the end of the first month, the cries of the infant change; parents are able to tell when he is angry, hungry, or simply tired.

Although the rate of growth and development will vary from one child to another, and although there are many patterns of development, the sequence will remain roughly the same. The infant will crawl before he walks or runs or jumps; this is related to the maturation of the nervous system. Overall care must take into consideration the fact that normal infants and children will develop motor control and skill with little or no help from their parents, but these skills can often be enhanced by providing incentives and toys that require imagination and coordination.

Exercise and play begin with the baby's first cry and grow in complexity as the child develops. In the infant years, the child will receive his exercise by crying, laughing, kicking, waving his hands, and turning his body; soon he learns to creep, stand, walk, and jump. The ultimate object of this exercise and play is to help the child grow properly and develop skeletal and muscular systems, and to furnish relaxation and enjoyment. Good care by those in charge will see to it that exercise and play are adapted to the child's age and his stage of development. Every child should be encouraged to play with other children, not only for his own emotional adjustment and development, but for his muscular development as well. When he reaches school age, he will automatically become part of a system in which exercise and play with other children are included.

At the same time, activity should be balanced by rest, and this balance is different for each child. Sleep is the most complete form of rest. By the time a child enters school he will have the kind of sleep pattern that has been set by his own internal mechanism plus that of his surrounding environmental experience. (*See* INFANT CARE.) From infancy to about ten years of age, the child is still in the process of learning to sleep and may make certain demands on the parents at bedtime. The amount of sleep generally decreases with age. Rapidly growing children may need more sleep, and adolescents may sometimes need a seemingly inordinate amount—which may be an inherent need of that phase of development. (*See* ADOLESCENCE.)

Another aspect of child care which must not be overlooked is the role of the school. Next to the home, school is the most important agency in society in the maturation of the child. Here, too, care must be shown so that no child will be categorized as slow in any way without appropriate evaluation. From nursery school onward, the child's experience—intellectually, socially, and emotionally—partially depends on teachers who respond and help to develop his physical, mental, and emotional horizons (though at a different pace in each child).

The attitudes toward one another of both privileged and underprivileged children, which are developed in these early school years, will have much influence on their emotional and social development. School is a place where the lower socio-economic status of some children, with their constant deprivations in proper food, shelter, and medical care, can create handicaps. Inadequate clothing and other evidences of "inferior" status may also deprive them of a feeling of personal adequacy and produce an attitude based on their own sense of reality and their own life situation. Nor is the privileged child without his own pressure, if success in school is demanded of him at every turn and if every goal of achievement must be immediate. Also, parents and teachers should not lose sight of so-called "deprived affluent" children for whom there is too much permissiveness, or protection, or supervision. In *any* school or group situation, parents and teachers should always be aware that in any physical activity the late-maturing child may be at great handicap when compared with those who mature early. Nutritional needs, too, should not be overlooked.

Care of the very young in day-care centers is a comparatively new idea in the United States. This type of care differs from nursery school and kindergarten in that its primary focus is on the care of children of working mothers, whereas nursery schools and kindergartens emphasize the educational aspect of care. Since the chief motive for many working mothers is economic, all-day, year-round facilities for child care have become a necessity. It may become important for communities to set standards and regulations for the bodily and health care of these young children (as they have in school-aged children).

Good child care also takes into account inherited characteristics. Many factors of hereditary origin (and for which genetic counseling is sometimes indicated) are fixed and not subject to modification. Modern techniques have made it possible to recognize many defects early and treat them before they cause chronic handicaps. Other, less permanent, disorders can sometimes be modified by efforts directed toward their control, or even by environmental influences. The object is to encourage the child to use his hereditary equipment so that he can develop desirable traits, while undesirable characteristics can be minimized.

The care of a child is an ongoing process and requires everyone's help—parents, teachers, playmates, etc. From the birth period, when he is completely dependent upon others and is uncontrolled in his movements, to the time when he will have learned to see, hear, touch, walk, and understand the language spoken to him, the child is forming a sense of trust. He is finding, through the care given to him, that there is order and stability in the world. With this sense, and the initiative that he inevitably develops, self-control and a sense of "self" will help him to achieve his full potential.

Society, in general, is now increasing its demands for improved and comprehensive child health care that will include guidance, developmental medicine, and help with

Presbyterian St. Luke's Hospital, Chicago

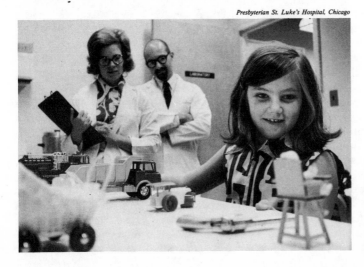

Child-testing for perception and awareness can alert physicians to physical or mental problems which may influence school work or emotional and social behavior.

emotional, behavioral, and school health problems. There is an urgency to have accessible, adequate, equitable, and continuous care. This may require new thinking, new public policy measures, community planning, and innovative financing. It certainly is not a simple matter, but if this kind of child care can be provided it will pay dividends for generations to come at all levels of society.

Child Health. Since 1909 the federal government has shown increasingly marked interest in child health: White House Conferences have been called since 1909; the Children's Bureau, with its manifold tasks, was established in 1912; Title XIX of the Social Security Act provides assistance to families with dependent children, the blind, aged, or permanently handicapped; the Maternal and Child Health Services have increased their grants since 1935 in a wide variety of child health services; the Handicapped Children's Program has administered funds through the states and provided a source of service for handicapped children. Federal and state funds have also provided child health conferences, maternity clinics, developmental clinics, and child-welfare services. The welfare services have been a source for homemaker services, protective services to abused children, foster care, adoption services, and social services to unmarried parents and their babies. Now, the Head Start program provides culturally and economically deprived children an opportunity to develop mentally and physically in a preschool setting, before starting formal schooling. Many voluntary agencies also contribute to child health, not to mention the preventive measures sponsored by many hospitals, such as prenatal clinics, parent education programs, well-baby clinics, heart clinics, chest clinics, cerebral palsy clinics, hearing and speech clinics, mental evaluation clinics, etc.

In the new approach to child health and

How to Reduce Drug Dosages for Children

Prescribing drug and vitamin doses should be handled by the family physician, but in an emergency or when the physician cannot be reached, the following formulas are standard and universal. Each recognizes the child's weight and age.

Fried's rule: for infants under two years of age

Divide the infant's age (in months) by 150, the weight of an average adult, and multiply by the adult dose.

Example: *Adult dose of 60 mg. reduced for an infant of ten months*

$$\frac{10}{150} \times 60 \text{ mg.} = 4 \text{ mg.}$$

Clark's rule: for children over two years of age

Divide the child's weight (in pounds) by 150, and multiply by the adult dose.

Example: *Adult dose of 600 mg. reduced for a 75-pound child*

$$\frac{75}{150} \times 600 \text{ mg.} = 300 \text{ mg.}$$

Young's rule: for children between 3 and 12 years of age

Divide the child's age (in years) by the child's age plus 12, and multiply by the adult dose.

Example: *Adult dose of 100 mg. reduced for a child of 8*

$$\frac{8}{8 + 12} \times 100 \text{ mg.} = 40 \text{ mg.}$$

its problems, community relationships have become increasingly important in the delivery and maintenance of good child care. Many physicians have now proven the value of knowing both the family and its social background, and have worked in close partnership with such related disciplines as psychology, sociology, social work, education, and economics. The field of pediatrics is increasing in both its scope

Height-Weight Averages for Boys and Girls from Birth Through Thirteen Years

AGE	BOYS						GIRLS					
	HEIGHT (inches)			WEIGHT (pounds)			HEIGHT (inches)			WEIGHT (pounds)		
	LOW	AVERAGE	HIGH	LOW	AVERAGE	HIGH	LOW	AVERAGE	HIGH	LOW	AVERAGE	HIGH
Birth	18¼	19½–20½	21½	5¾	7–8¼	10	18½	19¼–20	21	5¾	7–8	9½
3 months	22½	23¼–24¼	25	10½	11¾–13½	16½	22	22¾–24	24¾	9¾	11½–13¼	15
6 months	24¾	25¾–26¾	27¾	14	15½–18	20¾	24	25–26¼	27	12¾	15–17½	20
9 months	26¾	27½–28¾	30	16½	18¾–21½	24½	25¾	27–28¼	29¼	15	17¾–20¾	24¼
1 year	28	29–30¼	31½	18½	21–23¾	27¼	27	28½–30	31	16¾	19¾–23	27
1½ years	30½	31½–33	31½	21	23¾–27	27¼	29½	31–32½	34	19½	22¾–26¼	31
2 years	32½	33¾–35¼	34¾	23¼	26¼–29¾	31½	31½	33¼–35	36¾	21½	25¼–29¼	34½
3 years	35¾	37–38¾	37¼	27	30¼–34½	35	34¾	36¾–38½	40¾	25½	29½–34½	41¾
4 years	38½	39¾–42	40½	30	34–39	39¼	37½	39½–41¾	44¼	29¼	33½–39½	48¼
5 years	40¾	42¼–44¾	43½	33½	37½–44	44½	39¾	42–44½	47¼	32	37½–44¾	52¾
6 years	43	44½–47½	46½	37	41¼–49¼	50½	42	44½–47	50¼	35½	41½–49	57½
7 years	45	46¼–49¼	49	40½	45–54	57	43¼	46–48¾	52½	38½	45½–54	65½
8 years	47¼	48½–51½	51½	45¼	49¾–61	64½	45	48½–51¼	54½	43	50¾–62	76¾
9 years	49	50½–53¾	54	49½	55–68¼	73	46¾	50½–54	57	47	55¼–72¼	88
10 years	51	52½–56	56½	54	61–76¼	83	48½	52½–56½	59½	51½	61½–82	100
11 years	54¼	54½–58¼	58½	64¾	67¾–85½	94½	50	54¼–59	62	56	69¼–92	113½
12 years	54¼	56½–60¾	60½	64¾	74–95½	108½	51¼	56½–61	64½	61½	78–101¼	125¾
13 years	55¾	58¼–63½	66½	73¾	82–108½	139	52½	63–67	67	68	110¾–142½	142½

and complexity. The demand for high-caliber clinical care for everyone is increasing from all sides, and is assumed to be a basic human right. (*See* CHILD CARE; INFANT CARE; PEDIATRICS.)

Child Safety. Accidents kill and disable more American youngsters each year than all the dreaded children's diseases combined. Growing up is full of risks, with a lot of scrapes and bruises in the process. But if parents use common sense—and instill it in their youngsters—many of the risks of growing up can be reduced.

Parents and adults who work with children should be alert to potential dangers in the child's environment, including home, school, back yard, playground, or ball park. Being alert doesn't mean being neurotic. A parent shouldn't prevent his child from having a bicycle, for example, for the reason that "a bicycle is dangerous." That's neither logical nor fair. A parent should, however, when giving a child a bicycle, teach the youngster bicycle safety rules. The bicycle isn't dangerous by itself; the person riding it makes it that way.

Using the same example, when a child is given a bicycle he should be taught to enjoy it, but also to respect it. Respect doesn't mean fear. A child who participates in any activity with the fear of getting hurt is the very child most likely to be injured. But if he is aware of the potential danger in what he does, he is likely to be more cautious.

Parents should encourage their children to be curious, to try new things. This is an important part of every child's development. But at the same time youngsters must learn to be careful. Before they are coordinated enough, or mature enough to have good judgment, children should be supervised by an adult. Until a child is old enough to go to school, he is almost completely dependent on adults. Sometimes the best, and only, way to protect small children from getting hurt is to remove haz-

ards. In other words, "child-proof" his environment.

Home Safety. Put guards on windows that are low or on any window that a child might climb up to. Secure screens. Install gates at the tops and bottoms of stairways until young children have learned to climb safely. Cover unused electrical outlets and protect all electrical outlets by attaching a neutralizing device that is available at the hardware store.

If there is heavy furniture around that a child could tip over, secure it with small L braces. Put decals on glass doors or use frosted safety glass. It's not funny when someone walks through a glass door.

Use common sense when purchasing a child's first furniture. Low feeding chairs don't tip over as easily as high chairs. A crib should have slats close enough together that a child can't get his head wedged in. And keep the crib side up if you turn your back on the child. Don't use a crib pillow and never use plastic bags—such as dry cleaners use—as a waterproof sheet in cribs. Thin plastic can cause suffocation.

Train children early to pick up their toys. Objects scattered around on the floor are a danger to adults as well as to children. And when you buy toys, keep your child's safety in mind. Don't let a child play with toys that have sharp corners and edges, or that have loose parts that might be swallowed—such as animal eyes, marbles, buttons, and car wheels.

Bathroom. The bathroom is potentially one of the most dangerous rooms in the home. Make it safer by putting rubber safety mats in bathtubs and showers. The mat on the bathroom floor should have a skid-proof backing. Keep all medicines and drugs in a locked medicine chest. That's the best place for razors, blades, and scissors, too. Never throw razor blades or broken glass in a container that a child might get into. Use plastic containers and drinking cups instead of glass ones.

If the bathroom door can be locked from the inside, remove the lock so a child can't lock himself in. A hook installed high up on the outside of the bathroom door keeps children out before they are old enough to be trusted in the bathroom alone. And a hook high up on the inside assures adults of privacy.

Never put a small child in a full tub of water. Children can drown in just a few inches of water. Train children to use the water faucets and to know the difference between hot and cold.

Kitchen. This room can also be a danger area for small children. Teach youngsters to stay away from the hot stove. Put pans on the back burners, and keep handles turned away from the front of the stove so a child can't pull the pot and its ingredients down on himself. Keep electric cords from dangling over the counter where a child might pull a toaster or coffee pot down on himself. Young children must be taught to keep their hands off appliances such as the washer and dryer, garbage disposal, and dishwasher.

When a child is eating, stay with him in case he chokes on his food. You might not hear him in another room. Some doctors feel you should not let children under five eat popcorn, nuts, or candy bars with nuts.

If you have a gas stove, chances are your child will learn to turn on the gas just as he has seen you do. Prevent this by removing the knobs when you aren't using the burners.

Place cleaning solutions and poisons in an overhead cabinet out of the child's reach, and lock the cabinet.

Storage areas. Many people accumulate an assortment of old and little-used possessions in a closet, attic, or garage. Children like to explore, and such places should be off-limits. A child can find an old knife or gun years after his parents have forgotten they had it. Children also like to crawl into trunks and abandoned refrigerators. They

don't think about the fact that the lid or door may shut and trap them inside. For good reason, law requires that doors on discarded refrigerators and freezers be removed. Storage areas should be kept well ventilated and clear of refuse that could easily go up in flames.

Car safety. Never let children play in or around cars. Children should not be left alone in a car, especially if the engine is running. They should wear seat belts or, if they are too young, they should ride in a child's car seat. Babies should ride in a crib in the back seat, never on mother's lap. Keep doors locked as an added precaution. Drivers, when backing out of the driveway, should take special care to watch out for children playing.

When a teenager is old enough to drive a car, insist that he take driver education in school where he will learn rules, skills, and proper attitudes. If a youngster likes to show off, give him limited access to the family car until he proves his responsibility.

Bicycle safety. Most youngsters want a bicycle. Make sure that the bicycle is the right size for the rider: he should be able to put a foot on the ground while the bicycle is upright. A well-equipped bicycle should have a horn or bell, a light, reflectors on front and rear fenders, and a basket so that hands are free for steering. A bicycle should be taken care of, just like a car, to keep it in good running order. Replace parts that are worn out or broken.

When children ride their bicycles in the street, they must obey traffic rules and regulations: Don't run red lights. Ride on the right-hand side of the street. Ride single file and never weave in and out of traffic. Signal turns. Don't hitch a ride by hanging on to a car or truck.

Bicycles are a convenient means for getting from one place to another in a hurry. They can be used for play as well as transportation. Children who use their bicycles to perform stunts and to race should be kept off the streets and sidewalks, away from traffic and pedestrians. Caution young bicycle riders not to attempt stunts which could injure them or other people or someone else's property.

Sports safety. Parents should see to it that when their children participate in organized sports activities only proper equipment is used, there is adult supervision, safety is stressed, and rules are followed. In addition, see to it that children of similar age, size, and coordination are put in the same play groups.

Before a child participates in any activity, whether it be an individual sport like swimming, skiing, or ice skating, or a group activity like baseball or hockey, he should receive proper instruction in the sport. Along with learning the skills required for each activity, he should be taught safety rules and made aware of potential dangers.

For any sports activity: use proper equipment, wear appropriate clothing, follow the rules, don't show off, and rest frequently.

Chills. Episodes of shivering or shaking of the body with the sensation of coldness of the skin are called chills. Exposure to a wet or cold environment causing involuntary contractions of the body muscles can bring on chills. Muscle contraction results in heat production by the muscle cells, which serves to warm the body again. Chills are also, very often, the early sign of an infectious disease. Pneumonia (lung infection) and malaria frequently are accompanied by chills. (*See* MALARIA.) Nearly any disease that produces fever can also produce chills. The feeling of chilliness results from the clamping down of the blood vessels of the skin. A rise in body temperature (fever) almost always follows this phenomenon.

Chiropodist. In England, the specialist responsible for the care of the human foot is called a chiropodist. The term chiropodist has been replaced in the United States with the word podiatrist. (*See* PODIATRIST; PODIATRY.)

Chiropody. In England, the branch of the healing arts concerned with the care of the human foot is known as chiropody. This term was used many years ago in the United States, but now is considered obsolete, having been replaced by "podiatry." The specialist practicing podiatry is responsible for diagnosing, preventing and treating foot disorders by medical and surgical means. (*See* PODIATRIST; PODIATRY.)

Chiropractor. A person who is trained to treat diseases by manipulation of the spine and other body structures is called a chiropractor. His field, known as chiropractic, is believed to have been originated by physicians in ancient Greece and Rome. Its principles were revived in 1895 by Daniel D. Palmer of Davenport, Iowa, who founded a training school for chiropractors before the turn of the century.

The theory of chiropractic is that any change in the position of one or more vertebrae in the spine (due to pressure or strain) can impair the action of the nerves that are involved. Since nerves carry impulses throughout the body, the nerves that are impaired can produce disease symptoms, such as pain, in places sometimes quite remote from the spine. But when the affected vertebra is manipulated back into its proper alignment, the nerves will again function normally and the symptoms will disappear.

Chiropractors fall into two groups. One group limit themselves to manipulation. The second also make use of heat, water, light, and mechanical or electrical devices. Both groups use X rays as part of their diagnostic procedure. Chiropractors do not prescribe drugs or do surgery.

Chiropractic training is available at fifteen schools in the United States and Canada that are accredited by the International Chiropractors Association or the American Chiropractic Association. Entrants must be high school graduates and at some schools must have up to two years of college education. On completing their training, they are required to have a license, for which they must pass a state examination.

Chloasma. Abnormal pigmentation of the face and other parts of the body with yellowish or brownish patches and spots in known as chloasma.

The most common form is chloasma gravidarum, which occurs in pregnant women and disappears after the baby is born. It is due to increased activity of hormones which stimulate melanocytes, cells that produce skin pigment called melanin. (*See* PIGMENTATION.)

The condition may also result from the use of some oral contraceptives. Other types of chloasma may result from exposure to the sun or continuous heat, from excessive use of some drugs, from injury to the skin by friction or pressure, or from obscure metabolic disorders. (*See also* CAROTENEMIA; JAUNDICE.)

Chloral Hydrate. When an oily liquid called chloral combines with water to form a white, crystalline solid, it is called chloral hydrate. Refined in the early nineteenth century, this substance, like the bromide drugs, was used as a sedative and hypnotic. (*See* BROMIDE.)

In prescription doses, chloral hydrate has little effect upon heart action, respiration, and blood pressure, but it does depress the central nervous system, hence it is classified as a depressant drug. While it is usually irritating to the gastrointestinal tract, producing nausea and vomiting, it does allow sleep to come quickly.

An ingredient in "knockout drops," chloral hydrate is activated through combination with an alcoholic drink. This combination provides an added depressant effect on the victim. While this may be achieved by using any depressant drug and alcohol, chloral hydrate is most commonly used.

Regular use of the drug results in habituation (mental dependence), the development of tolerance, and, frequently,

death. Some users experience confusion, mental delusions, and disorientation after taking the drug. (*See* ADDICTION; DRUG ABUSE.)

Chlorine. This widely used gas is yellow-green in color, has a pungent odor, and can irritate the respiratory organs. It is used to purify water, to make bleaching powder and deodorants, and is the active principle in germicides. (*See* WATER PURIFICATION.)

Chloroform. Also known as trichloromethane, chloroform is a colorless, rapidly evaporating liquid used as a solvent, antispasmodic, and anesthetic. Ether is often used in its place in surgical procedures, as chloroform is too potent, irritating, and quick acting. (*See* ANESTHESIA.)

Chlorophyll. Many medical claims have been made for this green chemical substance produced in specialized cells of plants. In plants, chlorophyll is essential for the manufacture of carbohydrates from water and carbon dioxide, giving off oxygen in the process. Chlorophyll is itself produced by specialized cells called chloroplasts.

Various manufacturers have incorporated chlorophyll in their products with wide-ranging claims. Its benefit in reducing tooth decay and mouth odor has been generally disproven. Mainly, chlorophyll has been claimed as an odor remover, being used in mouthwashes, deodorants, and cat litters. Its benefit for such uses has not been substantiated, but neither is it harmful. Other boasts have included beneficial results when used to treat ulcerations, burns, and other tissue damage. There is no proof of this. In fact, the use of chlorophyll may keep patients from other drugs which could aid in the healing process.

Choking. The interruption of breathing by pressure or by an obstruction in the airway is called choking. The blocking usually occurs in the larynx, or voice box, which opens into the throat. The cause may be illness, injury, food, or a foreign body.

Disease affecting the respiratory tract can obstruct breathing in several ways. In a genetic disorder called "cystic fibrosis," for instance, respiration may be blocked by abnormally thick secretions in the throat. In some acute inflammations of the larynx, particularly in very young children, swelling of tissues in the larynx can cut off air. In some other disorders, such as infectious mononucleosis and Vincent's infection, a membrane, or film, forms on the surface of the throat and larynx, and a loose patch of membrane can catch in the larynx and lead to a block in breathing.

In a situation of this kind it is important to open a channel for air before breathing is too severely obstructed. Sometimes a flexible tube is inserted through the nose or mouth down into the larynx and the trachea, or windpipe, directly below the obstruction. This is usually a temporary measure. For longer use, a rigid tube is inserted into the trachea through an opening in the front of the neck. This procedure is called a tracheotomy.

Breathing may also be obstructed by an injury, such as a fracture of the larynx. This kind of damage commonly occurs in an automobile accident, when the front of the neck strikes the dashboard or some other part of the car. With an injury this severe, a tracheotomy is usually performed as soon as possible.

FOOD AND FOREIGN BODIES. Often the obstruction is a crumb of food, a little liquid, a small foreign body inhaled into the larynx, or a large lump of food or some other object caught in the throat above the larynx.

Many such accidents could be prevented. Food should be chewed thoroughly to eliminate large lumps that can stick in the throat. Children should not be allowed to run around while they are eating. If they are too young to chew, they should not be given nuts or popcorn, and the meat they eat should be ground or chopped fine.

If someone does choke on food or some other object, try to keep calm. You may be able to help by following these guidelines:

If the object caught in the throat or larynx is sharp or pointed, such as a bone or an open safety pin, breathing may become obstructed gradually as the points or sharp edges cause swelling. Eating bread or mashed potatoes won't help, and it may make the obstruction worse. Take the victim to a hospital to have the object removed.

An adult or older child can dislodge most obstructions by forceful coughing. Encourage him to cough. Don't distract him.

If the person can put his head down between his legs while he coughs, gravity may help dislodge the object. If he resists, however, don't insist.

A small child usually cannot cough with enough force to get an object out of his throat. Turn him head down, over your arm or over your lap, and slap him between the shoulder blades.

Do not slap an adult on the back while he is coughing. If the object is coming loose, you may jar it back into place.

If the victim becomes faint or unconscious, put him on a chair with his head between his legs and slap him on the back. The throat muscles will relax, and the slap may jar the object loose.

If you can see the object in the throat, you may try, very carefully, to grasp it with your fingers, or a forceps, and pull it out. However, there is a risk of pushing it further in.

If first aid is not successful, the victim should go to a hospital emergency room quickly. Call the police or fire department for help. They are trained in first aid and emergency driving. You may not be calm enough to drive safely.

If breathing returns to normal, but the object has not been expelled, a doctor should be consulted. If the object has gone down into the trachea or the bronchial tubes, it can cause serious consequences.

(*See* LARYNGITIS; LARYNX; THROAT.)

Cholangitis. An inflammation of the bile duct is known as cholangitis. (*See* BILE; GASTROINTESTINAL SYSTEM; JAUNDICE.)

Cholecystitis. Inflammation of the gallbladder is called cholecystitis. It usually is a complication of gallstones, but may result from other problems which interfere with the concentration of gallbladder bile or its evacuation.

The symptoms of cholecystitis resemble those of a gallbladder attack due to gallstones. There may be a sharp pain called biliary colic in the area of the gallbladder, and it may spread. There may be nausea and discomfort due to belching and flatulence, as well as gas in the stomach and intestines. (*See* GALLSTONES.)

The symptoms flare up after the person has eaten fatty foods. These trigger secretion of bile, which causes pressure on the sides of the gallbladder and ducts because it cannot flow out properly.

Treatment consists of putting the patient on a low-fat diet. It is particularly important to eliminate most cooked fats, such as those found in most fried foods and steak. Cooked fats do not emulsify at body temperature as uncooked fats do. That is, the cooked fats do not mix as well with body liquids, and therefore are harder to digest.

Immediately after an attack, the patient should be on a soft, bland diet relatively low in cooked or fried fats, until the patient has recovered from most symptoms. Then he can progress gradually to soft foods such as boiled eggs, cooked vegetables, or nonirritating cereals. (*See* DIETS.)

Most persons who have had attacks of cholecystitis must watch their fat intake permanently. Such diets must be planned by the physician. Gallbladder trouble is serious, and an unregulated diet can do great harm.

Sometimes cholecystitis, particularly when complicated by stone formation, may be cured only by removal of the gallbladder (a cholecystectomy). An almost normal diet may then be followed. The surgery is usually quite successful, with complications more likely to occur in aged patients.

Neglect of signs of gallbladder trouble is dangerous, as untreated cholecystitis can result in necrosis (tissue death) and even gangrene. If such complications are suspected, emergency surgery is necessary.

Cholecystitis may be associated with blocking of the duct from the liver, which will cause complications in that organ. (*See also* GALLBLADDER; LIVER.)

Cholelithiasis. This term refers to the presence of gallstones. Choledocholithiasis refers to gallstones lodged in the bile duct. (*See* GALLSTONES.)

Cholera. Cholera is caused by contaminated water or food supplies that carry the micro-organism Vibrio cholerae. Human infection results in diarrhea, muscle cramps, vomiting, dehydration, and sometimes shock. The disease is seldom mild,

During the European epidemic from 1840 to 1849, cholera victims died in the street and were carried off in both horse-drawn and hand-carried coffins, as depicted in this wood engraving by Daumier for Fabre's *Némésis Médicale Illustrée,* Brussels.

National Library of Medicine

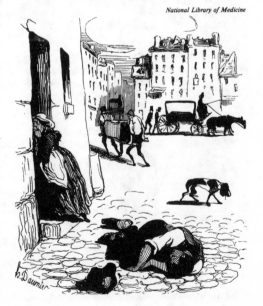

and resembles a severe case of food poisoning.

Treatment includes the restoration of lost fluids, replacement of lost potassium, elimination of acidosis, and glucose feeding. Tetracyclines and sulfa drugs are helpful.

The mortality from untreated cases is high, but the death rate among patients who receive prompt treatment has been reduced to about one in twenty.

Cleanliness is vital to prevent the spread of the disease through the patient's excrement, vomit, and eating utensils. Isolation is routine. Screening and pesticides can prevent flies from spreading the causative germ.

In recent years cholera has been largely confined to south central and southeast Asia.

Cholesterol. The fatty substance called cholesterol is essential to the cells of the body. It is also found in liquids of the human system, particularly in the blood.

Cholesterol has many functions. It is used by the adrenal glands, and male testes, and the female ovaries in the production of vital hormones. The liver uses it to form cholic acid, an ingredient needed to produce the bile salts that are important in digestion.

With other fatlike substances called phospholipids, cholesterol is also found in nerve tissue and in the corneum layer of the

Cholesterol

To understand the meaning and importance of cholesterol, it is first essential to understand the definition of the terms *saturated fats* and *unsaturated fats*. Chemically, *saturated fats* are full of (saturated) hydrogen atoms in their carbon atoms; *unsaturated fats* have carbon atoms that accept more hydrogen. More simply, this means that milk fat, coconut oil, cocoa fat, and meat fat are the primary saturated fats. The less saturated fats are found in veal, chicken, and turkey. Recently a new term, polyunsaturated fats, has appeared. These are the liquid vegetable oils such as soybean, corn, cottonseed, and safflower oils. They tend to lower the blood cholesterol.

While some research nutritionalists restrict heart patients to low cholesterol diets, others advocate the importance of maintaining a well-balanced diet to inhibit the buildup of cholesterol in the arteries. Some heart patients eat high cholesterol foods (eggs, liver, butter) with no apparent problems, reports state, because three B vitamins—cholin, inositol, and vitamin B_6—were added to maintain normal blood cholesterol. Other patients improved when lecithin (made up of fat, cholin, inositol, and essential unsaturated fatty acids) was added to the diet.

A knowledge of nutrition and the importance of each vitamin and mineral to the body's activity is necessary before going on any diet. Check with your physician. If he is aware of the importance of nutrition, you may still enjoy eggs and sour cream with your meals. Listed before each item are the unit grams of saturated fatty acid (includes oleic acid) found in foods. When T precedes an item, it means a *trace* (very small amount) of that food.

36	Whole milk
18	Evaporated milk
T	Powdered skim milk, instant
T	Skim milk
23	Fortfied milk
T	Skim milk, noninstant
4	Buttermilk
24	Powdered, whole milk
22	Malted milk, ½ cup ice cream
10	Cocoa (1 cup)
11	Baked custard (1 cup)
13	½ cup light cream
T	1 cup uncreamed cottage cheese
10	1 oz. cream cheese
10	2 eggs
10	1 tbsp. butter
92	½ cup lard
5	1 tbsp. corn, soy, peanut, **or** cottonseed oil
2	1 tbsp. salad dressing (French, 1000 Island)
7	3 oz. beef, chuck (pot-roasted)
35	3 oz. roast beef
9	3 oz. corned beef
7	3 oz. broiled chicken
0	Domestic duck
14	3 oz. braised lamb
21	3 oz. pork roast
8	3 oz. broiled veal cutlet
0	Braised kidney
0	2 slices lamb liver
0	2 oz. liverwurst

skin, where it helps retard evaporation.

Cholesterol is taken into the body's system from two sources. Most, called exogenous (from outside the body) cholesterol, is absorbed from food fats in the intestinal tract. But quantities of cholesterol called endogenous (from within the body) also are manufactured in various body cells, particularly in the liver.

ABNORMAL ACCUMULATIONS. One of the problems of civilized man, particularly in countries where meat products are consumed in large quantities, is a high level of serum or plasma cholesterol. Associated with this are deposits of cholesterol and other fatty material within the walls of blood vessels. The deposits are called

atheromas, or atheromatous plaques, and the general condition is known as atherosclerosis.

Hypertension, heart disease, and other circulatory problems follow atherosclerosis as the atheromas close greater portions of the arteries. At least half of the adult population of middle age or older in the United States have some degree of atherosclerosis, and many have turned to dietary lowering of their serum cholesterol levels in an effort to stem the disease.

Precise proof is lacking that cholesterol is the main culprit in causing atheromas in man, although it has been demonstrated in a few animals. Some authorities suspect that factors other than cholesterol alone

5 5 breaded fish sticks	17 ½ cup grated cheddar cheese	12 1 slice choc. cake, fudge icing
0 Broiled halibut	7 1 oz. swiss cheese	
0 ½ cup raw oysters	8 2 eggs, yolks only	6 2 oz. bar choc.
3 Yogurt	88 Hydrogenated cooking fat	9 1 cup tapioca pudding
16 Ice cream (1 cup)	(½ cup)	28 ½ cup unsalted cashews
42 ½ cup heavy cream	5 1 tbsp. mayonnaise	3 French-fried potatoes
5 1″ cube cheddar/American cheese	3 1 tbsp. safflower, sunflower, walnut oil	7 ¾ cup scalloped potatoes/ cheese
8 1 oz. roquefort cheese	7 2 slices crisp bacon	9 10 large green olives
14 2 eggs scrambled, omelet, fried	9 3 oz. ground lean hamburger	10 1 lb. whole wheat bread
80 ½ cup butter	11 3 oz. round steak	4 1 muffin/refined flour
76 ½ cup margarine	25 Beef pot-pie (4½″)	5 1 section pizza (cheese)
13 1 tbsp. olive oil	16 3 oz. roasted chicken	2 Sweet roll/refined flour
0 Salt pork	14 3 oz. roasted leg of lamb	3 1 cup wheat germ
15 3 oz. hamburger (commercial)	19 3 oz. broiled ham	2 1 cup chicken/turkey soup
	0 Roast turkey	2 1 cup veg. soup
25 3 oz. sirloin steak	14 1 cup chili with beans	6 1 2″ cube gingerbread
7 3 oz. corned beef hash	36 ″ without beans	4 1 cake-type doughnut
11 3 oz. fried breast, leg, or thigh of chicken	7 3½ oz. sautéed beef liver	31 ½ cup almonds (roasted)
	18 2 frankfurters	19 ½ cup shredded coconut
33 4 oz. broiled lamb chop	0 Sweetbreads	11 Mashed potato/milk, butter
18 3½ oz. pork chop	0 3 oz. cooked crab meat	4 10 potato chips
40 3½ oz. pork sausage, bulk	4 3 oz. fried haddock	12 10 large ripe olives
13 3 oz. roast veal cutlet	0 Canned mackerel	2 1 cup yellow cornmeal
0 1 slice calves liver	4 3 oz. canned sardines	2 1 cup noodles
0 2 slices pork liver	3 Canned, drained tuna	2 2 cups salted popcorn (oil)
13 3 oz. beef tongue	6 Pan-fried potatoes (¾ cup)	6 1 cup spaghetti/meat sauce
0 3½ oz. broiled cod	12 ½ large avocado	4 1 cup bean soup
0 Baked flounder	12 1 lb. loaf white bread	11 1 cup cream soup
0 ½ steamed lobster	24 1 cup macaroni/cheese	11 ¾ cup bread pudding/raisins
1 3 oz. canned salmon	2 1 cup oatmeal	3 5 caramel candies
9 Milk pudding (cornstarch)	11 1 large sweet roll	31 ½ cup unsalted brazil nuts
9 Ice milk (1 cup)	8 1 med. waffle	17 ⅓ cup commercial peanut butter
10 1 cup creamed cottage cheese	4 1 cup beef/veg. soup	
	6 1 cup tomato/milk soup	

may contribute to the development of atherosclerosis.

Nevertheless, in view of the known association of cholesterol with atherosclerosis, it is good advice for anyone over the age of forty to reduce his intake of foods which raise the cholesterol level.

Most persons with atherosclerosis or heart problems are put on low-cholesterol diets, and their serum cholesterol levels are tested from time to time to evaluate their progress. The measure of cholesterol levels is given in the number of milligrams (mg.) of cholesterol per 100 milliliters (ml.) of blood serum. A normal level is from about 150 to 260 mg./100 ml.

Cholesterol levels rise when the diet is high in saturated fats, which are usually derived from animals. Most cuts of meat, milk, butter, and many other dairy products are high in saturated fats. So is coconut oil.

An intake of largely polyunsaturated fats, on the other hand, will lower the serum cholesterol level. These fats are found in vegetables, nuts (except coconut), fish, shellfish, and fowl, as well as in liver, sweetbreads, and heart, all of which are recommended for low-cholesterol diets unless otherwise restricted. (Liver, sweetbreads, heart, and some fish, for example, are often not advised for gout patients.) Skim milk, vegetable oleomargarine, and peanut oil are excellent low-cholesterol substitutes for whole milk, butter, and conventional animal fat shortening.

It should be remembered that some cholesterol is essential to health. Drastic low-cholesterol diets should not be tried without reason or without a physician's recommendation.

Some patients seem to respond well to cholesterol-lowering drugs, either alone or accompanied by a low-cholesterol diet. Some of the drugs used are nicotinic acid, heparin, neomycin, dextrothyroxine sodium, cholestyramine, and clofibrate. Another, more drastic, method of reducing cholesterol levels is to cut out the part of the intestines which is responsible for the uptake of cholesterol from saturated fats.

Serum cholesterol levels are also used to evaluate and diagnose other diseases. The levels are high in patients with hypothyroidism (low activity of the thyroid gland) and severe diabetes.

Cholesterol sometimes forms crystals in the gallbladder that result in gallstones. When cholesterol levels are high but apparently unrelated to other disorders, the condition is known as hypercholesteremia (hypercholesterolemia). (*See also* ATHEROSCLEROSIS; DIETS.)

Choline. A nutritional factor with vitaminlike activity is the chemical compound choline. Because the body can manufacture choline, it is not a true vitamin.

Choline is an important agent in utilizing fat within the system. To prevent damaging accumulations of fat in the liver, fat must be changed within the liver from storage forms to forms that can move about. The role of choline may be important in some liver diseases.

Choline is found in many foods, usually in association with proteins. Good sources include egg yolk, meat, cereals, and legumes. There is very little choline in fruits and vegetables.

Chondrosarcoma. One of the several so-called connective tissues of the body is cartilage, which forms most of the temporary skeleton of the human fetus and remains in the adult throughout the body, usually in association with bone. A malignant tumor arising from this cartilage is called a chondrosarcoma. Its benign counterpart is called a chondroma. (*See* CANCER; MALIGNANT.)

Chordee. Sloping and bowing of the penis downward, due to a number of possible causes, is termed chordee. This may be the result of a congenital abnormality or a gonorrhea infection, affecting the urethra. (*See* PENIS; URETHRA.)

Chorea. A number of distinct diseases with entirely different causes but with similar symptoms, including involuntary and irregular jerking motions and mental difficulties, are collectively referred to as chorea. The types of chorea are based on age of onset, nervous symptoms, correlation with other diseases, and inherited predisposition to the disease.

Sydenham's chorea occurs in children and young adults. It is associated with rheumatic fever. Huntington's chorea occurs in older persons. (*See* HUNTINGTON'S CHOREA; SYDENHAM'S CHOREA.)

Choriocarcinoma. The human placenta has an epithelial cell covering. (*See* CELL; PLACENTA.) The malignant tumor which arises from this tissue is called a choriocarcinoma. Much research has recently been done on this kind of tumor, and excellent cure rates have been obtained. (*See* CANCER; CARCINOMA; MALIGNANT.)

Chorion. The outermost membrane of the two which surround the developing infant during pregnancy is called the chorion. Its inner surface touches the inner membrane, or amnion, and its outer surface touches the uterine lining, called the decidua vera. For further information *see* BAG OF WATERS.

Chorionepithelioma. This very rare disease involves a highly malignant uterine growth arising from certain cells of the placenta. This condition is also referred to as choriocarcinoma.

Although chorionepithelioma is regarded as a highly malignant tumor, it should by no means be considered uniformly fatal. This is one form of cancer where treatment has significantly improved a patient's chances of survival. According

to studies, apparently if a patient lives one year her chances of surviving for five years (the usual standard for being "cured" of cancer) are excellent.

Chorionepithelioma develops in the uterus from the cells usually associated with the placenta. In fact, it is considered a tumor of the fetal cells which has invaded the tissues of the mother.

Although chorionepithelioma may occur late in a regular pregnancy, more often it develops after delivery, miscarriage, or a hydatidiform mole or molar pregnancy. Fully 50 percent of all cases of chorionepithelioma are believed to follow molar pregnancies. Malignancy develops in probably less than 5 percent of molar pregnancies, however. The benign or noncancerous hydatidiform mole is by far the more common.

Symptoms of this disease can appear any time from a few weeks to many years after a pregnancy. Bleeding is the chief early symptom. Later a woman may have profuse and offensive vaginal discharge. Since such symptoms are also common to a number of other diseases, the woman should always consult her gynecologist and follow his advice.

Early detection of chorionepithelioma provides the doctor with more opportunity to effect a cure. As the disease progresses, the woman can develop weakness, anemia, and emaciation from frequent profuse bleeding.

Spreading of the choriocarcinoma can appear relatively soon. Frequently the vagina and the vulva become diseased, appearing with dark, clotted varicose veins or hemorrhoids. The lungs, brain, liver, bones, and even skin may become involved as well.

At times the disease has been known to disappear spontaneously. At other times the uterine tumor will disappear, but the patient may die of the damage the disease has done to other organs. Investigators are not certain what causes these changes.

Diagnosis of chorionepithelioma is generally made by microscopic examination of cells from the uterus. Curettage can remove growths from within the uterus, but surgery, including hysterectomy, is sometimes considered necessary. Recent therapy using drugs has been found to be particularly successful, however, and is being used more frequently. (*See* HYSTERECTOMY; UTERUS.)

Christmas Disease. A form of blood disorder, hemophilia B, is also known as factor IX deficiency, or Christmas disease. (*See* BLOOD DISEASES; HEMOPHILIA.)

Chromium. Recent studies have shown that chromium deficiencies in diet may cause a condition of abnormal glucose metabolism that resembles diabetes. Chromium apparently is needed for the proper remedial action of insulin. The concentration of chromium in Americans diminishes progressively with age, but not in citizens of several other countries that have been studied. This may be due to our extensive use of refined sugar and other foods from which chromium has been removed during preparation. Chromium is found most abundantly in dairy products, fish, and meat. (*See* TRACE ELEMENTS.)

Chromoblastomycosis. A variety of fungi, most of them belonging to the same genus, produce this uncommon infection. Though most cases occur in tropical and subtropical regions, the disease has been encountered on practically every continent except Asia. Warty, raised, rough, convoluted outgrowths entirely confined to the skin are the diagnostic hallmark of chromoblastomycosis, accounting for the common name "mossy foot."

The infection often follows abrasion or injury by an object contaminated with fungal spores. The fungi do not ordinarily invade man and become pathogenic only after being introduced traumatically into human tissues. Factors which contribute to infection include lack of shoes, poor living

standards, and indifference to injuries sustained on the extremities.

The infection usually begins on the leg or foot, but sometimes the inoculation may occur on some other exposed part. The early lesion is an itchy bump which enlarges irregularly and slowly forms a nondescript, superficial plaque, sometimes resembling a ringworm patch. The lesion is dull red and sharply defined, but painless.

The original plaque may continue to extend peripherally, subsequently acquiring the rough, warty appearance which characterizes the disorder. At intervals, new patches may appear and after many years most of the extremity becomes irregularly enveloped in masses of greatly elevated, hard lesions with a decidedly warty, rough surface. The multiple lesions fuse, form irregular masses with patches of normal skin in between. Progression is slow; the person's general health remains good. Sometimes, masses of elevated, hard, brownish or reddish nodules surmount the plaques, giving a cauliflowerlike appearance. Through secondary infection and neglect, older lesions may ulcerate and exude a foul-smelling discharge, but the lesions are characteristically dry and hard.

The treatment of chromoblastomycosis is still not well defined. When the infection is limited and the lesions are small, it is often possible to completely remove each of the lesions by cutting through the healthy skin around each lesion as deeply as necessary to avoid leaving behind any residual particles of pathologic tissue. The operation may be completed with plastic repair (grafting).

Lesions of limited size have also been effectively treated with amphotericin B and fluorouracil, but for many cases there is no effective treatment. Experience has shown that this disease may recur after long periods of quiescence and seeming cure. (*See* FUNGAL DISEASE.)

Chromosomes. The nucleus of a cell is made up primarily of chromosomes which direct the activities of the cell, maintain protein production, and control the reproduction of the cell and thus of the whole organism. Chromosomes cannot be seen except while the cell is dividing. (*See* MITOSIS.)

The information of heredity is written in the chemical DNA in genes in the chromosomes. (*See* DNA; HEREDITY.) Each plant and animal has an exclusive, individual set of chromosomes. This means that two distinct species can never together produce offspring. Man has forty-six chromosomes, arranged in twenty-three pairs. Each chromosome looks quite different under the microscope. The chromosomes together contain all the information which makes man what he is.

More and more research demonstrates that chromosomes can be damaged by a number of chemical, physical, and radiation factors. Such damage to chromosomes can in turn result in damage to offspring.

Chronic.
An illness or condition which is long term is referred to as being chronic. This is a relative term and is usually used in contrast to the term "acute," which indicates a sudden, fulminating, but short-duration disorder. Thus an appendicitis is an acute illness, but tuberculosis is a chronic one.

Many diseases are considered to be chronic. Cancer, tuberculosis, asthma, emphysema, stroke, congestive heart failure, cirrhosis of the liver, some kidney, infections, and ulcerative colitis are a few chronic diseases. These persist for years, causing disability and discomfort. Infections of the body in general are classified as acute or chronic, and the body response to each is different. Some chronic disorders may result from complications of acute diseases.

Chyle.
The milky fluid taken up by the intestinal lymphatic glands from food after digestion is referred to as chyle. (*See* DIGESTION; GASTROINTESTINAL SYSTEM; INTESTINES.)

Chyme.
The semifluid, creamy material produced by gastric digestion of food is known as chyme. (*See* DIGESTION; GASTROINTESTINAL SYSTEM; INTESTINES.)

Cilia.
Some of the cells that make up the mucous membranes of the body have tiny hairlike extensions. These are called cilia. Their function is to sweep along fluids or solid particles in the proper direction with whiplike motions.

Many cilia are found in the air passages of the lungs and trachea (windpipe). These help rid the lungs and trachea of dust and other materials that may enter through the nose or mouth. They also aid in evacuating the air passages of fluids and pus that may develop in the body as the result of disease.

When the material to be expelled is brought upward by the cilia through the larynx, it reaches the pharynx, where it may be coughed up or swallowed. (*See* COUGHING.)

Circadian Rhythms.
Just as the universe is in constant rhythmic motion, so are all of the physiological and biochemical processes of life. Modern techniques of collecting data on body processes have shown that nearly all body functions fluctuate over the course of a day. For this reason, the name "circadian" is derived from the Latin *circa dies*, meaning "about a day."

Perhaps even more remarkable is the fact that if all clues as to local time were to be removed, these circadian rhythms would continue to rise and fall with a period of twenty to twenty-eight hours. Body temperature usually decreases one or two degrees at night and then rises to a peak in the afternoon. This rhythm is so stable that it is often used as a synchronizing reference in the study of other body rhythms. Kidney function and the circulating components of blood also show a rhythmic cycle.

Unexpected fluctuations in man's bodily rhythms of temperature, blood pressure, levels of circulating hormones, and a variety of other metabolic substances usually

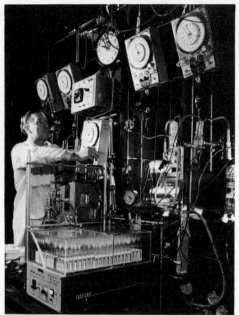

Equipment in an automated laboratory devoted to the study of circadian rhythms.

coincide with the onset of illness. Furthermore, various agents such as bacteria, anesthetics, vaccines, noise, hypnotics, muscle relaxants, and antibiotics exert their effects on the body with rhythmic characteristics. (*See* PINEAL GLAND.)

Circulation. The term circulatory system refers to the flow of blood through the body. This is described in the articles BLOOD CIRCULATION and HEART. Another circulatory system transports lymph. (*See* LYMPH.)

Circulatory System. Supplying the body's cells with fuel, water, and oxygen, and disposing of waste products, is the function of the circulatory system. It consists of the heart and blood vessels, and is responsible for the perfect functioning of the pulse, heartbeat, blood pressure, and blood supply.

The heart, which beats approximately seventy-two times per minute, is a hollow organ enclosed in a muscular wall (the myocardium), then surrounded by a fiber-like sac (the pericardium), and protected on the inside by the endocardium. It has four chambers: two at the top are called "atria," and two at the bottom are known as "ventricles." They are separated by a muscular partition known as the "septum."

After the blood has taken on waste products from the cells, and given up its oxygen, it flows into the right atrium of the heart. Here it gathers until entering the right ventricle through a small one-way valve, the tricuspid. The right ventricle then contracts and pushes the oxygen-poor blood (blue in

The human vascular system—the veins and arteries which carry the blood.

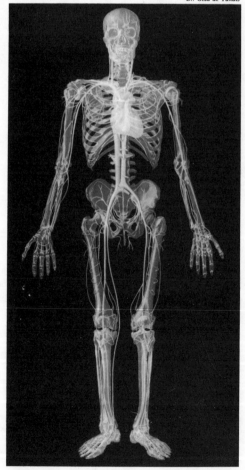

color) into the pulmonary artery. Its destination is the lungs, where it will take on oxygen.

After the blood has left the lungs, it returns to the heart through the pulmonary veins. It enters the left atrium, passes through the mitral valve and into the left ventricle. Once the left ventricle contracts, the fresh blood surges into the aorta and moves to all parts of the body.

When the blood leaves the aorta, it is at the speed of approximately fifteen inches per second. It then moves into the arteries which branch off the aorta. From the arteries it fills the arterioles, then the smallest vessels, the capillaries. Here it travels at 1/50th of an inch per second. The job of the capillaries is to carry blood fluid to cells through microscopic spaces in the capillary walls.

After oxygen and other products are diffused into the cells by capillary action, and receive, in return, waste matter, the blood carries the waste products from the capillaries into the venules. These tiny vessels belong to the return system which connects with the veins. From this point, the blood travels to the great venae cavae, large blood vessels, and then into the right atrium of the heart. (*See* BLOOD CIRCULATION.)

Circumcision.
Surgical removal of the prepuce (foreskin) from the penis is called circumcision.

The operation often is performed when the male infant is quite young, but it also is done on older boys and men. It is a preventive or treatment for various disorders of the foreskin and penis, though it is a common religious practice among Jewish people as well.

The prepuce is the loose, double, extra skin which folds over the skin of the glans at the tip of the penis. It does not extend back along the penile body, but is attached just behind the bulge or corona where the cone-shaped glans begins.

In circumcision, the outer and inner layers of skin on the prepuce are cut, parallel

to the edge of the corona, either with a surgical knife or scissors. Local anesthetic is used first, and the foreskin may be slit lengthways to make its movement easier during the operation.

In a redundant prepuce (long or excessive), it may be necessary to separate the foreskin from adhesions to the glans, and an extra inner mucous membrane must be removed.

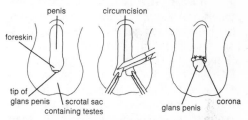

Before circumcision (*left*), the foreskin covers the glans penis almost completely. During circumcision (*center*), this loose foreskin is pulled tight, cut, and stitched parallel to the corona, the ridge where the glans joins the body of the penis. After circumcision (*right*), the glans is completely exposed.

Normally, only the surface skin and membrane are cut; the tissues underneath are left undisturbed. The edges of skin on the glans and body of the penis are sewed to each other to heal in a smooth line.

PREPUCE DISORDERS. A redundant prepuce is particularly subject to infection because of the difficulty in keeping the covered area adequately cleaned. The same is true of phimosis and paraphimosis.

In phimosis, the prepuce is too tight over the glans, making it almost impossible to pull back the skin for cleaning or other purposes. Paraphimosis is the reverse problem, when the prepuce becomes folded or rolled back behind the corona so tightly that it cannot be returned to its normal position covering the glans.

Edema can set in, inflaming the tissues so that they block blood circulation. Cracks (fissures) and ulcers may result, and eventually gangrene (death of tissue) may occur.

The skin turns dark in color. There is tenderness and severe pain. Drug injections may help reduce the swelling, but often a surgical slit is needed to free the foreskin enough to permit returning it to its proper condition.

Phimosis and paraphimosis tend to recur even after such corrective measures. Thus circumcision is the preferred treatment and preventive.

CLEANLINESS NEEDED. The tighter or larger the prepuce, the more difficult it is to keep clean. If it is not removed by circumcision, the area under the foreskin should be cleaned gently but thoroughly at least once each day—on infants as well as adults.

To do this, fold the foreskin carefully back over the body of the penis, wash gently with mild soap and water, then rinse. Be certain to return the prepuce carefully to its original position covering the glans, or edema can set in and cause paraphimosis and its complications.

Cautious cleanliness is needed because the area tends to accumulate foreign materials and its own secretions, such as smegma. This is a thick, cheesy, greasy secretion produced by the sebaceous glands to lubricate the area under the foreskin. Smegma is much like the oily sebum found on the forehead and nose. It is not related to the sperm and seminal fluids ejaculated during sexual stimulation. Smegma provides an excellent material in which bacteria can multiply, making the area highly subject to infections. This condition is corrected when the foreskin is removed.

In addition, the secretions and foreskin may increase irritation, sensitivity, or stimulation of the glans. This may affect a man's sex life by causing premature ejaculation. (*See* IMPOTENCE.)

GENITAL CANCER. Cancer of the penis and genitals is rare among men who have been circumcised, and extremely rare among those circumcised as infants.

Cirrhosis.
When we speak of cirrhosis we generally mean a liver condition. The word itself is derived from a Greek word meaning orange-yellow, and refers to the abnormal color of a diseased liver.

In fact, the term cirrhosis may be applied to any condition in which the working part of an organ (parenchyma) wastes away, while its nonfunctioning framework (interstitial tissue) tends to increase. In cirrhosis of the lung and cirrhosis of the kidney, for example, there is hardening and loss of function due to chronic inflammation. (*See* CIRRHOSIS OF THE LIVER; KIDNEY; LUNGS.)

Cirrhosis of the Liver.
Some persons believe that anyone who has cirrhosis of the liver must be an alcoholic, or at least a heavy drinker. It is true that in the United States a high percentage of cirrhosis patients are alcoholics, usually middle-aged or older. But no matter what the cause, long-continued damage to the liver may result in cirrhosis. It can occur in nondrinkers and even in young children.

In cirrhosis, functioning tissue (the cells that transform and store food materials or eliminate harmful materials from the blood) is replaced by useless scar tissue or by fat. The liver is the only organ that can replace damaged tissue, but in cirrhosis the process of repair is inadequate. The liver's reserves, great as they are, are eventually exhausted.

Some authorities believe that the malnutrition so often associated with alcoholism is what brings on cirrhosis. It is certainly true that people who "drink their lunch," and sometimes all other meals as well, are getting no real nourishment, only "empty" calories provided by the alcohol. Multiple vitamin deficiencies and severe protein deficiency are likely to result. Most heavy drinkers do not get cirrhosis, perhaps because they combine drinking with eating.

The relationship to malnutrition is confirmed by the occurrence of cirrhosis in many countries where malnutrition is a serious problem and alcoholism is not. The children's disease known as kwashiorkor, the result of extreme protein deficiency, is often associated with liver damage.

Some recent studies, however, show that alcohol *can* damage the liver, regardless of how well fed the drinker may be. A number of industrial solvents, some of them closely related to ethyl alcohol, have caused liver injury when their fumes were inhaled by unprotected workers.

Cirrhosis associated with Wilson's disease, a hereditary condition that interferes with the body's use of copper, is due to copper deposits in the liver. Hemochromatosis, a similar condition in which iron collects in various parts of the body, is often associated with severe liver damage leading to cirrhosis. (*See* HEMOCHROMATOSIS.) This disease, sometimes called bronze diabetes, is fairly common in some parts of Africa but is not widespread in the United States.

Infectious hepatitis, if properly treated, does not generally lead to cirrhosis. (*See* HEPATITIS.) But inadequate rest, poor diet, and use of alcohol may prevent the liver from healing and help to bring on permanent and even fatal injury.

Pathologists (experts in the study of diseased tissues) distinguish a number of types of cirrhosis of the liver. In some the liver is enlarged; in others it shrinks. Portal cirrhosis, the type usually associated with alcoholism, causes atrophy (shrinkage). The surface of the liver becomes bumpy and rough, a condition sometimes referred to as "hobnailed liver."

Because the liver influences or controls so many necessary functions, cirrhosis affects every part of the body. Early symptoms may be rather vague—tiredness, loss of appetite, indigestion. As the disease progresses, the patient may lose weight, vomit frequently, especially in the morning, and become jaundiced.

A characteristic sign of advanced cirrhosis is accumulation of fluid in the abdomen. The medical term for this is "ascites," and

the common word is "dropsy." It is one of the signs of obstruction of the portal circulation, an indication that the liver can no longer handle the blood that normally flows through it. Obstruction of the portal vein also leads to enlargement of the veins in the esophagus and of surface abdominal veins. This happens because blood that can no longer get through liver is diverted into new channels. The enlarged veins in the esophagus may break, causing bleeding that is very difficult to stop, often proving fatal. People with liver disease, especially when jaundiced, tend to bleed easily because the liver normally provides substances necessary for clotting. Even minor bleeding leads to anemia and further weakness. Another indication of impaired circulation is the appearance of "spider nevi" on the arms and face. A spider nevus is a red mark on the skin, centered by a tiny artery which is surrounded by broken capillaries that resemble the legs of a spider.

Enlargement of the abdomen may aggravate existing hernias or produce new ones, especially through the navel. In advanced cases of cirrhosis, toxic substances enter the bloodstream, affecting the nervous system and causing coma.

With proper care, a patient with moderate cirrhosis may recover lost liver function. Alcohol is, of course forbidden. A diet rich in protein and carbohydrate, moderate in fat, and low in salt is usually prescribed. The patient needs a great deal of rest. Supplementary vitamins to make up for past nutritional deficiencies are often necessary. Since disease of the liver tends to make people feel extremely depressed, a great deal of encouragement is needed. The liver, given a reasonable amount of help, is capable of repairing a great deal of damage. The patient should be reminded of this. (*See* LIVER.)

Citric Acid. Fruits such as oranges, grapefruits, and lemons contain citric acid, which gives "citrus fruits" their flavor. Citric acid is useful in the body's utilization of carbohydrates.

Commercial food manufacturers sometimes add citric acid to foods to add flavor. It keeps certain minerals in solution, and prevents the development of cloudiness in some beverages, but adds little nutritive value.

Claudication. The medical expression claudication, when used alone, refers to limping or lameness. Intermittent claudication specifically refers to pain that appears in the legs (and sometimes elsewhere in the body) only during exercise, and disappears during rest.

The calf muscles are most often involved. The pain is the result of insufficient circulation of blood to meet the nutritional needs of the muscles. If circulation is adequate, it may be the result of the blood being deficient in oxygen and other substances necessary for muscular activity.

In Buerger's disease, a problem of circulation, the intermittent claudication may be noticed in the arch of the foot or the palm of the hand. Intermittent claudication in various forms may also appear in some other disorders that restrict flow through blood vessels, such as atherosclerosis, in which deposits thicken the artery walls. (*See* ATHEROSCLEROSIS; BLOOD CIRCULATION; BUERGER'S DISEASE.)

Claustrophobia. A person who has a fear of being locked or shut in a small, enclosed space, such as an elevator, suffers from claustrophobia. It is quite a common symptom in psychoneurotic patients, and is usually accompanied by feelings of compression, suffocation, increased heartbeat, and severe panic. (*See* PHOBIAS.)

Clavicle. The two bones across the front of the chest (one on each side) at shoulder height are called the clavicles, or collarbones. (*See* COLLARBONE.) The space between the two clavicles forms the hollow at the base of the throat. (*See* BONES.)

Cleanliness. Keeping one's body and one's surroundings clean, or free from dirt or germs, is an important prerequisite for good health. (For related information, see DEODORANTS AND ANTIPERSPIRANTS; DETERGENTS; DISINFECTANTS AND ANTISEPTICS; HYGIENE; SOAP.)

Cleft Palate. About one in every eight hundred babies is born with a cleft palate (an opening in the roof of the mouth) or a cleft lip, sometimes called a harelip, or both.

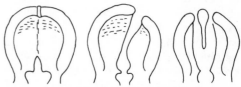

Three basic types of cleft palate are illustrated, looking up inside at the roof of the mouth behind the gums. *Left,* the pointed split up the middle (at bottom of drawing) shows division of the soft palate, which is only the rear portion of the palate. *Center,* split continues upward on one side, called unilateral complete cleft palate. *Right,* widened division straight up the middle is the full two-sided split, known as bilateral complete cleft palate.

In the normal development of a baby before birth, the lips, jaws, and palate grow from each side until they join in the center. Sometimes the two sides fail to join in a normal way, and a cleft is created. These defects vary in size and location.

The cleft may be in the soft palate, at the back of the mouth, or in the hard palate, leaving an opening into the nasal cavity. It may divide the upper lip or the bony alveolar ridge that holds the upper teeth. In more severe cases it cuts all the way through the top of the mouth and the upper lip, either on one side or on both. Occasionally a cleft is hidden by the membrane lining the mouth, and is discovered by X rays.

CAUSES. Scientists are not sure why these defects occur. Studies made with animals indicate that an inadequate diet in pregnancy may play a part. But human mothers who are well off, well educated, and presumably well fed seem to have babies with cleft palates and lips as often as those who are less fortunate.

Statistics do show that babies with these defects are more likely to be born to older parents, and they tend to weigh less than normal babies, even when they are not born prematurely. Figures also indicate that cleft palate and lip defects are more common among Japanese and rare among Negroes.

REPAIRING THE CLEFT. Correcting the cleft and the problems related to it is a long process and should be started early. Depending on the needs of the child, it may require collaboration by specialists in dentistry, surgery, speech correction, psychotherapy, and other fields.

A cleft lip is usually repaired in the first few months of life, as soon as the child is strong enough. A cleft palate is usually surgically repaired when the child is one and a half to two years old. It may take two, or even three, operations to close the cleft in the hard palate and to reconstruct the soft palate so that muscles can close off the airway between the nose and throat when necessary for speaking.

To prevent speech difficulties, a very young child may be fitted with a lightweight appliance, like an upper denture plate, to close off the cleft until he is ready for surgery. An older child with a cleft that cannot be successfully repaired by surgery can be given a similar appliance.

OTHER PROBLEMS. Closing the cleft solves only part of the problems for a child with this defect. As a baby, he must be fed in a special way. Later, he will need a great deal of special dental care, such as braces to bring his teeth into proper alignment. He is likely to need speech therapy so he can learn to speak more normally, with a less nasal sound. He may need to have old scars removed, a malformed nose straightened, or medical care for frequent middle-ear in-

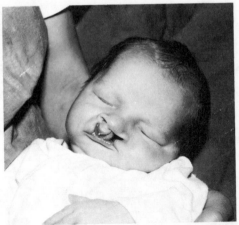

Armed Forces Institute of Pathology

This infant has congenital (present at birth) defects known as cleft palate and harelip.

fections which could lead to hearing impairment. He and his family may also need counseling or psychotherapy to help them accept the burdens that his handicap places on all of them. (*See* BIRTH DEFECTS; SPEECH; SPEECH DIFFICULTIES.)

Climacteric. The transitional period in a woman's life during which her reproductive power diminishes and, with menopause, finally disappears is known as the climacteric. It is often referred to as the "change of life."

The climacteric appears to span the years between the ages of forty-five and fifty, the time when about half of all women cease menstruating. There are wide variations in this, however, with one-fourth of all women continuing to menstruate after age fifty and another fourth reaching menopause before age forty-five. (*See* MENOPAUSE.)

Climate. The combination of weather conditions that characterizes a place or region over a season or longer is called climate.

There are some indications that man's activities may be affecting climate, particularly in cities, where air pollution may

Chart Showing Wind Chill Temperatures, Derived from Outside Temperature and Wind Speed

Outside Temperature (° F.)	WIND CHILL TEMPERATURE (° F.)							
46	44	36	31	27	25	24	23	22
42	39	31	25	21	19	16	15	14
37	34	25	18	14	12	9	7	6
31	28	18	11	6	3	0	−1	−3
27	24	13	7	1	−3	−6	−8	−9
22	18	7	1	−6	−10	−14	−15	−17
17	13	0	−8	−13	−17	−21	−23	−25
12	8	−6	−14	−21	−25	−29	−31	−33
7	3	−12	−22	−28	−32	−36	−38	−41
2	−2	−18	−31	−35	−40	−43	−45	−49
0	−5	−21	−36	−39	−44	−47	−49	−53
−2	−7	−24	−38	−42	−47	−51	−53	−57
−7	−12	−30	−42	−49	−55	−59	−62	−65
−12	−17	−36	−48	−56	−62	−67	−70	−73
−17	−23	−42	−54	−63	−70	−75	−78	−81
−22	−28	−49	−61	−70	−77	−82	−86	−88
−26	−32	−54	−67	−77	−83	−89	−93	−95
−32	−38	−61	−75	−85	−92	−97	−101	−104
−37	−44	−67	−81	−92	−100	−105	−109	−112
−42	−49	−73	−88	−99	−107	−113	−117	−120
−46	−54	−78	−94	−105	−113	−120	−124	−127
	5	10	15	20	25	30	35	40

(Wind Speed (mph))

cause climatic variations. Wind, however, is the basic factor that influences climate in cities. Tall buildings increase friction and thereby reduce the speed of moderate and strong winds, but increase turbulence in light winds. Heat is a climatic feature that can affect health, especially the health of ill or weak or aged persons. Four factors contribute to increased heat in towns: changes in thermal conditions on surfaces, caused by buildings and roads; changes in airflow patterns due to decreased diffusion of heat; lower evaporation rates and heat loss; and heat added by man's activities, as in industry. (*See* AIR CONDITIONING; TEMPERATURE; TEMPERATURE INVERSION.)

Rainfall, too, is related to health. Rainfall in cities is altered by (1) the presence of pollutants that serve as condensation agents; (2) increased turbulence caused by buildings; and (3) convection airflow caused by higher temperatures. (*See* HUMIDITY.)

On a global scale, there is some concern that two atmospheric components, carbon dioxide and dust, may be changing climatic patterns. From the 1880's to the 1940's the average temperature of the world rose by at least 0.7° F. (−14° C.). Some experts view this as a consequence of a greater carbon dioxide content in the atmosphere which, during the same period, rose by about 11 percent. This is the so-called "greenhouse effect." But after 1940 the world began to cool off, and by 1960 had cooled about 30 percent of the previous increase, even though carbon dioxide concentrations continued to rise. This phenomenon has been explained by the greater reflectivity of the earth caused by more dustiness. All these changes require adjustment and adaptation by the world's inhabitants.

Another manmade mechanism that may be influencing climatic changes on a global scale is an increased cloud cover caused by pollutants, such as contrails from jet planes. (*See* AIR POLLUTION; BIOMETEOROLOGY.)

More and more, scientists are beginning to discover the relationships between certain diseases and climatic conditions. Certain allergies and respiratory diseases, such as asthma, are either caused by or complicated by climatic factors. Doctors may frequently advise their patients who are sensitive to particular climates to move to other areas where the same set of conditions do not exist. (*See* ASTHMA.)

Clinic. Any institution which provides medical care to outpatients (patients not in a hospital) is known as a clinic. A clinic may be a group of individual doctors' offices in one building or a large building equipped with every conceivable piece of diagnostic and therapeutic equipment.

Some clinics are supported by universities, states, or cities and provide free care to whoever needs it. Many clinics are closely affiliated with hospitals. There are several large, privately owned clinics across the country which serve as referral centers for difficult medical problems. Among these are the Mayo Clinic, the Cleveland Clinic, and the Menninger Clinic. The number of clinics in this country will most likely increase since these structures relieve the burden on hospitals and provide medical care for large numbers of people.

The practice of medicine in a clinic is not new. This woodcut from Galen's *Opera Omnia,* Venice, appeared in 1550, and shows trephining (cutting open the skull), couching (displacement of the eye lens) for cataracts, dentistry, and treating of leg and abdominal wounds.

National Library of Medicine

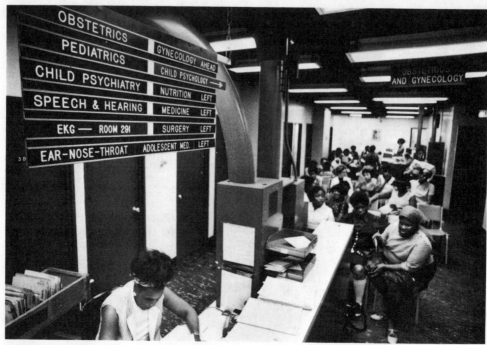

Presbyterian St. Luke's Hospital, Chicago

A clinic permits many patients to be cared for in a central location where a number of doctors share the same modern equipment and facilities. The modern clinic has many departments, each with its own staff of specialists.

Clinical Medicine. That aspect of medicine which involves the bedside care patients is referred to as clinical medici Physicians practicing clinical medicine deal directly with sick people either in the home, in the office, in a clinic, or in the hospital. Clinical physicians are patient managers and are referred to as clinicians.

Fields of clinical medicine include internal medicine and the medical subspecialties (cardiology, gastroenterology, endocrinology, etc.), general practice, pediatrics, surgery and the surgical subspecialties (urology, orthopedics, plastic surgery, etc.), obstetrics, and gynecology. Psychiatry is also a field of clinical medicine. Medical research and specialty fields such as pathology which do not deal directly with patients are not included in clinical medicine.

Clitoris. This is a highly sensitive female organ similar to a tiny male penis. It is found just in front of the introitus or opening to the vagina. (*See* FEMALE ANATOMY.)

The clitoris is almost hidden in small folds of tissue called the frenulum and prepuce, almost completely covered with only its tip visible. It is near the front of the external female organs, at the junction of the labia or fatty-tissue folds between the legs.

The clitoris contains erectile tissue that, during sexual activity, massage, or irritation, swells and stiffens.

Nerves in the clitoris are especially sensitive in creating sexual feelings as well as in responding to impulses relayed from the brain. The clitoris is believed to be the main point of sexual stimulation in the woman. (*See* FEMALE SEX ACT.)

Clonus. Normally, when the examining physician taps a tendon with his rubber hammer, the patient responds with a single muscular twitch. If the doctor taps the patellar tendon, the quadriceps muscle contracts briefly, and there is a knee jerk. Similar jerks can be elicited by striking the tendons at the ankle and the elbow; these are called tendon reflexes. In some abnormal situations, instead of a single muscle twitch, there will be a succession of twitches, and a rhythmic response called ankle-clonus, jaw-clonus, and so on. When this occurs, the physician searches further to determine the cause.

In convulsive seizures like those of epilepsy, there is commonly a tonic phase followed by a clonic phase. In the former, the patient's body is rigid and comparatively still. In the clonic phase, the body is shaken by tremors that become slower and more extensive until the whole body is tossed by a succession of violent contractions alternating with relaxations. Similar convulsions are seen in a great variety of nervous and metabolic diseases and intoxications. (*See* COMA; CONVULSIONS; DIABETES MELLITUS.)

Clot. Blood flowing from a wound or greatly slowed in its movement through the circulatory system forms a thickened mass or clot. Various names are used for clots formed inside the heart and blood vessels. The general term is "intravascular clot." More specifically, such a clot is called a "thrombus" (plural, thrombi) if it is stationary, that is, if it is caught at one point in the circulatory system, or an "embolus" (plural, emboli) if it breaks away and moves with the bloodstream. (*See* BLOOD; BLOOD CIRCULATION.)

Blood clots are rather jellylike, midway between a liquid and solid in substance. Mainly they are the cells of the blood, caught in a network formed from fibers of a protein substance. This interlaced network is the structure that gives strength to the clot, somewhat like the iron reinforcing bars in a concrete dam. And, like those bars, this network makes up only a small fraction of the total clot structure—about 1 percent.

The protein is *fibrin,* which is not a substance in the blood but is formed when a protein substance that is in the blood contacts air or is affected by injury to a blood vessel. That substance is *fibrinogen.* An interrelated chemical process of several steps leads to the formation of the fibrin fibers from fibrinogen.

At the time of the injury, the damaged tissues give off an enzyme called thromboplastin. This enzyme then reacts with calcium ions and other proteins in the blood to form a new material, prothrombin activator. They, in turn, cause other chemical changes that form another new substance called thrombin, and it is thrombin that reacts with fibrinogen to form the fibrin fibers.

This process of clot formation takes about two to six minutes. Important as it is, though, in preventing blood loss, it is fortunately not the only means of closing a wound. If it were, we could bleed to death. For enough blood can be lost from some wounds in twenty seconds to be fatal. An even faster process of hemostasis (stopping blood loss) is *spastic contraction.* When a blood vessel is damaged, the shock or trauma to the vessel tissue causes impulses in the smooth muscle of the vessel walls to crimp together spastically, constricting the broken ends of the vessel.

Complete closure of the vessels comes after the clot has fully formed. Then the fibrin fibers slowly pull together, causing two effects. First, the liquid part of the blood, serum, is squeezed out, leaving the formed bodies such as erythrocytes (red cells) and platelets. The clot then begins to take on its familiar drier appearance. Second, the contracting fibers pull together the broken edges of the blood vessels, completing their closure.

The fibers continue growing together until they have formed the tough cells of connective tissue on the exterior surface of the vessels. At the same time, smooth tissues (endothelial cells) grow back to form a new lining for the repaired vessels.

Clots form inside the blood vessels as one effect of several types of heart and vascular disease. Such clots are a problem particularly in atherosclerosis (hardening of the arteries), myocardial infarction, and coronary artery disease.

In the arteries, such clots form at plaques which are hardened growths on the inner artery walls. These clots are called thrombi.

In atherosclerosis, the formation of many thrombi impedes blood flow and may completely block it at certain points. In coronary artery disease, thrombi may block the critically important arteries that feed blood to the heart. If a clot completely shuts these arteries—total coronary occlusion—it can starve the heart muscle for oxygen, causing myocardial infarction which results in death or immediate incapacitation until treatment.

Thromboembolism is the formation of further clots in the roughened, injured inner surfaces of the cardiovascular system. It is one result of serious heart and vascular disease. Reduced heart action after a serious myocardial infarction may result in clots forming in the interior of the heart. These are called mural thrombi because they cling to the walls.

A great danger in thrombus formation is the possibility that it will break loose and move through the arteries with the bloodstream. This can happen any time from two days to three weeks after a heart attack. Then thrombi become emboli and can cause serious damage and death when they reach a restricted point in the vascular system and impede or completely stop circulation. In the brain this stoppage is called a stroke. In the heart, as noted, they can cause a coronary heart attack. When such a moving clot reaches the abdominal organ, kidneys, or limbs, it may demand emergency surgery.

Emboli also develop in the veins, as in a patient who has been bedridden for long periods. A danger here is the development of clots in the legs which then move through the veins to the pulmonary blood circuit and may cause a pulmonary embolism.

In addition to blood, lymph and spinal fluid also form clots.

Cloves. These aromatic spices are often used in medical preparations to relieve gastrointestinal discomfort or nausea. They are also used in pain-relieving medicines. (*See* DRUGS; PRESCRIPTIONS.)

Clubfoot. One of the most common congenital deformities of the foot is clubfoot. The medical name for clubfoot is *talipes equinovarus.* The word "talipes" refers to the ankle; "equino" indicates that the toes are pointed down as if to stand on tiptoe, and "varus" indicates that the toes point inward. The severity varies from minimal to so great that the toes touch the inner edge of the leg. The Achilles tendon, or heel cord, is always shortened. The foot may be so tight that it cannot be moved to a normal position. Bone changes vary with the severity of the deformity. Clubfoot usually affects just one foot, but it can affect both. Twice as many boys as girls are affected.

The cause of congenital clubfoot is not known, but there are three main theories. The first is that the foot develops abnormally during the first three months of pregnancy. Part of the support for this theory is that other abnormalities are frequently found elsewhere in the body of a person who has a clubfoot. A second theory is that the deformity is due to muscle imbalance. The last theory—that the deformity is due to improper position of the foot while the child is in the uterus—is generally disregarded.

In an infant, it is easy to decide that club-foot is congenital. Clubfoot diagnosed later in life, however, may be caused by paralysis, especially spina bifida, cerebral palsy, poliomyelitis, or muscular dystrophy. In long-standing cases there is often knock-knee, as the body tries to rebalance its weight. A child with clubfoot has difficulty learning to walk because the muscles in the affected leg tire quickly. A person with clubfoot on one side will limp. If clubfoot is present on both sides, there is a characteristic waddling or reeling gait.

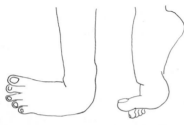

Deformities of the foot are called talipes, or clubfoot. In talipes varus (*left*) the foot is markedly twisted. In talipes equinus (*right*) the Achilles tendon is contracted, preventing the person from placing his foot flat on the floor. Plaster casts, stretching of muscles, and cutting of tendons are some of the measures used to correct clubfoot.

The earlier treatment is started, the better the outlook. If treatment begins before the age of three months, full correction can usually be obtained without surgery, but it may require several years. In cases where treatment begins after the first year, there is seldom complete correction. If the condition goes untreated, it becomes worse as the person continues to walk on the outer border of his foot. Correction after the age of ten years requires surgery on the bones of the foot. It is important to overcorrect the deformity since there will be some undoing of the correction. The person must then be carefully watched for several years. Some people require a second period of treatment.

In infants, clubfoot can be corrected with a series of plaster casts, changed every three to fourteen days. Each cast obtains a bit more correction than the last. An alternate treatment is a Denis-Browne splint. This consists of two padded metal plates which are attached to the feet with adhesive tape. They are connected by an adjustable metal bar. Surgery may be required to lengthen the Achilles tendon with either type of correction. It may be necessary to wear a cast or splint at night for many months in order to maintain the correction. Special shoes are needed, with the toes turned outward and a wedge along the outer edge of the sole. Walking is encouraged to strengthen the involved muscles.

Coagulant. In the body fluids, including blood, lymph, and spinal fluid, the substances that cause thickening or coagulation are called coagulants. (*See* BLOOD; BLOOD CIRCULATION.)

Clotting action in the blood, for example, is an interrelated sequence of processes. The coagulant substances that mainly interact in this sequence are, in order of their clotting action, thromboplastin, thrombin, and fibrinogen. But they are not the only coagulants or clotting-related substances. Medical scientists have identified at least ten clotting factors in the blood. They include proteins, lipoproteins (combinations of fatty-waxy lipids and proteins), and calcium ions. (*See* CLOT; COAGULATION.)

Coagulation. The process of forming clots in the blood, plasma (including lymph), and spinal fluid is known as coagulation. It is a process in which the fluid is thickened.

Once this process has started, it usually cannot be stopped. It can be prevented from starting, however, by chemicals called anticoagulants, and sometimes internal clots that have formed in the blood circulatory system can be dissolved. (*See* BLOOD; BLOOD CIRCULATION.)

Coagulation of blood consists of the step-by-step formation, in precise sequence, of substances from the blood that finally form what appears to be the jellylike mass of a clot. Total time for clot formation is about two to six minutes.

This sequential process is by no means as simple as A, B, C, but it *is* easier to visualize if broken down into three major steps:

First, after an injury, processes form a fatty-waxy protein substance called thromboplastin. Second, thromboplastin acts in processes that form another protein material, thrombin. Third, thrombin acts on a blood protein ingredient called fibrinogen to form fibrin, and fibrin forms the framework or tough reinforcement of the clot.

A CONTRADICTION. Blood coagulation can be comprehended best if it is understood as truly a contradiction in terms. It is stating that blood, a fluid, can become something it is not, namely a semi-solid material. And this change does not actually begin in external causes. An injury triggers coagulation, but the blood must produce it.

The basic cause of the change is in the blood itself, but obviously in such forms that it cannot coagulate the blood at just any time. Otherwise circulation could be stopped erratically by clotting within the vessels. The blood substances that cause coagulation, therefore, must be in some pre-coagulant form that requires chemical or physical changes before they can cause coagulation. This is, in fact, the nature of the substances that coagulate the blood. They are there all the time but not as coagulants.

FRAGILE CELLS BREAK. When the body is injured, both the blood and the tissue at the point of the injury release the complex protein thromboplastin. At the same time, the smallest of the blood-formed bodies, called platelets and thrombocytes, spread around the injury as the blood comes out. These bodies measure only one to four microns in diameter. There are normally about 250,-000 to 300,000 platelets in one cubic milli-

meter of blood. They are shaped like flat plates (as indicated by one of their names) and have an important job in clotting (as indicated by their other name; Greek, *thrombos:* clot, *kutos:* hollow vessel). And that, in fact, is what they are—not true cells but hollow, fragile containers.

There are at least 13 factors known to be involved in the clotting of blood. They are given numbers—factors I to XIII. Factors I to IV are fibrinogen, prothrombin, thromboplastin, and calcium ions. The remaining factors are more recent discoveries, and their activity and function have been the subject of controversy for many years. Each year some investigator presents a new outline of the complicated events which lead to blood clotting. The most recent is as follows:

Factors XII, XI, IX, VIII, and X are present in inactive form in the circulating blood. When blood is placed in a glass vessel, the clotting process begins with the activation of XII by the wettable surface of glass. Activated XII activates XI, which activates IX, which activates X. (In blood shed from a cut or wound, a tissue factor activates VII, which activates X, thus at least partly bypassing XII, XI, IX, and VIII.) It is the combination of activated X, V, calcium ions, and a specific fatty material from disintegrated platelets which becomes the thromboplastin (factor III) of the older medical literature.

This thromboplastin combination converts prothrombin to thrombin, which in turn quickly converts soluble fibrinogen into the insoluble strands of fibrin. The latter become enmeshed, and hold together the blood cells and serum in the form of a gel, quite like a fruit gelatin mold.

Factor XIII is involved in transforming the loose clot into the final firm clot. Factor VIII is the antihemophiliac factor. Its congenital absence from blood is the cause of hemophilia. The absence of factor IX produces a milder bleeding disease, sometimes called hemophilia B.

Cobalt. This trace element, found primarily in green, leafy vegetables, is thought by some scientists to be an essential element for humans. This is because it serves as one of the components in the vitamin B_{12} molecule, an anti-anemia factor found in the liver. (*See* TRACE ELEMENTS.)

Cocaine. The leaves of the coca plant, found in South America, yield an often misused drug called cocaine. Referred to as "coke," the drug is a stimulant that causes euphoria when sniffed or injected. It is often mixed with heroin to speed up the effect of H (heroin), or to cut the stimulating effect of cocaine.

Cocaine is a short-lived drug and requires repeated daily usage to maintain a "high." Because of this characteristic, overdosage is common and death is swift, since there is little time to reverse the effects of cocaine poisoning.

Repeated usage develops no physical dependence but a strong psychological need. Paranoia, delusions, hallucinations, and hearing distortions occur with continued heavy use. (*See* ADDICTION.)

Cocarcinogenesis. Most physicians believe that many cancers require more than a single factor to initiate their growth. That process by which cancer is induced by the action of two or more agents working together is called cocarcinogenesis. Many investigators feel that hormones may play the role of cocarcinogen by changing the chemical environment of certain cells, thus making them more susceptible to carcinogens. (*See* CANCER; CARCINOGENS.)

Coccidioidomycosis. A relatively common disease, in desert areas of the United States and throughout the world, where persons are exposed to the fungus *Coccidioides immitis,* is coccidioidomycosis. The fungus is breathed into the lungs and from there spreads through the blood to the skin, bones, central nervous system, and other organs. The severity of the disease varies widely, depending mainly on degree of exposure; only one out of a thousand cases is fatal. Those most afflicted are workers in the deserts who breathe dust that carries the fungus.

Respiratory symptoms are similar in many respects to pneumonia, with congestion due to the inflammation caused by the spores of the fungus. After seven to twenty-eight days following exposure, the patient develops headache, backache, fever, cough, fatigue, and chest pains. These initial symptoms greatly resemble those of influenza. One of the largest problems with the disease, in fact, is that most persons do not seek medical attention since no distinct symptoms are present that would lead one to suspect other than routine illness.

In some instances, the fungal infection develops in the skin. This may be due to introduction of dust into wounds in the skin. Swelling and irritation follow.

Diagnosis is made by response to skin tests and to laboratory cultures of the fungus taken from the patient. Suspicion of the disease generally follows a return from an area where the fungus is known to exist. In this country the desert areas of California, Arizona, New Mexico, Texas, Utah, and Nevada produce a large number of cases.

Coccidioidomycosis is locally known by a number of common names, including desert fever, San Joaquin Valley fever, and valley fever. (*See* DESERT FEVER.)

Coccyx. The four vertebrae at the base of a child's spine fuse as the child grows older to become a single bone in the adult, called the coccyx. The coccyx is the only remnant man has of a tail after millions of years of evolution. The coccyx normally curves forward between the buttocks. It can be fractured in a fall if the person lands on it, or it can be bent slightly more forward. This can cause muscle spasms and pain and must be corrected by a physician. (*See* SPINE.)

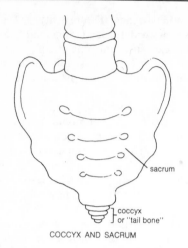

COCCYX AND SACRUM

Cockroaches. Although cockroaches do not present any physical harm to humans through direct contact, as do lice and mites, they do feed on food and human feces. Because of this, they often become infected with disease-producing organisms which they later excrete on to food, thereby spreading disease.

Cockroaches are found world-wide. They are agents in spreading cholera, dysentery, and many species of parasitic worms.

Codeine. One of the drugs obtained from the juice of an unripe white poppy is codeine. It is chemically similar to morphine, also an opium derivative, but milder. Codeine is commonly used in cough medicine and as an analgesic (pain-killer) in tablet form.

When abused, codeine produces a mild "high" and sedative reaction. Withdrawal symptoms are likewise mild. Like many other drugs, codeine causes the body to build up a tolerance which stimulates the user to need more and more of the drug to achieve desired effects. (*See* ADDICTION; DRUG ABUSE.)

Cod Liver Oil. A rich source of vitamin A and vitamin D is cod liver oil, obtained from the livers of codfish. It is an ingredient in many vitamin preparations and is often prescribed by itself for certain vitamin deficiencies. (*See* VITAMIN DEFICIENCIES; VITAMINS.)

Coffee. To begin their day, or to gain relief from a stressful situation, many people rely on a cup of coffee. Coffee has almost no nutritive value and is primarily a stimulant. The stimulating ingredient is caffeine. Coffee also contains a small amount of tannic acid, with percolated coffee having more than drip coffee.

Some people say that coffee has the effect of waking them up or giving them a feeling of instant energy. This is because, as a stimulant, coffee affects the central nervous system, considerably increasing the heart action in rate and in strength. This results indirectly in increased activity of the kidneys. Respiration is deepened, and the brain centers become excited. For this reason, coffee is often used in reviving a person who has had too much alcohol to drink.

Many students, watchmen, and others who must remain alert for long hours drink considerable amounts of coffee because they think it takes away their feelings of fatigue. This feeling occurs because of coffee's stimulating effect on the brain.

Individuals can tolerate different levels of caffeine in coffee. Certain persons, particularly those who have cardiac conditions or hyperthyroidism, in which the heart is already overstimulated, should reduce their coffee intake.

For the benefit of persons who cannot tolerate caffeine, decaffeinated coffee is available. The coffee beans are softened by steaming them under pressure. The caffeine is then extracted with alcohol, and the extracting solvents are removed by resteaming. After this treatment, the coffee beans are roasted, packed, and sold like standard coffee.

The method of preparing coffee affects its caffeine content. Drip and vacuum coffee contain the least amount of caffeine, percolated coffee contains slightly more caffeine than does drip coffee, and "boiled" coffee contains more caffeine than either drip or percolated. The caffeine contained in a cup of instant coffee is generally high compared with the amount in regular coffee. Usually, the average cup of coffee contains about 1.5 to 2.5 grains of caffeine. This depends, however, on the amount of coffee used and the resulting strength of the brew. (*See* CAFFEINE.)

There is caffeine in tea, and a similar substance in cocoa.

As with all other stimulants, moderation in drinking coffee is advisable for all persons.

Coitus. Sexual intercourse is also known by the term coitus. Also called coition, the word derives from a Latin word meaning "to come together." (*See* FEMALE SEX ACT; MALE SEX ACT.)

Coldness. A common symptom of many conditions is a feeling of coldness. Such a feeling is normal when a person is exposed to low temperatures. It is pathological (disease connected) when it is experienced independently of the temperature of the surrounding atmosphere.

The feeling of coldness is usually caused by a diminished flow of blood in the skin; the endings of the nerve fibers which convey coldness are stimulated when the skin temperature falls. The sensation of coldness depends on skin temperature and not on the internal temperature of the body. A person may feel cold on going to bed and remain so for a long time; but this is not so after a warm bath. In each case, the internal temperature of the body remains about the same.

Coldness may be felt in one part of the body only. Local lesions of blood vessels of an obstructive nature—such as embolism, thrombosis, or temporary arterial spasm cutting off the blood supply—will cause coldness of the affected part, usually a limb. Cold, sweating hands and feet sometimes occur in rheumatoid arthritis. The cause is sluggish circulation. General coldness of the body occurs in surgical or traumatic shock.

Some people believe in taking an alcoholic drink to "keep out the cold." This may make a person feel warmer, but actually it may increase heat loss from dilated skin vessels unless the person is well wrapped. When a person is covered with blankets, alcohol can cause him to pick up heat. (*See* CHILLS.)

Colds. Everyone knows what a cold is, and has his own pet remedies. But even this statement, like almost everything else you can say about the common cold, is subject to some question. Just how do we distinguish, for example, between a severe cold and a mild case of influenza? There is no precise line between the two.

Some medical authorities feel we should abandon the term "common cold" and make it clear that this so-called disease is really a set of symptoms which are caused by many agents. A cold is the result of viral infection. But most diseases are caused by one or a few specific viruses, while common cold symptoms may result from perhaps a hundred different viruses.

If the common cold could be blamed on one virus, perhaps we could develop a vaccine for long-lasting immunity. But how to cope with a whole army of viruses? The problem is one of the most difficult for medical science. Some vaccines seem to impart a slight degree of immunity, but apparently only against infection by a few of the many viruses that may cause a cold.

There is no real cure for a cold. Available remedies sometimes seem to work, because they make you feel better or are active against bacterial complications rather than the virus culprit itself. Some progress has been made in research with a substance called interferon, which helps body cells

Questions and Answers About Colds

Q. What should you do when a cold strikes?

A. The prescription is to ease cold symptoms, not cure them. Take aspirin, drink fluids, keep warm, and go to bed. Antihistamines will neither cure your cold nor prevent infection from cold viruses. They simply reduce the amount of secretion that occurs from cold symptoms, thereby making you more comfortable.

Q. Does the wind make you catch cold?

A. Possibly, as cold viruses are airborne and spread more easily during windy weather.

Q. Does bad weather make you susceptible to a cold?

A. Wet, cold weather is conducive to catching a cold, especially if it is windy. Dry weather, hot or cold, does not encourage colds, nor does it make a cold victim as uncomfortable as does cold, wet weather.

Q. Is a cold the same thing as an allergy?

A. No, in most cases. When a victim is suffering from an allergic inflammation of the nose, his symptoms may parallel those of a cold. Only a physician can diagnose which it is.

Children who have allergies that affect the upper respiratory tract get colds more frequently than do nonallergic children.

Q. When can you tell if you're getting a cold?

A. Ordinarily not until symptoms appear. An inflamed throat, a runny nose, and watering eyes are the usual signs.

Q. Are colds contagious?

A. Yes. So wear a mask and keep your hands washed if you are caring for a child or preparing meals while you have a cold. After coughing into a tissue or blowing your nose, always destroy the tissue and wash your hands to prevent the spread of germs.

prevent invasion by viruses or stops them from reproducing within the cells.

Antihistamine preparations have been strongly advocated as cold remedies, but they are effective only if the cold symptoms are caused by an allergy. (*See* ALLERGY.) Some persons may be allergic to the viruses themselves or to the by-products the body produces in response to them.

Allergies, influenza, chickenpox, some types of pneumonia, whooping cough, rheumatic fever, and a number of other diseases may first manifest themselves with symptoms identical to those of a simple cold. (*See* ALLERGY; CHICKENPOX; PNEUMONIA; RHEUMATIC FEVER; WHOOPING COUGH.) The lesson here is that you should never take your cold for granted. Watch it carefully, and if complications develop, call your physician for advice.

DEFINITION OF A COLD. What is a simple cold? We need to define it before we can tell what to do about it. It is a virus infection of the upper respiratory passages, with resulting inflammation and blocking of the nasal passages, a thick or watery discharge from the nose, a scratchy or tickling throat, uncomfortable breathing, and itchy or watery eyes. The sufferer may have aches in various parts of his body, a moderate headache, and a mild fever. (*See* FEVER; HEADACHE.)

Each person seems to have his own special pattern of symptoms for a simple cold. The degree of discomfort also differs from one person to another. Presumably the type of virus may also determine the severity of the symptoms.

Here's a good rule: For a simple cold, take simple precautions. *Avoid* drastic remedies. Get extra rest—in bed, if you can. Relieve your discomfort with aspirin in conservative doses. Drink plenty of fluids. Eat carefully, not because diet will cure your cold, but to avoid adding digestive irritation to your discomfort. Avoid getting chilled or too warm. A hot bath may make you feel better and the steam may help relieve nasal congestion. Keep your home well humidified.

Don't take laxatives for your cold. But if you happen to be constipated as well as having a cold, there is no harm in a mild laxative. If you have a *simple* cold, avoid nasal decongestant sprays. While they may open up your nasal passages, they also may dry and expose your mucous membranes so that they are more vulnerable to complicating bacterial infections.

There are only two purposes in treating a simple cold. One is to relieve the symptoms. The other is to prevent complications. If you can do this, your cold will run its course in some five to ten days. If the cold lasts longer than two weeks, you should suspect that your simple cold has been complicated by bacteria. Or the symptoms may be a sign of some other problem.

If your throat is not just slightly irritated but raw and sore, if your headaches are severe and persistent, if your sinuses are involved, if your ears ache, or if you have a high or constant fever, then you no longer have a simple cold but a complicated one, and should take precautions. Your doctor may prescribe antibiotics to combat bacterial infections, and recommend decongestants; and you had better avoid pushing yourself through your normal day's activities and get to bed.

If you are careful, chances are your cold will go away without making you seriously ill and with a minimum of complications. There are about 250 million cases of the common cold in the United States each year, and only a relative few have serious complications.

You will risk developing sinusitis, otitis media (middle ear infection), bronchitis, flu, and pneumonia if you get overtired, fail to get proper nutrition, or otherwise contribute to lower resistance while you have a cold.

AVOIDING A COLD. Scientists have conducted experiments to see if volunteers can catch colds on purpose by getting chilled, sitting in drafts, or exposing themselves to persons with colds. They have found it hard to infect someone with a cold virus deliberately. Probably the reason is that it may be a combination rather than a single factor that makes a person susceptible to attack by a virus.

Persons who cut themselves short on sleep and experience a period of stressful living tend to catch colds more easily than others. Some of these same people also have poor eating habits. There is little doubt that improper nutrition will make you more vulnerable not only to colds but to most other diseases.

If you catch cold readily, try taking things a little easier during the cold season. Get plenty of rest, eat balanced meals, and don't let the pace of modern life get you down.

Do not overdose yourself with vitamins. Vitamin C tablets, for example, may well help you avoid a cold, but only if you happen to be deficient in this vitamin in the first place. Your body has certain daily needs for vitamins, but loading yourself with more than you need is a waste of money and exposes you to possible harmful side-effects. (*See* VITAMINS.)

The viruses that cause colds are chiefly airborne. Sneezing, coughing, blowing the nose, and talking help spread these viruses. So avoid crowds when many people have colds. If you isolate yourself as much as possible when you do have a cold, your cold will not go away any faster, but you will be doing your family and friends a favor by keeping your viruses to yourself.

Youngsters are more susceptible to colds than are most adults. Crowded classrooms, close contact with playmates, and poor habits, such as neglecting to wipe noses and wash hands, may be the reason.

The use of disposable tissues instead of cloth handkerchiefs will help prevent the spread of cold viruses, but not if you toss the soiled tissues into any handy wastebasket or leave them lying on chairs and dressers. Put them into a paper bag for disposal or flush them down the toilet.

It is a good health precaution not to let your body get chilled, but it is doubtful that chilling alone can cause a cold. Physical exercise in itself is a good healthful habit, but there is no evidence that it will help you ward off colds. In fact, many athletes often get colds. This could be due to the fact that many infective organisms become airborne in steamy locker and shower rooms during the changing of sweaty clothes and as body dirt is scrubbed off.

Low humidity, common inside homes and offices in the winter, tends to dry out the mucous membranes of respiratory passages, making them more vulnerable to infection. (*See* INFLUENZA; VIRUSES.) Try to keep the relative humidity in your home at a level of at least 45 percent. If a member of your family is particularly subject to respiratory complications, buying an automatic humidifier may be well worth the expense. In other cases, home remedies may be sufficient. (*See* HUMIDITY.)

Cold Sores. The common fever blister, or cold sore, as it is sometimes called, is a virus infection called herpes simplex. (*See* HERPES SIMPLEX.)

Colectomy. The surgical removal of part or all of the colon is referred to as colectomy. (*See* COLON; GASTROINTESTINAL SYSTEM.)

Colic. Extreme, sharp abdominal pain, particularly in the area of the large intestine—that is, lower in the tract—is *colic.* Rather than being a specific disease, colic is more often a symptom of other disturbances. Often the cramping, spasmodic pain is fleeting and recurrent. Colic is generally treated by removing the actual cause of the ailment, rather than by treating its symptoms.

Colic may be the result of poisonings involving lead, zinc, or excessive eating or drinking. Similar symptoms can result from buildup of gas in the intestinal tract, as is often the case with infants; this latter instance can generally be prevented by proper feeding and burping of the child.

Other difficulties leading to colic include menstrual cramps, parasitic infestation of the bowels, obstructions in the intestinal tract, and constipation. Colic may occur when there are stones in the gallbladder or the urinary tract, or when the urinary tract is inflamed due to infection. (*See* CALCULI.)

Colitis. Specifically, colitis means inflammation (itis) of the colon, a portion of the intestines. There are many diseases in which this can occur as a symptom. Only certain disorders, however, are commonly given the label of colitis.

One is ulcerative colitis. It is typified by diarrhea, often bloody and mucous. In severe cases, the patient may have twenty or more bowel movements in a day. Sometimes, however, the person may be constipated instead of having diarrhea, or alternate between these extremes. Ulcers are the source of bleeding. But these are ordinarily smaller and not as deep as the common peptic, duodenal, or jejunal types usually referred to when one speaks of ulcers. (*See* ULCERS.)

Loss of weight and anemia may result from the impairment of the uptake of nutrients from the intestines during colitis. Fever and abdominal pain are also common during acute (sudden) attacks. Toxemia—poisonous body or bacterial by-products—may also occur.

The problem may be chronic, that is, it may be long-lasting with periods of remission (freedom from symptoms) and exacerbations (return of symptoms). Complications may be varied, including hemorrhoids, abscesses, prolapse of the colon (doubling over of the intestinal wall), fistulas (abnormal passages), and strictures (narrowing of the colon in places.)

Ulcerative colitis often starts in the lower, or sigmoid, colon. But it may include the entire large intestine and even extend to the ileum, the part of the upper, or small, intestine which joins the large. Some physicians call this "backwash ileitis." (*See* ILEITIS; ILEUM.)

Diagnosis is often made by examination by a sigmoidoscope, an instrument for looking into the lower colon, or by similar instruments designed for other parts of the intestinal tract.

POSSIBLE CAUSES. Most cases of ulcerative colitis occur without the determination of a specific cause. It is suspected that infections may sometimes be to blame, but in most instances no abnormal bacteria (some are normally in the intestines) or viruses are found.

In dysentery, which causes inflammation of the colon, microorganisms start the disease process, but this problem is not usually classified as colitis. (*See* AMEBIC DYSENTERY; DYSENTERY.)

Children often develop ulcerative colitis, and it is suspected that the tendency may be inherited. Statistics show that the disease does run in families, particularly among younger adults, and in women more so than in men.

Emotional factors in ulcerative colitis have been the subject of many studies. The patient is often depressed, with a feeling of hopelessness and helplessness, and is inclined to rate his life as a failure. The same pattern fits many persons with mucous colitis. This is a variation in which there is much mucus and no blood, or little blood, in the stool.

Spastic colitis is another term, used more by patients than doctors, to describe general irritation of the lower intestines. Physicians often class it with what is called the "irritable bowel syndrome," which covers disturbances of the intestines believed to be largely emotional in cause. (*See* BOWELS.)

Allergy to specific foods is another possible cause of colitis.

TREATMENT. The person with ulcerative colitis is usually kept in bed during acute attacks, given sedatives, and put on a bland low-residue diet. Raw fruits and vegetables;

fruit juices, coffee, and alcohol; and highly spiced foods are not recommended for colitis patients, as they may be irritating to the already sensitive colon.

Psychotherapy often helps. This is treatment aimed at relieving tensions, frustrations, and resentments that may have contributed to the onset of colitis. In some persons it is found that the onset of colitis will follow a distressful circumstance, such as the loss (by death, divorce, and so forth) of a loved one, or discharge from employment. Antibiotics, sulfa drugs, and corticosteroids such as ACTH have aided some patients, although it is not clear exactly why. In severe cases, removal of a portion of the intestines may be the only means of obtaining relief.

Cancer of the intestinal tract occurs more often among persons with colitis than among those with a normal colon. (*See* CANCER.)

For other problems which involve the colon or which may have symptoms resembling that of colitis, *see* DIARRHEA; ENTERITIS; INTESTINES.

Collagen. The protein responsible for most of the support in our skin, bones, cartilage, tendons, ligaments, and other connective tissues is collagen. The proper amount of collagen in these tissues is necessary to provide just the right degree of support. Too much of the albuminlike protein results in stiffness; too little decreases resilience.

The digestive system contains an enzyme called collagenase which breaks down the collagen in meats so that they can be digested and used by the body. Collagen is also used industrially in the production of gelatin for dessert foods.

Collagen Diseases. Several diseases which are grouped together on the basis of a similar characteristic—an involvement of connective tissue—are called collagen diseases, or connective tissue diseases. The most common of these are systemic lupus erythematosus, dermatomyositis, polyarteritis, and scleroderma. Interest in and knowledge of these diseases has increased markedly in the last twenty-five years, though their cause is not yet known.

The connective tissue system, located between the various body cells, provides support and lubrication. There are two parts to connective tissue: fibers and a shapeless matrix, or ground substance, that contains the fibers. There are two types of fibers, collagen fibers and elastic fibers.

In collagen diseases, connective tissue throughout the body becomes inflamed and damaged. These changes in the connective tissue can be detected microscopically by staining each of the components of connective tissue with a different dye, making identification of the various parts easy. Some of the fibrous material loses shape and is deposited in the ground substance.

Another form of connective tissue damage shows that gamma globulin is involved in some of the diseases. (*See* GAMMA GLOBULIN.) The presence of abnormal gamma globulins has led to the theory that these are "auto-immune" diseases—that is, the person reacts to certain parts of his body as if they were foreign substances, and tries to destroy them.

All the collagen diseases show individual characteristics as well as a common involvement of joints, blood vessels, heart, skin, and muscles. Certain characteristics of all the diseases respond to treatment with steroid medications.

Systemic lupus erythematosus, or SLE, is a kind of collagen disease which affects the blood vessels, the skin, and the serous and synovial membranes. The disease usually shows exacerbations and remissions. It is most common in young women and may have a hereditary component. A sign peculiar to SLE is the appearance of a butterfly-shaped rash on the face after exposure to sunlight. The skin and joints are usually the first parts of the body to be affected. Occasionally, the complaints may be local in-stead of generalized. (*See* LUPUS ERYTHEMATOSUS.)

Dermatomyositis commonly involves the muscles and skin, although skin involvement may be minimal or occasionally absent. There is muscle weakness in the area of the shoulders and hips, the upper arm and thigh, and the neck and throat. The onset of dermatomyositis often follows an infection or some other disorder, particularly cancer. In fact, it may be a result of the body's reaction to the malignancy. Symptoms can be of any intensity from very mild to very severe. (*See* DERMATOMYOSITIS.)

Polyarteritis, formerly called polyarteritis nodosa, involves the arteries of muscles throughout the body. Often there are nodules, or small lumps, on the arteries. Similar changes are seen in allergic reactions, but there is usually no history of allergic reactions in patients with polyarteritis. It is now believed that several different diseases produce the changes of polyarteritis. (*See* POLYARTERITIS NODOSA.)

Scleroderma, or progressive systemic sclerosis, causes widespread changes in the skin. The skin becomes leathery and highly pigmented and begins to atrophy. Arteries become constricted, and the tissue they nourish dies. There may be loss of fingertips. The skin becomes tight and stretched. The face loses expression and the lips tend to be tightly drawn together. There is often general weakness and weight loss. Later there is difficulty in swallowing. Function of the thyroid, pancreas, pituitary, and adrenal glands is affected. The heart and lungs can also be involved. Scleroderma affects women more than men, usually striking during middle life. There has also been a high incidence of the disease reported among workers exposed to silica dust. (*See* SCLERODERMA.)

Some researchers consider rheumatoid arthritis to be a collagen disease. It is a systemic disease which affects the joints, particularly the small joints, and is charac-

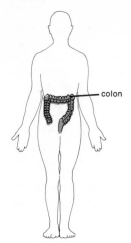
colon

terized by a chronic inflammation of the synovial membranes. (*See* SYNOVIAL MEMBRANES.) Joints become stiff and painful and are eventually deformed by the inflammation. Systemic signs are fatigue and weight loss. (*See* ARTHRITIS.)

Collapse. When a person is in a condition of extreme prostration, with failure of blood circulation, he is in a state of collapse. The term collapse also applies to an abnormal falling in of the walls of any organ or body part. (*See* CIRCULATORY SYSTEM; FAINTING; LUNGS; PTOSIS; SYNCOPE.)

Collarbone. One of the bones most frequently fractured is the collarbone, or clavicle. (*See* CLAVICLE.) There are two of these bones in the body, located on either side across the front of the chest, just below the neck. The purposes of the collarbone are to transmit forces from the arm to the trunk, to hold the arm up and slightly away from the trunk, and to provide a place for muscles to attach. The weakest point, and therefore the place where most fractures occur, is two-thirds of the way from the middle of the chest to the shoulder. The usual cause of fracture of this bone is a fall in which the person lands on his hand or arm. When the collarbone breaks, the muscles are unable to support the weight of the arm.

A person who has fractured his collarbone is thus often seen holding up his sagging arm. A plaster cast is not usually used in treating the fracture, but a sling is used to support the arm until the bone heals. (*See* BONES.)

Colon. The part of the large intestine between the cecum and rectum is called the colon. (*See* INTESTINES.)

Color Blindness. The inability to recognize any colors, or certain colors, is usually inherited as a genetic defect. The problem lies in defects in the cones, small color-sensitive cells in the retina of the eye. Defects in the various types of cones determine the kind of color blindness. A protanope is a person who has little or no sensitivity to red. A tritanope is blind to the violet colors, and a deuteranope is blind to green. Some deuteranopes, able to detect blue clearly, may confuse red and green, seeing yellow instead. There are other combinations of color blindness as well.

Some persons who are color blind may be unaware of the defect. They confuse color changes with dark and light shades, and have no way of understanding the nature of colors they have never seen. How would you describe the color red to someone who has never seen it?

Disorders of the eye other than inherited defects may also result in temporary or permanent color blindness. Color vision loss may result from degeneration of the optic nerve due to neuritis, anemia, and infectious diseases such as syphilis, tuberculosis, or malaria.

Malnutrition and swallowing of poisonous chemicals or drugs are other causes of color blindness or a limited perception of colors. Cataracts and other eye diseases that result in opacities (nontransparent areas) of the lens and cornea will reduce color vision.

If the underlying disease can be cleared up, better color vision may return. But some color blindness, such as that which is inherited, cannot be corrected. (*See* EYE.)

A person may not be aware he is color blind until his eyes are examined. If he finds he cannot see colors properly, he should train himself to use other clues to vision. Examples are the standard arrangement of stoplights with the red at top, and the shapes of various warning traffic signs.

Colostomy. When part of the lower intestine is removed because of cancer or other condition, the cut end of the colon (largest part of the large intestine) is sewed to an opening in the abdomen for the removal of feces (waste digestive material).

The individual wears an attached appliance with disposable bags for receiving the discharge of material.

Details are described in the article ILEOSTOMY. An ileostomy is similar to a colostomy except that the ileum, rather than part of the colon, ends at the surface of the abdomen.

Colostomy. The normal path of waste matter through the colon is indicated by the arrows. If the colon is diseased beyond repair, it may be necessary to cut off the lower portion of the colon (see dotted line) and make an artificial opening, or colostomy, so that waste material may pass out from the abdomen into a bag worn on the surface of the body.

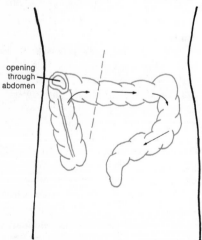

opening through abdomen

Colostrum. Several months after a woman becomes pregnant, her breasts begin to secrete a thick, yellowish fluid known as colostrum. This liquid is not true milk.

For approximately two days after delivery, the breasts continue to produce colostrum before the mother's milk comes in. Newborn infants should be allowed to suckle the colostrum, however, since it contains valuable antibodies from the mother that will help protect the infant from disease. This first food also contains more protein and more minerals than breast milk, but less sugar and fat. (*See* BREAST FEEDING.)

Colpotomy. An incision made into the abdomen through the cul de sac of the vagina is known as colpotomy. This cut allows a physician to explore the abdominal cavity for possible disease or other abnormalities. The technique is especially useful for diagnosing ectopic pregnancies.

Coma. When a disease process blots out the function of the cerebral hemispheres so that the cortex of the brain cannot be aroused, a person is said to be in a state of coma. A tremendous number of syndromes can potentially bring on a comatose state. These include cerebral hemorrhage, large cerebral infarction, blood clots in the brain, tumors, failure of oxygen supply, nutritional deficiency, poisonings, concussion and other trauma, and electrolyte disorders.

Tumors in the brain cause coma by growing to such a size that pressure is placed on those parts of the brain which are responsible for consciousness. (*See* BRAIN.) This is usually a progressive condition, beginning with a sluggish feeling, leading to stupor and, finally, loss of consciousness.

Brain lesions caused by a number of difficulties bring on coma by blocking or destroying normal neural pathways. The transmission of impulses is stopped and consciousness ceases.

Metabolic problems impair function in the brain and, since nerve impulses are abnormal, a state of coma ensues. Diabetic coma is one of the metabolic coma-producing diseases. (*See* DIABETES MELLITUS; INSULIN.)

If the acid/base balance, or pH, of the body fluids falls below about 7.0 to 6.9, a diabetic person develops coma. This is due to the acidosis which is a result of changing from carbohydrate to fat metabolism for energy. (*See* KETOACIDOSIS.)

Treatment of diabetic coma begins with massive doses of insulin. Instead of the usual amount, 20 to 80 units, injections of several hundred units at a time may have to be given. The totals may occasionally be as high as 2,000 units. Dehydration and acidosis are treated by intravenous administration of salt solution containing added sodium bicarbonate or sodium lactate; the amounts are determined by frequent assays of the blood and urine.

In other types of coma, measures are first taken to ensure that no further damage will be done to the brain. This means making certain breathing is normal and that the heart is functioning properly. Glucose is given intravenously to assure sufficient nutrition to the brain. The next step is to definitively determine the cause of the coma. Each kind requires specialized therapy.

The physician may seem to be delaying treatment of coma when he asks a number of questions, but this is vital. In fact, headstrong treatment without knowing causal factors can be dangerous. Has the person had a fall lately? Has he been drinking heavily? Is there a chance of drug abuse? Does he have a history of kidney, liver, or heart disease? Cooperation of all persons involved with the patient is essential in developing the most comprehensive history.

Once the causal factors have been determined, action is taken to correct the immediate problem. Drugs may be given to counteract other drugs taken. X rays may be used to locate a tumor or lesion. Medication is often necessary to combat an infection in another organ which has led to the coma.

Communicable Disease. If the bacteria or viruses that cause a disease can be passed or carried from one person to another, either directly or indirectly, that disease is said to be communicable. (*See* CONTAGIOUS DISEASES; INFECTIOUS DISEASES.)

Communication. The interchange, transmission, or sharing of knowledge, thoughts, and ideas between two people or more is communication.

Communication varies from group to group and from culture to culture, but it basically takes the form of language. It is how man relates to his immediate environment and to the outer world, and is essential to his psychosocial development. Lack of communication and its effect on the personality are one of the main causes of personality disturbances.

Communication takes many forms other than precise language. Ideas, thoughts, and emotions can be conveyed by the senses, the tone and quality of the voice, by body gestures, and by facial expressions. Everyone should be aware that as others are listening to him, they are also observing him and looking for hidden meanings in the tone of his voice, in his body postures, and in his facial expressions.

In infancy, the baby quickly learns the difference between a harsh voice and a cooing voice. A toddler knows that a slap on the hand means he has done something wrong. The wink of an eye or the wrinkling of a nose can sometimes convey more than words can. Gestures and posture can convey arrogance, fear, sadness, joy.

In relationships within the family group or outside it, adequate and honest communication is essential. Without it, resentments, hostilities, rage, and suspicion result

Communicable Disease Information

Disease	First Symptoms	Incubation Period	Quarantine Period	Comments
Chickenpox	Fever, tiny water blisters on red spots.	14 to 21 days	About 1 week, or when surface scabs have fallen off.	Others in family may attend school or work.
Diphtheria	Sore throat with gray-white patches, moderate fever, croupy cough.	2 to 5 days, sometimes longer	Until two successive cultures, taken not less than 24 hours apart, are negative for diphtheria bacilli.	Others in family may attend school or work if nose and throat cultures are free of diphtheria bacilli. Immunization usually required for entrance to school.
German Measles	Signs of cold, swollen glands, fever, rash.	14 to 21 days	4 days or more, until well.	Others in family may attend school or work. Immunization usually required for entrance to school.
Measles	Signs of cold, running nose, cough, red eyes, fever.	10 to 14 days	5 days or more, until all catarrhal symptoms are absent.	Others in family may attend school or work. Immunization usually required for entrance to school.
Meningococcal Meningitis	Sudden fever, headache, vomiting, sometimes convulsions, followed by higher fever and stiff neck and back.	2 to 10 days, usually 3 to 4	Until 24 hours after start of chemotherapy.	Others in family may attend school or work.
Mumps	Sore throat, fever, nausea, pain and swelling about jaws.	14 to 21 days	Until all swelling has disappeared, about 9 days.	Others in family may attend school or work.
Poliomyelitis	Sore throat, headache, vomiting, fever, stiff neck and back.	7 to 14 days	1 week or more from date of onset and until at least 24 hours after fever subsides.	Immunization usually required for entrance to school.
Smallpox	Sudden high fever, headache, backache; skin eruption (red spots) on third or fourth day.	7 to 16 days, usually 9 to 12	Until all lesions have healed and scabs have fallen off.	All persons in contact with patient must be promptly vaccinated or re-vaccinated, then quarantined for 16 days from last exposure.
Streptococcus Infections ("Scarlet Fever," "Strep" Throat)	Sore throat, fever, rash, vomiting.	2 to 7 days	7 days after fever, or until two consecutive cultures, 24 hours apart, are negative.	Others in family may attend school or work.
Whooping Cough	Signs of cold, cough with whoop, vomiting.	7 to 28 days	3 weeks.	Immunization usually required for entrance to school. Immunization recommended by 2 months of age or as soon afterward as possible.
Infectious Hepatitis	Fever, nausea, fatigue, headache, abdominal discomfort.	10 to 40 days	7 days or more until well.	Others in family may attend school or work.
Infectious Mononucleosis	Fever, sore throat, fatigue, general discomfort.	14 to 40 days	Until symptoms are gone.	Others in family may attend school or work.

in severe emotional conflicts which may lead not only to a rupture of relationships but to severe disturbances of personality as well. Being able to talk out problems and worries and occasionally being able just to "blow off steam" help resolve problems and keep lines of communication open. (*See* MENTAL HEALTH.)

Complex. A group of ideas that are linked together and related to repressed experiences form a complex. For example, a person who has suffered early experiences that have made him feel inferior may have an inferiority complex. He may react by being very timid, or he may do just the opposite and act very aggressive, giving the impression that he feels superior.

The reasons for such feelings or complexes are usually repressed in the unconscious mind. (*See* MENTAL HEALTH.)

Complexion. The skin of the face, including its color and appearance, is usually referred to as the complexion. (*See* COSMETICS; HYPOALLERGENIC COSMETICS; SKIN; SKIN CARE.)

Complication. Ailments secondary to the original complaint, which may have developed because of the first illness or because of weakened resistance of the body, are *complications*. For example, if a patient with influenza is not treated and given proper rest for recovery, his resistance to bacteria may be lowered. Thus a complication of flu may be pneumonia.

Surgical complications may occur if the psychological state of the patient is low. Although not understood, the will to recover is considered very important. Another example of complication in surgery is the proximity of a tumor to a vital organ. Complete removal may result in damage to that organ.

Similarly, any abnormal difficulty in routine treatment of disease is called a complication.

Compress. In cases of severe bleeding a compress, or pad of clean, folded cloth, should be applied with pressure directly over the wound to slow the blood flow and let normal clotting occur. A compress also can be soaked with medication or hot or cold water and used to ease soreness or inflammation. A hot compress should be used with caution, however, because there is danger of burning the skin.

A hot water bottle, another form of compress, is helpful in relieving menstrual pain, arthritis, and lower back pain caused by pulled muscles. But a hot compress should not be used on a stomachache. If the pain is caused by appendicitis, the application of heat is likely to induce rupture.

Compression. When a deep-sea diver is submerged, quantities of nitrogen dissolve in the tissues of the body under compression; if he comes up too quickly, nitrogen

Severe compression of the twelfth dorsal vertebra of the spine. The front-seat passenger in an automobile crash may suffer this injury along with other spinal injuries.

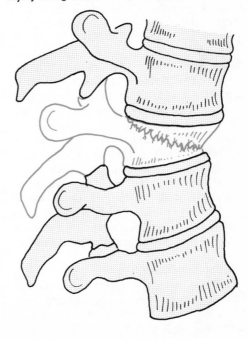

bubbles form in his blood through rapid decompression. This problem is called decompression sickness, compressed air sickness, diver's paralysis, or the bends. (*See* BENDS; DECOMPRESSION.)

Beneath the sea great pressures keep the dissolved nitrogen in the tissues. When the pressure is removed, the nitrogen escapes into the fluids inside and outside the cells. This can be avoided by gradual ascent, allowing the respiratory system to rid the body of the nitrogen.

Symptoms of the sickness include local pain in the legs or arms, dizziness, paralysis, shortness of breath, and, in more advanced cases, extreme fatigue, pain, and possibly collapse.

Compulsion. Sometimes a person has an irresistible impulse to perform a certain act, such as constantly washing his hands. Such a person knows what he is doing and may not want to, but he has a compulsion to continue it.

This compulsion usually is the result of an obsession—in this example, an obsession with cleanliness. A person usually is unaware of the underlying reasons for his compulsion. (*See* MENTAL HEALTH.)

Computerized Medicine. Storing standardized data on symptoms, diseases, diagnosis, and treatment on tapes for later consolidation and retrieval may some day put us into an era of computerized medicine. This branch of electronic medicine has the potential of aiding physicians in making a diagnosis for a particularly difficult case, finding the most up-to-date information on treatment, and providing a prognosis of what can be expected to happen. In addition to the purely clinical end of medicine, many other possibilities can be seen on the horizon.

Computers have been used in a number of other sciences. They offer the advantage of being able to store vast quantities of data for infinite periods of time and give the information back in many forms whenever it

is needed. But computers can spew out only what they are fed. If you program a computer that Shakespeare wrote *Hamlet* and *Julius Caesar*, it can answer the question, "Who wrote *Hamlet?*" But it can offer no information to the question, "Who wrote *Romeo and Juliet?*" Nor can it offer a clue to the author of a play dealing with a Roman general unless that extra information is provided it. Though simplistic, these examples offer insight into the problems facing computerized medicine.

In chemistry, the word *iron* is a specific thing—a chemical element with a certain molecular weight and physical and chemical properties. But in medicine, human qualities enter the picture, making concepts less clear-cut. Pain may be a very different thing for two different persons. Is it throbbing pain or sharp pain? And what do those words in turn mean? Even the names of diseases vary greatly, perhaps due to regional colloquialisms or tiny but important differences.

It has been estimated that today there are about 28,000 names for 3,262 distinct diseases. And when you begin to talk about symptoms, the enormity of the problem is magnified. Think again of the ways the word pain could be described. When you finish making your list remember that other persons could make another just as extensive, with no duplication.

Nevertheless, researchers are confident that eventually these difficulties will be overcome and that information will be standardized to enable medical data to be fed or programed into computers. If so, the possibilities are endless.

In fact, some application of the computer to medicine is already being made. The Scientific Information Exchange at the Smithsonian Institution in Washington uses a computer to avoid duplication of scientific research projects. Hospitals are beginning to store information about their patients. A bit of tape can hold entire case histories of not only the individual but also his family. These records are not likely to be lost and can be obtained quickly when necessary, providing data that may simplify later problems. And correlations can be drawn by the computer, giving clues which may aid a diagnosis and perhaps save a life. Eventually, hospitals may be hooked up together so they can obtain information of a patient thousands of miles from home.

Computers are currently being used to aid in examinations. Additional machinery tied to the computer can provide twelve pieces of information about a single sample of blood. Not only do such advances save time for medical personnel, but they save money for individual patients. What can be done in the area of chemical examinations in the near and distant future can only be speculated upon, but the gap between fiction and science is constantly narrowing.

Computer banks are being established in medical centers so that doctors can query the computer about the latest medications and treatments for a particular disease. Eventually, it is anticipated that there will be a computer center servicing the whole country, which will link doctors with experts in various fields. Prerecorded information on specific diseases can be obtained by dialing a certain telephone number. So far, over several hundred telephone numbers have been assigned, and up to five thousand are anticipated for the future. One of the obvious advantages is for the country doctor who is a great distance from available consultation.

The biggest dream yet to be realized, but almost certain to occur, is the computer's ability to diagnose disease. After examining a patient, the physician may be able to give the symptoms to the computer, which will in turn correlate them and produce a disease diagnosis. As mentioned earlier, however, the biggest drawback here is the lack of uniformity in terminology. Such an advance will not eliminate the need for doctors, as trained medical personnel will still be needed to determine symptoms. And the computer will doubtless be used only for especially difficult cases or where two dis-

ease entities may be similar. Regardless of advances in electronics and machinery, the human element of disease will still require the human attention of physicians.

Conception. A new child is created and pregnancy begins when the father's sperm fertilizes the mother's ovum (egg) in a process called conception or fertilization.

Within about five minutes after sexual intercourse, some of the sperm travel upward through the woman's uterus and out through her uterine tubes to the abdominal cavity near the outside of the ovaries. If this is near enough to the time when an ovary releases an ovum (during ovulation), fertilization will take place.

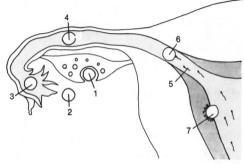

Steps in the conception process are pictured numerically above: 1 through 4. Mature ovum is released from ovary and travels through uterine tube. 5. Sperm swim rapidly up through uterus to uterine tube. 6. Conception: a sperm meets and enters ovum. 7. Fertilized ovum attaches to surface of uterine endometrial lining.

Although each spermatozoon can swim very rapidly through bodily fluids with a whipping motion of its tail, it needs additional speed. This extra impetus, it is believed, comes from contractions of the uterus (womb) and uterine tubes. The contractions are caused by a hormone, oxytocin, which is released as the result of stimulation initiated by coitus (intercourse).

It is believed that a mature ovum remains capable of being fertilized for about twenty-four hours after being released from the ovary. Sperm are thought to remain highly fertile and healthy in the female genital tract for twenty-four to seventy-two hours.

Thus, for conception to take place, coitus must occur during the period which permits both ovum and sperm to be fertile at the same time, but there may be great individual variations in this timing.

Only one sperm is needed to fertilize an ovum. As soon as the first sperm enters, the ovum automatically prevents penetration by other sperm, and any that come near are immediately made inactive. It is not yet understood how this process occurs.

Each sperm is formed by half of a cell from the father's body, and each ovum derives from half a cell from the mother. The two halves form one complete cell. Since each complete cell, male or female, contains twenty-three pairs of chromosomes, the resulting sperm contains twenty-three individual chromosomes from the father and the ovum has twenty-three from the mother. (*See* OVUM; SPERM.) The sex of the child is determined by which of the father's sperm happens to fertilize the ovum. The father's pair of sex chromosomes consist of XY (both a female X chromosome and a male Y), and when each cell divides, one sperm gets the X and another gets the Y. Female cells contain an XX pair; thus, both ova formed from each cell will receive a female X chromosome. If one is fertilized by a male X sperm, the baby will be a girl; if it is fertilized instead by a male Y sperm, the infant will be a boy. (*See* GENETICS.)

As soon as the sperm fertilizes the ovum, each set of twenty-three individual chromosomes begins to merge into the appropriate twenty-three pairs. At the same time, the ovum is being propelled along its path by a slow current of fluid, from the point where it was released into the peritoneal cavity of the abdomen into and through one of the uterine tubes toward the uterus. (*See* IMPLANTATION; PRENATAL DEVELOPMENT.)

When two or more embryos are developing in the mother's uterus at the same time, this is known as multiple pregnancy. If they are identical twins, triplets, quadruplets, etc., they originate from one ovum fertilized by a single sperm; all the resulting children will be identical in sex and appearance. Nonidentical twins are formed by two separate ova which are fertilized by separate sperm; they may be of different sex and appearance. (*See* MULTIPLE BIRTHS; QUADRUPLETS; TRIPLETS; TWINS.)

Concussion. A violent shaking or shock to any part of the body because of a severe blow or fall is called a concussion. When it occurs in the skull and brain, unconsciousness and other symptoms follow, and it is called brain concussion. There also can be concussion to other parts of the body, such as the spinal cord or the passages (labyrinth) of the inner ear. (*See* BRAIN; SPINAL CORD.)

Wherever concussion occurs, its symptoms and effects to a great degree are due either to hemorrhaging (bleeding) or edema (watery swelling) of the damaged tissues. These in turn cause a shortage of usable blood in the adjoining tissues and more distant areas supplied by the same vessels. There may or may not be fractures of the bones involved, and there may be no serious damage to the tissues affected.

SPINE CONCUSSION. In concussion of the spine there usually is pain in the back and sometimes in the legs or arms. There may also be loss of feeling in some parts of the body, muscular shrinking and weakness, and occasionally even mental or physical disability.

Initially, the areas affected will depend on the pathways of nerves and blood vessels located in the injured portion of the spine. Later, however, much more distant areas can become involved. Damage can even reach the brain. This is because pressure spreads upward inside the spinal column as the result of increasing hemorrhage and continued swelling of the tissues that surround both the spinal column and the brain.

EAR CONCUSSION. Deafness and tinnitus

(ringing, roaring, or hissing in the ears) can result from damage to the inner ear due to a blow, fall, or explosion. There also can be damage to the middle ear.

Ear concussion is due to the extremely high outgoing air pressure and returning air suction caused at the time a blast occurs. Such a blast can result from an ignited gasoline tank, or accumulated cooking gas in the home or in pipes.

Deafness is not unusual as the result of a head blow or injury which is sufficient to cause unconsciousness. But minor injuries in which there is neither a fracture nor unconsciousness also can result in deafness. In either case, if the deafness does not clear up within one or two months, it is likely to be permanent. This is also true of tinnitus, and the resulting uncontrollable ear sounds can be a disturbance to sleep as well as a frustration during waking hours. (*See* DEAFNESS; EAR.)

The vertigo (dizziness) which often accompanies or follows a brain concussion or head injury may be due to inner-ear damage, especially when a blow from the back forces the head forward rapidly. This can be a recurring problem in which even slight movements of the head can bring the dizziness back. Or the patient may often feel as if the ground were rolling under him like the deck of a ship at sea.

If this dizziness persists, a series of exercises (Cawthorne-Cooksey) may help relieve the condition. Preferably, they should be started as soon as possible and supervised by a physician trained in such procedures. (*See* DIZZINESS.)

These exercises include movements to slowly loosen muscles and other tissues of the head and shoulder by moving the head while the eyes are focused on objects which are near and far away, and moving the head and arms while the eyes are closed. Other exercises are walking up and down stairs with the eyes open and then with the eyes shut, bouncing and catching a ball with the body bending and turning, and alternating slow movements with fast ones.

BRAIN CONCUSSION. In brain concussion, the brain itself may be bruised—not only on the side where the skull was bumped, but also on the opposite side. This is because the brain is not fastened securely to the skull but is suspended in tissues called "meninges," which resemble a sponge filled with water. Normally, these tissues protect the brain from being damaged seriously by a mild bump, but they are not sufficiently rigid for adequate protection in severe cases. If the blow is hard enough the brain can bounce back and forth inside the skull like a ball in a cage.

This also can happen in a few cases where the head does not even hit a solid object, but is thrown about or snapped like a whip, such as when a car stops suddenly or collides. This so-called "whiplash" injury to the head and neck is more likely to occur in women with long, slim necks, rather than in men with short, more muscular necks. It is also more likely in cars without headrests.

Brain concussion is a clear possibility whenever a person falls, bumps a solid object, gets hit by a hard ball or bat, is in a car accident without the seat belt securely fastened, or is close to an explosion.

CONCUSSION SYMPTOMS. The symptoms, and the speed with which they set in, depend on the severity of the initial injury—except that a head bump which at first seems mild can later become quite serious because of increasing damage. Any patient who has sustained a blow to the head should be watched carefully for at least two days. During this time, if head pain or any other symptoms persist at all, the patient should be awakened every hour during sleep to make certain he is merely sleeping and is still conscious.

The patient may be unconscious only a few seconds or minutes, then get up and walk around, claiming that he is all right. Or he may lose consciousness for hours, days, or weeks—or regain consciousness in a very short while, only to lose it again later.

Before, after, or between periods of unconsciousness, the patient may be confused. This may be barely noticeable, and for only a short while. Or he may merely remain quieter than usual, possibly without answering questions or initiating comments.

Other significant early symptoms include vomiting or nausea, and toilet accidents or loss of control of other bodily functions and movements. The patient can have cold skin, goose pimples, or chills; a slow, full, or weak pulse; unusually heavy, labored, or weak breathing; or a purple, red, blue, or grey face.

Dizziness and headache are the most common symptoms of concussion. In mild bumps there may be pain only at the surface where the skull tissue is bruised, or the pain may spread inward. More severe cases may have generalized headache or possibly pain in two areas on opposite sides of the head.

The eyes also are important. They may simply have a blank stare or they may roll around, a condition called nystagmus. The pupils may become dilated (widening of the center black spot), constricted (narrowing), or be different in each eye. (*See* EYE.)

Bleeding may not be visible unless the external skin is cut. Broken bones often remain in place so well that only an X ray can detect a fracture. But internal tissues may still be damaged and bleeding.

If the blow was behind the ear there may be disturbance of hearing as well as dizziness. The ear drum may even be damaged. A few drops of blood inside the ear may indicate fracture of the skull underneath the back of the head.

FIRST AID. After a head injury, the patient should lie down and remain completely quiet no matter how he feels. Have him do this even though he acts all right and insists that you leave him alone.

Cold packs are excellent immediate first aid in any blow to the head. They slow down the bleeding and swelling of tissue, thus helping to prevent or reduce damage that can set in later. Even if the bump seems mild, keep putting new cold packs on it periodically for a day or two.

It does not matter whether you use ice wrapped in a washcloth or an ice bag. You can also fill a strong plastic bag with ice water, twist the top shut after squeezing out the air, fold it over, and bind it tightly with a rubber band.

Keep a cold pack over each spot on the head that aches or was bumped for at least a half-hour at a time or longer. Then leave it off a short while and put another one on.

Keep the patient flat on his back (or face down if he is vomiting) if his face is grey, blue, or pale. But if his face turns red or purplish, raise his head and shoulders with pillows or a rolled-up coat. (An old Navy first-aid rule is: Face is pale, raise the tail; face is red, raise the head.) Maintain him in this proper position especially if you are taking him to the hospital in an ordinary passenger car. It helps control the amount and kind of blood circulation to and from the head.

Give no medicine, pain-killers, or stimulants of any kind, particularly not whiskey, unless they are prescribed by a doctor. The patient may actually need the opposite of what you think you should give him.

Many of the symptoms of concussion are those of shock. If the patient feels chilled, has cold skin or goose flesh, or is using an ice pack, be sure to keep his body wrapped in a warm blanket or someone's coat. (*See* SHOCK.)

You should also give him something warm to drink—but only if he is conscious and alert. Coffee should not be given because it is a stimulant.

Never pour any kind of liquid down the throat of a person who is unconscious, drowsy, or confused. He could choke on it or literally drown if the liquid gets into his lungs.

The same danger is present when a person is vomiting while unconscious. Watch carefully, and turn him over on his side or face, possibly with the head over the side of the bed temporarily, to make sure the liquids drain out of his mouth and nose.

Quick medical care is required for any cuts or openings in the skin on the skull, because there is serious danger of infection spreading through the circulation from there to the brain. Such wounds may require antibiotics as well as other treatment.

Do not treat these recommendations lightly. Learn them thoroughly if you have children or work near youngsters. Unless treated promptly, bleeding inside the brain, which you cannot see, can cause severe and possibly permanent damage to nerves and brain tissue nearby. (*See* FIRST AID.)

Condom. Any device which fits over part or all of the penis and is designed to prevent sperm from entering the vagina during sexual intercourse is called a condom. Commonly used slang terms are practically limitless. Some of these are rubbers, skins, prophylactics, safes, safeties, and peels, as well as generically used brand names. Although condoms are not as effective as female mechanical birth control methods, they are still in widespread use. An additional advantage of a condom is that it helps to prevent venereal disease, since actual contact between the penis and the vagina is not made. Unlike some birth control methods, condoms do not require a physician's prescription for purchase. (*See* BIRTH CONTROL, MECHANICAL MEANS.)

Congenital Defects. Malformations or other bodily disorders that are present at birth are called congenital defects. Most of these defects are detected at birth or shortly thereafter. Some, however, do not manifest themselves until years later. When stillborn and liveborn births are analyzed, it is found that the incidence of congenital defects is about 10 percent. Essentially, every organ and biochemical system is subject to developing an abnormality. Although thousands of types of defects have been reported, only the more common congenital defects and their causes are considered in this article.

Many disorders present at birth are due to known and often detectable alterations in the hereditary material. The human germ cell (sperm or egg) contains genetic material in the form of genes arranged in units called chromosomes. The human infant and adult has forty-six chromosomes in each body cell. Since half of these come from the mother and half from the father, the sperm and egg each contain twenty-three chromosomes (twenty-two autosomes and one sex chromosome). During the process of meiosis in the human gonad (testicle or ovary), mistakes sometimes occur resulting in an abnormal number or structure of the chromosomes placed in the germ cell. Embryos resulting from such germ cells are usually defective. Many syndromes have been described. Down's syndrome, Turner's syndrome, and Klinefelter's syndrome are all due to such abnormalities. (*See* GENETIC DEFECTS.)

Other disorders which result from genetic abnormalities can be passed on from parent to child through many generations. These are referred to as hereditary diseases and are quite numerous. Chromosomes occur in pairs in the human organism. Genes located on the chromosomes are also in pairs and are referred to as alleles. Genes dictate body characteristics and biochemistry by being responsible for the production of proteins used by the body. (*See* GENE.) One or more pairs of alleles usually determine a given body characteristic, such as eye color or blood type. Hereditary diseases result from abnormalities in the structure of the gene, which can be passed on from parent to child. Dominant disease traits appear when the child receives the defective gene from either the mother or the father (the heterozygous state). Recessive traits must be passed from both mother and father to the child before expression is possible (homozygous state). Such abnormal genes may be present on ordinary chromo-

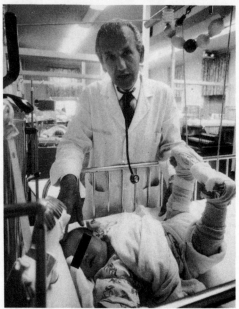

Presbyterian St. Luke's Hospital, Chicago

A congenital (present at birth) hip deformity, such as in this baby, requires surgery and immobilization. Many such defects can be corrected with leg braces worn at night to keep the legs and feet in their proper position.

somes (autosomes) or on sex chromosomes. (*See* CHROMOSOMES.)

Dominant pathologic traits are somewhat rare. If one of the parents has the disorder, there is a 50-50 chance of passing it to a child—that is, approximately half of the children are affected. Among the dominant autosomal traits are achondroplasia (dwarfism), Huntington's chorea, multiple polyps of the bowel, muscular dystrophy, night blindness, adult polycystic kidney disease, and spherocytosis. A recessive pathologic trait on the autosomes can be passed through a family for many generations and not reveal itself until the homozygous state is attained. Marriages between cousins and other family members, such as occurred in the royal families of Europe, predisposes to these forms of hereditary disorders. Recessive autosomal traits include albinism, cys-

tic fibrosis, galactosemia, muscular dystrophy, phenylketonuria, sickle cell anemia, and Friedreich's ataxia. The sex chromosomes, usually the X chromosome, can also carry pathological traits, most of them recessive. Among these disorders are hemophilia, color blindness, a type of gargoylism, and progressive muscular dystrophy.

Almost any organ system or body structure can form abnormally in the human. The cause for most of these defects is unknown. Some occur as part of the genetic and hereditary abnormalities considered above; others result from damage to the developing embryo by physical trauma, birth difficulties, or mutagenic agents. (*See* MUTAGENS.)

The digestive tract (esophagus, stomach, intestine, pancreas, liver, and gallbladder) is frequently the site of a congenital defect as a lone disorder or in association with defects in other systems. The anus sometimes fails to develop properly, thus providing no way for fecal matter to leave the body. Atresia (obliteration) of the bile duct system, which drains the liver and gallbladder, is somewhat rare but does occur. Intestinal or esophageal atresia is also reported. Stenosis (narrowing) of the pyloric valve between the stomach and duodenum may cause vomiting in the infant. Constipation in a child may be due to congenital absence of certain nerves in the large bowel. This disorder is called "aganglionic megacolon," or Hirschsprung's disease. Occasionally the abdominal organs may occupy the umbilical cord at birth. This developmental abnormality is called an "omphalocele."

Many defects are possible in the cardiovascular system (heart and vessels). Slightly less than 1 percent of live births suffer from such a disorder. Coarctation or stenosis of the aorta (the main arterial outflow tract from the heart) is seen quite frequently. Stenosis of the aortic valve of the left ventricle is also a rather common defect. (*See* HEART.) The pulmonary valve of the right ventricle is also frequently stenotic (narrowed). The walls (septa) which separate the heart chambers sometimes fail to form properly, leaving abnormal openings. Such a hole in the wall between the two atria is called an "atrial septal defect." A similar disorder in the ventricles is called a "ventricular septal defect." Such septal defects may occur in association with other heart abnormalities, as in the tetralogy of Fallot and the Eisenmenger complex. Fairly commonly the aorta emerges from the right ventricle and the pulmonary artery emerges from the left ventricle. This disorder is called "transposition of the great vessels." One of the commonest defects of the heart results when a communication normally present in the fetus, which connects the pulmonary artery and the aorta, fails to close after birth. This is referred to as a "patent ductus arteriosis" and can be surgically repaired.

The chest and lungs (respiratory system) are also subject to congenital defects. One lung or lobe of a lung may fail to develop (agenesis) or may be decreased in size (hypoplasia). Defects in the diaphragm (muscular septum between the chest and abdomen) allow abdominal organs to bulge through (herniate) into the chest. This may cause breathing problems or obstruction of the bowel. Pigeon breast (pectus carinatum) and funnel chest (pectus excavatum) are abnormalities of the sternum (breastbone) which rarely cause symptoms.

Abnormalities of the kidneys, bladder, and genital organs are rather common and are often seen in association with defects in other systems. Absence or greatly diminished size of one kidney is relatively common. Abnormal position of a kidney occurs in about one of eight hundred people. Fusion of the two kidneys, called "horseshoe kidney," is seen in one of every thousand people. Extra arteries to the kidneys are found very commonly. The tubular structure that drains urine from the kidney into the bladder is called the ureter; the most common disorder of this structure is the presence of two instead of one ureter per kidney. This is commonly called "double ureter." The bladder is only rarely congenitally defective. Occasionally the pelvis and lower abdomen fail to form properly, resulting in the eversion of the bladder wall. This is referred to as "exstrophy of the bladder." One of the most common defects in the urinary system is known as hypospadias. In this defect, the urethral opening of the male occurs underneath the penis rather than at the tip. This is seen in about one of every four hundred males. Anomalies of the female uterus are quite common and often complicate delivery.

Several defects are commonly found in the head and facial areas. A defect in the upper lip is seen in about one per thousand births; it is called "cleft lip" and can be surgically repaired. Often associated with this is "cleft palate." Cleft palate is an opening in the roof of the mouth that often interferes with eating and speaking; surgical repair is possible. Low-set ears are commonly seen in association with mental retardation syndrome. Complete absence or partial absence of the upper part of the brain is called "anencephaly" and is seen in one of every thousand births. A fairly common defect results from abnormal development of the fluid-containing cavities (ventricles) in the brain. This results in a large head and is called "hydrocephalus." Improper formation of the vertebral column is called "spina bifida." The spinal cord with its covering layers may herniate through the abnormality; this is called "myelomeningocele."

Lastly, congenital defects are seen in the musculoskeletal system (bones and muscles). Arms or legs may fail to develop (agenesis) or may be small (phocomelia). Extra fingers or toes (polydactyly) are rather common. Fusion of fingers or toes (syndactyly) is also frequently seen. The fetal bones sometimes—though rarely—fail to have calcium deposited in them; this results in a type of dwarfism known as achondroplasia. The clubfoot (talipes equinovarus) is seen in one of every thousand births. Congenital dislocation of the hip joint occurs in one of every fifteen hundred children.

Congestion. Excessive accumulation of blood at a particular site in the body is called congestion. This medical definition excludes the congestion of mucus in the nasal passages and elsewhere. Pulmonary congestion can occur when blood and fluid collect in the lower extremities while a person is standing and then rush to the heart when he is in a prone position. Because the lungs are not capable of handling this abnormal amount of blood, respiratory function is made difficult. (*See* HEART; LUNGS.)

Congestive Heart Failure. When a person's heart becomes inefficient and too much blood remains (congests) in the heart chambers, the problem is medically named congestive heart failure.

The term failure simply means that the heart is unable to pump blood efficiently enough to meet all the body's normal needs; it does not mean that the heart has stopped. For further information see the article HEART FAILURE.

Conjunctivitis. Inflammation of the conjunctiva is known as conjunctivitis. The conjunctiva is the thin mucous membrane which lines the underside of the eyelids and a portion of the anterior part of the eyeball. The disease is one of the most common eye problems.

Infection by bacteria or viruses, or both together, is the most frequent cause of conjunctivitis. Rarely, a fungus or a parasite may be responsible. Conjunctivitis may occasionally be the result of an infection from *Leptothrix,* a bacteria sometimes spread by cats. General allergic disorders, such as hay fever, or local allergic reactions to drugs,

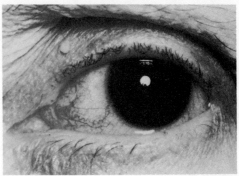

J. B. Kahn

Reddened blood vessels in the eye are symptoms of conjunctivitis, which in this case resulted from a reaction to soap.

cosmetics, or chemicals are other causes.

Some drugs, such as methoxsalen or phenothiazine, are photosensitizing—that is, they cause the conjunctiva, and other parts of the eye, to be especially sensitive to sunlight or other ultraviolet rays.

When conjunctivitis occurs in the newborn infant, it is known as ophthalmia neonatorum. Silver nitrate solution or a penicillin preparation is usually applied to the eyes of the infant at birth to prevent bacterial eye infection. Care is required because too strong a solution of silver nitrate may also cause irritation of the conjunctiva.

Trachoma involves inflammation of both the conjunctiva and the cornea. It is a common worldwide disease, although rare in the United States. (*See* TRACHOMA.)

Conjunctivitis, like other eye problems, may be related to systemic diseases such as herpes simplex, herpes zoster, Sicca syndrome, polycythemia, and various collagen (connective tissue) disorders. When conjunctivitis occurs along with inflammation of the cornea, it is termed keratoconjunctivitis. Viruses often are the cause. Inclusion blennorrhea is a type of conjunctivitis in which there is a heavy discharge of mucous fluid. Infection of the eye with the gonococcal organism, the cause of the venereal disease gonorrhea, results in blennorrhea.

In most conjunctivitis there is little or no pain or visual problem. The discharge may be thick or watery. The eyelid may be red, as in the common type of conjunctivitis, pinkeye. (*See* PINKEYE.)

If there is an underlying systemic disease, it should be cleared up with appropriate treatment while the eye symptom is treated. Bacterial conjunctivitis usually will clear up within a few days if an antibiotic ointment is used, but may last several weeks with insufficient or no treatment. Sulfa drugs also are used.

Steroid drugs sometimes are employed. Extreme care is needed, however, as this medication may cause severe eye complications if infection is present.

Infective conjunctivitis may be easily spread from one person to another through unwashed hands and common towels. (*See also* EYE; EYE CARE.)

Constipation.

If a person is unable to expel solid waste material from his body (have a bowel movement), he usually refers to himself as "constipated." The doctor may not agree with him, however. The word constipation, as used in this article and by most physicians, indicates a medical problem resulting from an inability to move the bowels. It is confusing to use the term simply to mean a person's lack of power to have a bowel movement when he decides he should.

Some people believe that their bowels must perform every day, and think themselves constipated if they do not. Actually, you may not have a movement for several days or even a week and suffer no ill effects. You certainly do not have "autointoxication," a fictional disorder in which even doctors once believed.

Today part of the confusion on the subject of constipation is the result of laxative advertising, which makes a great point of "irregularity." Regular habits are fine, but occasional breaks in the pattern have little significance.

And what is a regular habit? It is normal for most persons to have one movement a day, normal for others to have several daily, and normal for some to have only one every couple of days. The time of day for the act also varies widely from individual to individual. It is largely a matter of habits developed during childhood, modified by demands of work, school, or other routines of later life.

TYPES OF CONSTIPATION. Constipation may be classified according to the cause, of which there are many. Emotional factors, such as tension, resentment, frustration, or uncertainty, may result directly in constipation. The tensions may cause the muscles of the intestines to tighten, or contract, in what is called spastic constipation. This is often a part of the picture of the psychosomatic disorder called the "irritable bowel syndrome." (*See* BOWELS.)

Children sometimes react to emotional conflicts by becoming "holders." They do not obey the normal instinct to defecate, but retain fecal matter in the rectum long enough for it to form a large ball, sometimes the size of a grapefruit. This mass loses moisture as it remains in the rectum, becoming dried and hardened and difficult to evacuate. The child with this problem soon fails to feel normal signals which indicate it is time to evacuate the bowels. He must be gradually trained again to establish regular visits to the bathroom.

Sluggishness, with hard, dried feces, is a form of constipation. It is often a result of an atonic (without tone) condition of the intestinal muscles, which cannot move the material normally toward the anus. As the fecal material remains in the intestines, it loses water and thus becomes harder.

Atonic constipation may be the result of constant use of laxatives and enemas. These do not require the intestinal muscles to work normally. The lack of normal use causes the muscles to weaken, making the individual even more dependent on laxatives or enemas than before.

OTHER CAUSES. Obstructions along the digestive pathway may result in constipation. These may be in the form of benign or malignant (cancerous) tumors, distortions of the colon, and pressure from other organs in the body. A common example of the latter occurs during pregnancy, when the uterus (womb) enlarges and crowds the abdominal organs.

Some persons, particularly children, develop megacolon, or may have the condition from birth. This is a greatly enlarged colon that fills up with feces. Although the child may have regular bowel movements, evacuation is never complete. This is a different problem from the "holding" described above, and often requires corrective surgery.

Diseases that upset the chemical balance of the body may result in constipation. Examples are hypothyroidism or deficiency of the thyroid gland, and diabetes mellitus, in which there is insufficient insulin for proper utilization of carbohydrates.

Another example is hyperparathyroidism, in which the parathyroids (glands near the thyroid) do not function properly. This causes loss of calcium from the bones and other symptoms, including constipation.

Poisoning, particularly by metallic substances such as lead or arsenic, results in constipation as well as more serious reactions.

Another cause of constipation is lack of sufficient intake of fluids and bulky foods, which respectively help keep the material in the intestines moist and pliable, characteristics necessary for easy passage.

Constipation may occur in some women just before or during the menstrual period, because of the pressure of the enlarging uterus or an imbalance in body fluids. This is often complicated by emotional tension or premenstrual tension.

Aged persons often suffer from constipation, partly due to the diminishing tone of intestinal and other muscles, as well as the slowing down of the body signals from reduced efficiency of the nervous system. But old people who are without any chronic disease—and who eat nutritious foods, drink sufficient liquids, exercise moderately, and keep themselves emotionally in balance—seldom will find constipation a serious problem.

LAXATIVES AND PURGATIVES. If you ask the average man on the street how to treat constipation, he will echo what advertising tells him: "Take a mild laxative." He may also suggest an enema, a dish of stewed prunes, or bran flakes. These pat answers have danger in their very simplicity. A mild laxative now and then should harm no healthy individual. But too often laxatives become a habit which is harmful and hard to break. Habitual use of cathartics and purgatives—stronger agents for "cleaning out" the intestinal tract—are even more hazardous. Even prunes eaten day after day, or daily enemas, can be a crutch that you cannot easily throw away. Suddenly stopping the prolonged use of laxatives, cathartics, enemas, and so on, will inevitably result in constipation.

Some persons become as addicted to laxatives and cathartics as a person "hooked" on heroin. Common sense should tell you that the intestines cannot extract nutrients from food material if it is regularly hustled through with such agents.

Persons who use laxatives constantly or frequently are prone to hypovitaminosis, or vitamin deficiency, and some have serious body shortages of potassium. Their intestinal linings also are damaged, interfering with the body's chemical breakdown of poisonous substances in the material passing through. The unaltered toxic substances may then be taken up by the system. Sadly enough, this can happen to people who started the laxative habit to fight off the imaginary "autointoxication" of "irregularity."

Some purgatives (strong cathartics) work because they irritate the inner lining of the intestines. Castor oil, for example, produces ricinoleic acid, an irritant, in the digestive tract. The even older remedy, cascara sagrada, is seldom used today because of such irritation.

Some of the milder remedies such as milk of magnesia, phosphates, and epsom salts produce their effect by limiting the absorption of water by the intestine, thus producing a more watery and more easily passed feces. These may also irritate the intestines of some individuals, however, and, if used repeatedly, can start the patient on laxative dependency.

Mineral oil is intended to lubricate the digestive tract and does work as a remedy to constipation. But it has disadvantages, such as possible discomfort and reduction of uptake of nutrients by the intestines. From time to time the oil may also pass unexpectedly from the anus in small quantities, soiling the clothing.

Finally, laxatives taken by persons with unknown gallbladder trouble or appendicitis can do great harm, even endangering the person's life.

Laxatives and similar agents are valuable to the physician, who can prescribe their use by evaluating factors of which the layman is seldom aware. A good rule is this: If you must take laxatives in order to avoid constipation, then you are hiding a problem which should be corrected—and you need professional medical advice.

TREATMENT AND PREVENTION. Enemas, or irrigation of the colon with warm water, are generally safe treatment for constipation—provided they do not contain soaps, detergents, or other substances that may irritate the intestines. Like laxatives, they should not become a habit or substitute for normal bowel movements. Instructions on how to give yourself or another person an enema are given in the separate article, ENEMAS.

Following are some simple instructions on how to avoid constipation and help clear up mild existing problems.

Establish a regular habit of going to the bathroom at the same time every day. After breakfast or another time shortly after eating is preferred, as the early process of digestion starts the wavelike muscular movement (peristalsis) of the intestines, which force matter downward in the entire tract.

Relax at this time. Reading a book is often helpful. A portable radio, playing music to relax you, may be an aid. Avoid straining, but increase the pressure on the abdominal area, if necessary, by placing your feet on a footstool.

Again, remember that you may miss a natural movement on some days. Don't strain, but leave and go about your daily business. In most cases you will be back on schedule in a day or two.

Proper eating is as essential to proper elimination, as it is to good health generally. Digestion starts with the flow of saliva in the mouth, so take your time when eating and enjoy your food.

Avoid a diet high in fats. When fats are the largest part of the diet, there is insufficient roughage for the intestines, and constipation can result. (Too much consumption of fats is also hazardous in many other ways. See FATS.)

The soft (or low-residue) foods, which compose a large part of the fare in so-called civilized countries, also contribute to constipation problems. The intestinal muscles can more efficiently move food that has more bulk or solid substance in it. These are found in the high-residue foods such as leafy cooked vegetables, salads, and fruits.

Cereals and bread—particularly those made of whole grain—provide good bulk. Highly refined and soft-processed cereals are of little value for this purpose.

A word of warning on bran. This was once widely advocated to prevent or treat constipation. However, it can irritate the intestinal tract and produces gas and other discomfort.

Fruits such as apples, pears, raisins,

dates, figs, and prunes balance out the diet and help you avoid constipation. But do not eat just one kind of fruit. Vary your menu.

Sufficient fluid intake will help you avoid constipation. Drink six or eight glasses of fluid daily. But if you drink water during meals, don't use it to wash down food. You may inhibit proper mastication and saliva flow in the mouth. For other suggestions on dietary intake, see the article NUTRITION.

Moderate daily exercise is necessary for general health as well as an aid in avoiding constipation. It will keep your muscles in good tone. Ten minutes of setting-up exercises in the morning, or a walk of a mile or two, will help you after middle age. If you are younger and well, more active exercise will do you no harm. (*See* EXERCISE.)

If you have a sedentary occupation, by all means get up and stretch or walk to the drinking fountain once in a while. This will aid your general muscle tone. The combination of lots of sitting, too little exercise, and a diet heavy with fats and soft foods is very likely to result in constipation as well as other problems.

Since we know that constipation also is very often due to emotional stress, or a combination of this and physical factors, adjust your life to a sensible pace. Get rid of suppressed feelings of guilt and resentment, have distracting recreation, and learn how to relax. (*See* MENTAL HEALTH.)

Remember that our bodies were created to have normal bowel functions without the need of medicine or other special treatment. Unfortunately, constipation among children is often the result of family conflicts and improper training based on outmoded notions of modesty and fear, as well as of poor diet. (*See* TOILET TRAINING.)

If you have problems of constipation, you would do well to learn more details of the functions of digestion and elimination from the articles on DIGESTION; INTESTINES; STOMACH.

Consumption.   For many years, pulmonary tuberculosis was referred to as "con-sumption." The word derives from the Latin and means "a wasting away." (*See* LUNGS; TUBERCULOSIS.)

Contact Lenses.   Many persons who need eyeglasses to improve their vision choose to wear contact lenses.

Contact lenses and regular eyeglasses have many things in common. The lenses of both are constructed to improve the patient's vision and do this primarily by focusing images on the retina of the eye. It is estimated that more than seven million people of all ages wear contact lenses in the United States today. Young children and cataract patients in their late eighties are successfully fitted with contact lenses.

Contact lenses are made of plastic that is harmless to the eye. They are lighter in weight and proportionately thinner than a similar spectacle lens. Contact lenses allow a greater field of vision because they become part of the optical system of the eye and move with the eye. They change position as a person rolls his eyes. This means that he is always looking through the center of the lens, and his vision is not distorted. Because spectacle lenses are rigidly fixed in place and do not move with the eye, a person often must look through the outer edges of lens area, which usually causes a distorted view. Contact lenses do not fog up with moisture, and they have no heavy frames. Many athletes find them preferable to regular eyeglasses for these reasons.

Almost anyone who wishes to wear contact lenses can do so. Many persons find that the initial adjustment period may involve discomfort and adaptation but that after a short period of time, vision, as well as the lenses, is comfortable.

To be fitted for contact lenses, you should have your eyes examined by an ophthalmologist or optometrist, who will prepare the correct prescription for you. When your lenses arrive from the laboratory, they are checked against the original prescription to make sure that they will give you the desired correction of vision. Then they must be fitted to your eyes to assure you comfort and all-day wearing time.

The contact lenses float on a thin layer of tears on the surface of the eye. Special solutions for storage of the lenses when not in use also have antiseptic qualities to prevent any contamination of the eye.

Lenses should be handled carefully at all times. If the surface is scratched or the edges nicked even slightly, discomfort and reduction of wearing time, even eye damage, may result.

Because a contact lens fits directly on the surface of the eye, it can do some things that a spectacle lens can not do, including providing a tough plastic shield over the area it covers. Sometimes a contact lens is used to reshape the eye in cases of irregularities. Keratoconus, a noninflammatory disease that results in a conical reshaping of the cornea, can often be controlled with contact lenses. The contact lens actually presses the eye back into its proper shape. In such cases, contact lenses restore eyesight to people who cannot be helped by any other optical means.

Contact lenses are available in different colors which can be used to enhance the color of your own eyes. There are also cosmetic contact lenses available to change the color of your eyes completely. Bifocal contact lenses can be prepared when necessary.

Contact lenses are not easily broken, and

Hints for Wearers of Contact Lenses

1. Always wash your hands before inserting contact lenses. Hypo-allergenic soap is fine for removing surface dirt and excess skin oils because it leaves no film on the hands. Medicated soaps are not recommended by eye doctors for use before inserting contacts as they contain many different medicaments which often irritate the eyes and the sensitive surrounding skin area.

   If your contacts burn and sting immediately after you insert them but feel better as the day progresses, this is often an indication of cosmetics on the lenses. The lessening of the discomforting symptoms is due to the tears washing away some of the foreign particles.

2. Insert contact lenses before applying any makeup. By following this rule, you will be able to see better and more expertly apply your eye makeup too, and at the same time you will avoid getting any makeup in the eyes or on the lenses.

3. Eyeliners should never be applied on the lower lid as they may stop up the sensitive glands. There is also the chance that the liner will get in the eye and sensitive skin will be inflamed.

4. Use great care when applying mascara regardless of the type you prefer—the roll-on or cake.

5. Many eye doctors instruct patients not to wear contact lenses in the beauty shop. Sitting under a hair dryer dries both the tears and the plastic of the lens—the lens then rubs the eye instead of floating properly. Fumes from permanent waving liquids are also very irritating to contact wearers.

6. Avoid applying heavy facial creams, particularly those containing lanolin, around the eyes. These are often so greasy that they can coat the lenses with an oily film. Creams should never be used before inserting lenses.

7. Avoid getting hair spray in the eyes by covering them with a plastic shield. Hair spray can build up on lenses, and sometimes can be removed only by polishing the lens in the laboratory.

AR-EX Products Company

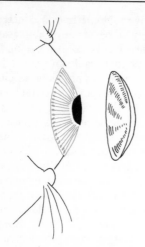

A contact lens fits over the cornea of the eye, with its outer rim under the eyelids. Like the lens of an eyeglass, the contact lens bends the incoming light rays to compensate for an abnormality in the eye's capacity to focus.

are insurable. Often, prescription changes are required less frequently for contact lenses than for ordinary spectacle lenses. Many persons can wear the same contact lenses for ten years. Annual—or, better, semiannual—examinations should be scheduled with your contact lens practitioner to assure you of the continuous good fit of your lenses. Also, he should clean and polish your lenses. This is especially necessary in urban areas where pollution is high, or if the woman wearer has the habit of handling them after applying greasy cosmetics. Should your lenses give you discomfort at any time, remove them and see your practitioner.

Contagious Diseases. Illnesses that are spread from person to person are called contagious diseases. These diseases were early thought to be caused by tiny germs, but the idea was not proven until the latter half of the nineteenth century, largely through the work of Louis Pasteur and Robert Koch. The knowledge of the natural history of contagious diseases led to the realization that they could be prevented. This stimulated hygiene and sanitation practices, as well as the organization of health and sanitation departments to combat these diseases.

Contagious diseases are most often spread by microbes or microparasites that are found in or around the mouth and nose. Among the best known are bacteria that cause scarlet fever, whooping cough, diphtheria, pneumonia, tuberculosis, and cerebrospinal meningitis. Other contagious diseases are caused by viruses, and include smallpox, chickenpox, mumps, measles, and influenza. (*See* BACTERIA; VIRUSES.)

The actual transfer of the disease agent is not always clear and varies from disease to disease. Direct contact by touching with finger and lips, as well as inhalation of airborne particles, are the usual means of transmission. Other maladies are spread largely through bowel discharges. These include cholera, typhoid fever, and dysentery. Venereal diseases, another group of contagious diseases, are spread by sexual contact. A number of diseases are clearly contagious, but the way they are spread is not clear. Poliomyelitis, infectious and serum hepatitis, leprosy, and trachoma are examples of this group.

The term "contagious" is often replaced by the broader term "communicable" by those who mean to include also those diseases that are transmitted by an intermediary host, such as insects or animals. Yellow fever, malaria, typhus, rabies, anthrax, undulant fever, tetanus, and the plague are examples of this broader classification of disease. (*See* EPIDEMIOLOGY; INFECTIOUS DISEASES; QUARANTINE; ZOONOSES.)

Contraception. The deliberate prevention of conception and pregnancy is known as contraception. Though contraception usually refers only to temporary methods of pregnancy control, it is sometimes practiced for long periods of time. (*See* BIRTH CONTROL.)

Contraction. The tightening of a muscle is known as a contraction. This is the term used to describe the action of the uterus leading to the delivery of a child. Uterine contractions during labor are usually very painful. So are the colicky contractions in the colon, ureter, and bile ducts.

During pregnancy a woman sometimes experiences irregular, painless contractions known as Braxton-Hicks contractions. These occur sporadically after the first three months and are not true labor. (*See* CHILDBIRTH; LABOR; MUSCLES.)

Contracture. When a joint of the body remains in one position for a long time without being moved as far as it can go, deformity often develops. This deformity is called contracture. It can be due to a shortening of the muscles around the joint, or it can be due to changes in the joint itself. Contracture most often develops in cases of paralysis or in the disease rheumatoid arthritis. (*See* PARALYSIS; RHEUMATOID ARTHRITIS.) The contractures usually develop in a bent rather than straight position of the joint. The joints most likely to become contractured are the shoulders, fingers, hips, knees, and ankles.

Although most contractures can be stretched back to normal, this is a long, sometimes painful, process. A much better way to deal with contractures is to prevent them. Moving every joint of the body through its full range of motion each day will prevent most contractures. Such exercises can be taught by a physical therapist. (*See* PHYSICAL THERAPY.) In diseases such as arthritis, the exercises should be done by active muscle contractions. If a part of the body is paralyzed, it should be moved passively—by the person himself or by someone else.

Contusion. The scientifically correct term for a bruise is *contusion*. (*See* BRUISE.) Contusions are caused by injuring underlying tissue without necessarily damaging the surface. The dull, aching pain associated with contusions may be due to the trauma itself, formation of blood clots, or fluid buildup that causes pressure. (*See* ACHING; INFLAMMATION.)

Convalescing. A patient who is recovering from a surgical procedure, illness, or injury is said to be convalescing. During the convalescent period, the medical, psychological, and social condition of the patient must be monitored and treated. Doctors, nurses, social workers, physical therapists, and family members can all help the patient through this trying time.

The convalescent patient only rarely requires hospitalization, the intense and costly care provided by the hospital being unnecessary. Recently, the concept of a facility that provides adequate care but a more suitable environment for convalescence has become popular. These are referred to as extended care facilities. An extended care facility may be a wing of a hospital or a completely separate structure. Here, nurses provide around-the-clock supervision and assistance for the patient. Drugs and certain treatments can also be administered. The present Medicare system covers most of the expense of such an extended care facility. (*See* EXTENDED CARE FACILITY.)

Other patients may be able to convalesce at home. During this period the services of a private nurse for drug administration and supervision may be beneficial. Occasional nursing help can be obtained through a visiting nurse association. A visiting nurse can come to the house several times a week and monitor or aid the patient's recovery. (*See* NURSES.)

The first consideration during convalescence is the disease process itself. It is this and the possible complications which concern the physican most. Signs of disease recurrence must constantly be watched for during the convalescent period. Surgical complications such as wound infection, pneumonia, and thrombophlebitis with pulmonary embolism (blood clot to the lungs) are always a threat. Confinement to bed, though often necessary, may threaten the convalescing patient. Bedsores (decubitus ulcer), thrombophlebitis, and pulmonary embolism are complications of constant bed rest. Early ambulation (walking) not only minimizes these complications but improves the patient's mood. (*See* AMBULATORY PATIENT.)

Long periods spent convalescing after an illness often lead to mental disorders. The patient often feels isolated, discouraged, separated from help, and even punished. The male who normally works and provides for his family often becomes frustrated by his inactivity and dependence on others. The mother who usually cooks, cleans house, and tends the children often thinks of herself as inadequate and burdensome during her convalescence. Anger or irritability may be early manifestations of these feelings. Other family members who fail to recognize this mood may react in ways which only worsen the situation. Depression may later develop as a mental complication, and may be treated with drug therapy or may require psychiatric care. (*See* PSYCHOTROPICS.)

Elderly people make up a large percentage of patients who are convalescing from an illness or injury. The period of convalescence for the geriatric patient is generally long, because his body does not heal as rapidly. Complications occur more frequently in the elderly, particularly when other diseases such as diabetes, cancer, and heart disease are already present. Senility, with its atherosclerosis and chronic brain dysfunction, may predispose to depression during a long period of convalescence. (*See* GERIATRICS.)

The housing and social setting for a convalescent patient can be important in his recovery. Patients recovering from various types of heart disease are not able to walk up or down stairs and thus may be forced to change their place of residence. Some nursing homes in this country are of such poor quality that they may actually hamper convalescence. The home situation for many children is so poor that adequate recovery from disease may be impossible. These kinds of problems must be considered and dealt with by the physician or by specially trained social workers who are employed by most hospitals to handle just such problems.

Conversion Reaction. When an emotional conflict is transformed into a physical symptom, it is called a conversion reaction. Usually the emotional problem is too painful for the person to face consciously, so the conflict is converted into a motor or sensory disability.

Sometimes the person may have what appears to be a real paralysis of an arm or leg, or may be blind, when there is no organic cause for the disability.

In hypochondriasis, a form of this conversion, individuals are able to constantly shift mental conflicts to organic areas.

Convulsions. In a convulsive attack, or fit, some of the patient's muscles move involuntarily—that is, outside of his control. Convulsions may occur for a number of reasons related to other diseases, such as in poisoning, childhood worms, fever, lockjaw, rabies, and anemia. Among small babies, teething, diarrhea, rickets, or other disorders may bring with them the disturbing symptoms of convulsions.

Among children, convulsions usually are of short duration, and the attacks finally diminish. They should give parents less concern than the underlying cause.

Primary first aid for someone with convulsions is to keep him quiet with just enough restraint to keep him from injuring himself. Loosen his clothing and place a rolled-up handkerchief or other soft, clean article between his teeth so that he will not bite his tongue.

Convulsions may take many forms.

There may be complete unconsciousness, drooling, foaming at the mouth, and cyanosis (the skin turning blue from lack of oxygen). Convulsions are the predominant symptom of epilepsy, which results from either a temporary or long-standing disorder of the brain. (*See* EPILEPSY.)

Coordination. The process of the brain that enables different groups of muscles throughout the body to function together and interact is known as coordination. (*See* BONES; JOINT; MUSCLES.)

Copper. A dietary source of copper is essential for the body's proper utilization of iron in building red blood cells. Animals on experimental diets low in copper develop anemia. Copper appears to be present in the enzyme systems that are involved in some step of hemoglobin formation. Recent investigations have also shown that the absence of copper in trace amounts may lead to bone defects and aortic aneurysms. "Wilson's disease" is an inborn or genetic disorder in which copper cannot be properly metabolized and excreted by the body. Reserves of copper build up in the liver, causing it to degenerate, and a copper ring forms in the iris of the eye. Also, deposits in the brain produce degenerative changes. (*See* TRACE ELEMENTS.)

Throughout the ages, copper has been thought to have mysterious healing qualities when held close to the body. Copper bracelets have been worn by people who believed this, but their beliefs are completely unfounded.

Copulation. The joining together in sexual relations is sometimes referred to as copulation. This is but one of a number of terms used to describe the coming together of male and female and the deposit of male sperm into the female vagina. (*See* COITUS; INTERCOURSE; SEXUAL RELATIONS.)

Cornea. The tough, transparent window covering the iris and the pupil of the eye is called the cornea. It protects the eye and acts as a magnifying glass. If it becomes opaque, and light cannot get through, particularly in the center, vision is impaired if not destroyed completely.

The cornea can develop many disease conditions. Keratoconus, which usually appears during the early teen years, is a condition in which a change in the shape of the cornea occurs. The cornea becomes slightly pointed at the center, and vision becomes increasingly impaired as the cornea changes. A corneal transplant or contact lenses may restore vision to persons with this disorder. (*See* CONTACT LENSES; CORNEAL TRANSPLANT.)

Another disease of the cornea is interstitial keratitis, in which the cornea becomes increasingly gray and opaque. This condition most frequently occurs in persons with congenital syphilis. This too may be corrected in some cases by corneal transplantation.

Corneal Transplant. When a portion of the patient's defective cornea is removed and a corneal disc from another person is substituted, the surgical procedure is called a corneal transplant. In recent years, advancements in this technique have given new hope to many victims of corneal disease whose sight was endangered.

Thousands of persons in the United States may be helped by corneal transplants, but the operation can only be performed where eye surgeons trained in the technique and facilities for obtaining the cornea to be transplanted are available. If the patient has a condition that can be corrected by the operation, he has an excellent chance of regaining his vision. Patients whose corneas have been scarred by injury or burn usually are good candidates for corneal transplants.

The other parts of the eye must be in good condition for the corneal transplant to be successful in restoring sight. The eye must also be free of infection. Chances for success are decreased if there is increased pressure from the fluids within the eye (glaucoma). In some cases, however, glaucoma will respond to treatment, and a surgeon can later perform the corneal transplantation.

When a large area of the cornea must be replaced, corneal transplantations are not usually successful. Conditions involving only parts of the cornea are most likely to respond well to this type of surgery. If the entire cornea has become opaque, and especially if the blood vessels are visible within the opaque portions, corneal transplantations are not usually advised. They are of little use when the cornea is opaque at birth.

Sometimes transplantation of the cornea will result in only temporarily improved sight. The ophthalmologist can usually determine the possibility of a return to blindness. He may advise the operation knowing that sight will be temporary, because it will result in improved vision for a period of time, possibly years. (*See* ARTIFICIAL EYES; CORNEA; EYE BANK.)

Corns and Calluses. Local pressure and friction on the skin can result in corns and calluses. A corn is a circumscribed, conical mass of thickened, hardened skin with a central core. It lies on a thin dermis (lower layer of skin) and is sensitive from compression. Corns appear over bony prominences such as joints of the toes and under the weight-bearing areas of the foot. Calluses are like corns but broader, and the skin beneath is not atrophic and sensitive. Calluses have no central core. They may appear on any area of the skin that is subjected to chronic friction or pressure.

The location of calluses is often determined by occupation, enabling one to identify the fingertips of a violinist or the hands of a mechanic. Slight callus can be considered normal in women when it affects the nonweight-bearing portion of the heel overlying the Achilles tendon. The friction caused by the border of the counter of modern women's shoes is undoubtedly responsi-

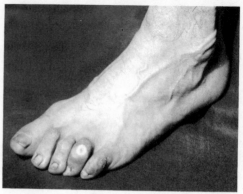

Scholl Manufacturing Company

A hard corn on the fourth toe caused by friction rather than pressure.

ble for this common abnormality. Other frequent sites for calluses on the feet include areas where bones are prominent, over arthritic joints, on the dorsa (posterior part) of hammertoes, and on the fat pads of the soles.

A callus is cured only by eliminating the cause. This may not be necessary in some areas, for the lesion is protective. Most of them, for example calluses on the palms, do not cause trouble and do not require medical attention. But in other locations calluses may cause pain. If its thickness and inflexibility result in fissures, which are painful and make infections likely, the excess tissue may be pared away and a soothing ointment applied. This treatment is best performed by a podiatrist. Calluses such as those on the back of the heels can be smoothed down by rubbing them with a pumice stone after soaking.

Corns appear almost exclusively on the feet, where they are caused by improperly fitting shoes that constantly rub against the skin, over bony prominences. Corns cause severe pain by downward pressure on the nerve endings in the dermis. Corns may be either soft or hard depending on whether or not maceration of the skin occurs from warmth and moisture. Soft corns develop in the webs between the toes, most commonly between the fourth and fifth toes where maceration is common. The most common site for hard corns is the top of the fifth toe, which is abnormally exposed to pressure and friction from shoes.

Successful treatment of corns, like that of calluses, depends on eliminating the cause. Properly fitting shoes are essential. Other treatment measures are best carried out by a podiatrist or a chiropodist. Soft corns can be given "first aid" by applying Vaseline and a Band-aid and by separating the toes, as with a small pad of cotton.

The various preparations promoted for the treatment of corns and calluses generally act by softening the hard mass of thickened tissue. They should be avoided, since most of them contain salicylic acid. This chemical can separate the tissue, cause pus to form, and thus start a serious infection. Corn and callus pads help to relieve pressure and pain.

Coronary Attack. Chest pain and shortness of breath resulting from the blockage of an artery supplying the heart (coronary artery) is called a *coronary attack*. The common name for this is *heart attack*. The lack of blood supply to the heart muscle (myocardium) results in damage to this tissue, so the proper medical term is *myocardial infarction*. The diagnosis is made by noting the common symptoms and by typical changes in the electrocardiogram (EKG) and elevation of certain enzyme levels in the blood. Treatment includes strict bed rest, close observation, and treatment of common complications such as abnormal heart rhythm. (*See* CORONARY OCCLUSION; HEART; HEART ATTACK.)

Coronary Heart Disease. Various closely related disorders of the heart, caused by insufficient blood flow through the arteries serving the muscles of the heart, are called coronary heart disease. Other names for the same problem are ischemic

heart disease, coronary insufficiency, and coronary artery disease. The arteries themselves are called coronary arteries.

The arteries carry blood rich in oxygen, vital fuel for the heart muscles. If the flow is reduced, the heart's efficiency is lowered. If it is stopped completely (occluded), or almost so, we have coronary occlusion—a heart attack. The most common reason for the inability of coronary arteries to carry enough blood is their narrowing by deposits of fatty substances, a condition called atherosclerosis. (*See* ATHEROSCLEROSIS.)

Blocking of the coronary arteries by a clot of blood or other material is called coronary thrombosis or myocardial infarction. The word "infarction" refers to an infarct, which is an area of tissue that dies because its supplying blood vessel is blocked, a serious problem when located in an organ so vital as the heart. (*See* MYOCARDIAL INFARCTION; THROMBOSIS.) The stoppage of the arteries, and resulting infarct, may also be due to an embolus. This is a clot that has traveled to the site of the blockage from another part of the circulatory system. (*See* EMBOLISM.)

Depending on the underlying disease—atherosclerosis, thrombosis, or whatever—the symptoms of developing coronary heart disease will vary. Often there will be edema (accumulation of fluids) and other complications of heart failure. (*See* HEART FAILURE.) Chest pain (angina) may appear. (*See* ANGINA PECTORIS.) Treatment also will be in accord with the basic cause of blocking of the arteries. (*See also* HEART ATTACK; HEART CARE; ISCHEMIA.)

Coronary Occlusion. The obstruction of blood flow through an artery supplying the heart (coronary artery) is called a coronary occlusion. The source of this obstruction is usually fatty deposits in the arterial wall which occur in atherosclerosis. (*See* ATHEROSCLEROSIS.) The blockage of arterial blood that normally feeds the heart muscle (myocardium) results in damage to this muscle. Severe chest pain and shortness of breath occur when this happens, and the term *heart attack* is commonly used to describe this condition. The proper medical term is *myocardial infarction.* (*See* HEART; HEART ATTACK.)

Coronary Thrombosis. Sometimes an artery supplying blood to the heart muscle becomes blocked by a blood clot or a clump of other material in the bloodstream. This is called coronary thrombosis. (*See* CORONARY HEART DISEASE; MYOCARDIAL INFARCTION; THROMBOSIS.)

Corpulence. Obesity or excess fat on the body is sometimes referred to as corpulence. (*See* OBESITY; WEIGHT.)

Cor Pulmonale. A disorder of the heart in which there usually is hypertrophy (enlargement) of the larger right chamber of the heart (right ventricle), due to an underlying lung disease, is called *cor pulmonale.*

The term often is used synonymously with *pulmonary heart disease,* which describes any heart problem related to a lung disorder. (*See* PULMONARY HEART DISEASE.)

Corpuscle. An old term for a blood cell is corpuscle. The word really means any small, rounded body. It also refers to an encapsulated sensory nerve ending. (*See* BLOOD; LEUKOCYTES; NERVES; RED BLOOD CELLS; WHITE BLOOD CELLS.)

Corticosteroids. The cortex of the adrenal glands secretes a group of hormones called corticosteroids. These are of two types: mineralocorticoids and glucocorticoids. The former affect the electrolyte balance—the amount of sodium, potassium, and chlorides—in the fluids outside the cells. The latter help to control carbohydrate metabolism, as well as that of fats and proteins. (*See* ADRENAL GLANDS.)

The adrenal cortex also secretes other steroids that act as male sex hormones. This secretion is exaggerated in certain diseases. (*See* ADRENOGENITAL SYNDROME.)

Three corticosteroids are particularly important. Aldosterone is largely responsible for mineralocorticoid activity; cortisol exerts most of the glucocorticoid function; and corticosterone has some of both effects. Cessation of production of the corticosteroids can have disastrous, even fatal, results. (*See* ADRENOCORTICAL INSUFFICIENCY.)

The two major actions of the mineralocorticoids are to increase reabsorption of sodium by the kidney and to increase the excretion of potassium. Proper balance of these electrolytes is essential to life.

The glucocorticoids control blood concentration of glucose, cellular protein levels, amino acid increases, fat metabolism by mobilization or storage—in general, what the body does with its nutrient level.

Production of the corticosteroids is controlled by secretion of glucocorticotropic hormone (ACTH) by the pituitary gland. Such production may be stimulated by various stress factors, including trauma, intense heat or cold, surgical operations, and debilitating diseases. Production of aldosterone is controlled by secretion of renin by the kidneys in response to changes in blood volume and potassium concentration.

The corticosteroids also have an effect on other hormones. Production of thyroid hormone drops when corticotropin secretion increases, and the converse is also true. Lack of corticosteroids causes degeneration of male and female gonads.

Cortisone. An adrenal cortical hormone which has important functions in the body's carbohydrate metabolism is cortisone. It is also an important drug administered in allergy and inflammation cases. This hormone increases blood glucose levels. (*See* ADRENAL GLANDS; ADRENAL HORMONES; CORTICOSTEROIDS.)

Cortisone is given for temporary relief of rheumatoid arthritis, rheumatic fever, traumatic inflammatory conditions, lupus erythematosus, and many allergic problems. Along with other agents, it is used to inhibit rejection of transplanted organs. (*See* ALLERGY; TRANSPLANTS.)

Excessive doses or prolonged use may produce side effects similar to excessive adrenal secretion. (*See* CUSHING'S DISEASE AND SYNDROME.) One feature is tissue swelling, often called moon-face.

Coryza. Any inflammation of the membrane inside the nose, marked by sneezing, discharge of watery mucus ("runny nose"), and watering of the eyes is referred to as coryza. (*See* INFLAMMATION.) Sometimes this term is used as a synonym for the common cold. (*See* COLD.) The common cold, caused by a virus, is more properly called acute infectious coryza. Repeated episodes of the common cold may lead to persistent

inflammation of nasal passages and nearby sinuses called chronic coryza. People who are allergic to various substances such as pollen, hairs, feathers, or dust develop what is called allergic coryza when they are exposed to these items. The symptoms of allergic coryza can usually be relieved by drugs known as antihistamines.

Cosmetics. Everyone—women and men alike—uses at least a few cosmetics. These products, which are intended to "beautify" the skin, hair, and nails, have been used since antiquity. It is said that the primary motive behind cosmetics is to attract the opposite sex. Perhaps it all began when a cave-dwelling beauty found that a little berry juice on her lips was intriguing to her boyfriend. Soon men too were using cosmetics—clay, ashes, grease, and other handy materials to paint their bodies, scare their enemies, and ward off evil spirits.

As civilization progressed, so did cosmet-

Allergies to Cosmetics: A Quick Quiz

	Yes	No
1. Do lipsticks dry, crack, burn, sometimes even blister your lips?	___	___
2. Do mascaras and eyeliners irritate your eyes (eyes water easily, hurt and itch, the lids become irritated)?	___	___
3. Do certain perfumes and perfumed cosmetics (including scented hair sprays) cause sneezing spells which seem to be hay fever all the year round (sometimes even coughing, watering eyes, respiratory problems)?	___	___
4. Do you occasionally break out in a rash around your eyes, mouth, and neck (particularly after you've applied nail polish)?	___	___
5. Is your skin sensitive and quick to anger when in contact with certain creams or face powders?	___	___
6. Is your skin temperamental and prone to "break out," even with the greatest of care in protecting it from the sun, wind, and weather?	___	___

If the answer is *yes* to one of these, you probably are allergic or sensitive to one of your cosmetics.

AR-EX Products Company

ics; by the time of the ancient Egyptian empire, they were widely used. Kohl, a black pigment, was used as eyeliner; green pigments were applied to the lids as eyeshadow; and the fingernails, palms, and soles were dyed with the vegetable dye henna. Fragrances such as frankincense and myrrh were used copiously. Even the poorest Egyptians used oils and ointments to protect their skin from the desert sun and dry air.

Through the ages the use of cosmetics has waxed and waned, but they have always been important, even though they have been considered luxuries and often available only to the rich. One of the factors leading to the French Revolution, it is said, was the peasants' dissatisfaction because the rich used flour to powder their wigs instead of to feed the poor.

From the Reformation through Victorian times, cosmetics—along with such sinful practices as dancing, card playing, and the theater—came to be frowned upon in certain countries as being artifices of the devil, immoral, and something no respectable person would tolerate.

Now times have again changed. Americans spend more than $8 billion a year on a multitude of skin and hair preparations. Modern chemistry and technology have put a wide selection of moderately priced cosmetics within the reach of most people.

Cosmetics for the eyes include liquid, cream, and powder eye shadows to color the eyelids with a frosted, matte, or shiny finish. Eye liners are available in cakes, pencils, and liquids. Eyebrows can be penciled or brushed on. Mascara can darken the lashes or make them appear longer.

The lips can be colored with lipsticks that range from white to pale pink to fire-engine red. Lip-liner brushes and pencils can be used to shape the lips.

The variety of face makeups is enormous. Makeup base is available in matte, frosted, and even "invisible" finishes, and as creams, liquids, or aerosols. Undermakeup gels can change the complexion color and

even add a fake tan. Rouge has appeared in the form of brush-on blushers, gels, and sticks.

Hair dyes can color the hair just about any shade desired. Wave-setting preparations in liquid, gel, and spray forms provide temporary curls. Permanent waves can either add "body" to the hair, or wave it slightly, or make it kinky curly. Chemical hair straighteners or curl relaxers do just the opposite. Hair conditioners, creme rinses, hair groomers, hair sprays, and numerous other products can temporarily change the texture, luster, and manageability of hair or keep it in place.

Creams, lotions, foams, and oils are available to help relieve dry or rough skin. Astringents and fresheners can remove excessive oil. For "problem" skins there are facials, masks, and other products. Special masking cosmetics are available to conceal blemishes and camouflage skin discolorations such as the birthmark called "port wine stain."

Finally, the old standbys such as powder, perfume, and cold cream are still with us, though they have undergone many changes.

The number and variety of cosmetics promoted for men are steadily increasing. Along with such standard preparations as after-shave lotion and cologne, new products include bronzers to add a tan to office pallor, sprays to hold the hair in place, hair dyes to cover gray hair, deodorants, and even night creams and facial masks.

The vast majority of these cosmetic products are safe and perform the job for which they are intended. The number of people with allergic reactions to cosmetics is very low in comparison with the number who use them, since allergenic ingredients are for the most part omitted from today's cosmetics. For those persons who are allergic to certain regularly used ingredients, special hypoallergenic cosmetics may solve the problem. These products generally exclude substances known to be sensitizers—that is, to produce allergic reactions. But it is impossible to exclude every ingredient to which someone, somewhere, might be allergic, and a few individuals may not be able to tolerate cosmetics at all.

In addition to their adverse effects on allergic persons, many cosmetics do have other irritating qualities, especially when misused. (See the accompanying chart for specific information about cosmetic allergens and irritants.) When trying to choose among the many brands of cosmetics available, at so many price levels, keep in mind that it is frequently difficult to detect differences in quality between most brands of cream, lipstick, nail polish, eye shadow, hair dye, shampoos, hair conditioners, mascara, makeup, and powder. Thus the selection of one particular brand depends largely on your personal preference. Remember, price is not always the best guide to quality. Several low-priced brands of cosmetics have proved satisfactory through years of use. Differences in price may simply be due to how much money is spent on advertising. On the other hand, they may mean that inferior, less expensive grades of ingredients are used or that methods of manufacturing are inadequate. This is a chance you take when purchasing unfamiliar brands, expensive or inexpensive.

Properly used, cosmetics can make a great difference in personal attractiveness. They accomplish this through their basic properties: color, fragrance, and emollient (skin-softening) effects. But there are no miracle cosmetics comparable with the so-called miracle drugs which have been developed in the past quarter-century to fight disease. So when you buy cosmetics, select those which make reasonable claims and avoid products containing "wonder" ingredients which are supposed to perform miracles. (*See* DEPILATORIES; HAIR CARE; SKIN CARE.)

Coughing. One of the most common symptoms of disease, particularly of the respiratory system, is a cough. It is caused by a reflex—an automatic effort of the body—to rid the lungs, air passages, or upper food passages of material that should not be there. You cough when you have a cold because you need to expel mucus or phlegm. Or you cough when you inhale dust, fumes, or anything to which you personally may be particularly sensitive or allergic.

When you cough, you first suck in air, then momentarily hold it in your lungs until you build up pressure. Next, you suddenly open the valve-like glottis in the larynx and permit the air to rush out with tremendous force. The speed of this air has been measured at close to one hundred miles per hour. The foreign matter explodes upward and outward with the air, and may relieve your congestion. But is also pollutes the air with viruses or bacteria that in turn can spread disease to others and start *them* coughing.

The cough reflex is set off by irritation of the trachea, the bronchi, and other air passages by foreign matter. Irritating gases bring on the cough reflex when they reach the bronchioles and the alveoli of the lungs.

Sneezing is similar to coughing in many ways, but is set off by irritation of the nasal passages and expels air by a different mechanism. (*See* SNEEZING.)

Coughing is treated by medication for the infection or other cause. Some coughs may also be relieved by antihistamines or corticosteroids. Drugs that loosen thick and sticky sputum are also helpful. Codeine phosphate is among the medications used to relieve coughing. (*See also* CILIA.)

Cowper's Glands. A pair of grape-sized glands which secrete additional mucus into the seminal fluids via the male urethra are called the Cowper's glands. Because of their location, they also are sometimes known as the bulbo-urethral glands. (For their counterpart in women, *see* BARTHOLIN'S GLANDS AND DUCTS.)

Mucus from the Cowper's glands precedes ejaculation of semen during sexual stimulation. This protects the semen by removing any urine that remains in the urethra.

In addition, mucus from the Cowper's and peri-urethral glands is added to the semen itself, giving it bulk, a milky appearance, and viscous consistency. Its alkalinity also counteracts the acidity of other seminal secretions.

For the first few minutes after ejaculation, the sperm are relatively motionless. It is theorized that the mucoid gumminess may help inhibit mobility until the mucus is dissolved by enzymes also carried in the semen.

The Cowper's glands are attached to the male urethra a short distance below the prostate gland. They are embedded in the sphincter muscle which surrounds the urethra and are emptied by its squeezing peristaltic action during emission and ejaculation. One of the glands is located on either side of the membranous or middle portion of the male urethra. Each has a short, thin duct which angles down into the beginning of the lower section of the urethra or corpus spongiosum at the internal bulb of the penis. (*See* MALE ANATOMY.)

When a Cowper's gland becomes infected, it can inflame large enough for a physician to locate the lump between the perineum and rectum. The gland also may be painful and sensitive to any contact. Cowper's infections can either cause, or result from infections in the adjoining urethral tract. In rare cases, there may instead be a tumor or cancer.

To remove these growths before they spread, or in cases of extremely persistent infection, occasionally one or both Cowper's glands are removed surgically. Since these contribute only part of the mucus in semen, their removal does not harm the male patient's sexual functions.

Cowpox. If a cow is infected with the cowpox virus, the results are often fatal. Yet the contents of the cowpox pustule on the cow's skin can immunize a human being to smallpox. Smallpox vaccine is medically prepared from the virus-laden pustules on the infected cow. (*See* SMALLPOX.)

Coxitis. An inflammation of the hip joint is known as coxitis. (*See* HIP; JOINT; RHEUMATOID ARTHRITIS.)

Crabs. The body lice which can infest the pubic hair (hair in the genital area) are called crabs, or pubic lice.

Crabs are shorter and fatter than head and body lice. They are square in shape, with well-developed, clawed extremities for clinging to hairs. The rear pair of clawed legs dig into the epidermis. These parasites feed from the skin near the hairs to which they cling, leaving pinpoint marks on the skin. Itching is the primary complaint, and secondary infection is common.

Ordinarily, crabs are limited to the pubic area, but they have also been found on eyelashes, eyebrows, underarm hair, and scalp hair. Crab infestation may be acquired from toilet seats, but close bodily contact is the usual source.

Cure is accomplished by shaving and applying DDT or other insecticides in whatever form (i.e., ointment) the doctor prescribes. (*See* LICE.)

Cramps. Tightening or knotting of the muscles produces a condition known as cramps. Abdominal cramps are not uncommon in women just before or during menstruation. These spasms are often painful. Cramps can also occur in the muscles of the calves, thighs, and buttocks, particularly in pregnant women.

Cramps are generally considered to be caused by chemical imbalances in the body's calcium, sodium, or potassium levels. Usually these conditions are only temporary. Very rapid breathing can also lead to such imbalances and cause cramps. A cramp can also develop if there is pressure on a nerve.

Cranial Nerves. Twelve pairs of nerves connected to the brain are called cranial nerves, or cerebral nerves. Among their many functions, these nerves are essential to our senses of seeing, hearing, smelling, tasting, and feeling. (*See* BRAIN.)

Cranium. The upper part of the head and the skeleton of the head is called the cranium. (*See* HEAD.)

Cretinism. When a thyroid gland is missing or fails to function adequately at birth or shortly afterward, the condition is called cretinism and the person who suffers from it is called a cretin. He becomes physically and mentally dwarfed. For further information, see the article HYPOTHYROID-ISM.

Crisis. In a disease condition, the turning point toward recovery or death is often referred to as the crisis. A sudden change may mark improvement or intensification of symptoms. Also, crisis may pertain to a psychological state, in which a person must make a decision based on uncontrollable circumstances. (*See* ANAPHYLAXIS; ASTHMA; BLOOD DISEASES; HEART; MENTAL HEALTH.)

Cross-eyes. When we see someone whose two eyes do not seem to look toward the same direction, we are inclined to call him cross-eyed, or crossed-eyed. The vision of the "bad" eye may indeed result in a crossed pattern of the lines of sight of the two eyes if the deviation of the eye is inward (esotropia or cross-eyed). But the eye may also abnormally turn outward (exotropia or wall-eyed), upward (hypertropia), or downward (hypotropia). The term "cross-eyes" is commonly used to include all of these variations.

Such deviations, when they cannot be consciously corrected by the patient, are known as strabismus. (Some persons can cross their eyes at will, but this is a harmless

activity and not what we are referring to as strabismus or cross-eyes.)

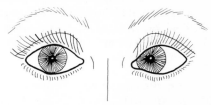

In cross-eyes, or strabismus, the two eyes do not focus together, and the person cannot control them properly. A person with normal eyes may cross his eyes deliberately, but this does not indicate a problem, as he has his eyes under control.

Most problems of cross-eyes involve a defect in one eye only. The defect usually is present at birth, and will not progress to a marked loss of vision unless treatment is neglected or the condition overlooked. The child is so disturbed by double vision (diplopia) or an otherwise fuzzy image that he mentally or subconsciously may shut off vision from one eye, usually the weakest one, so that he can see clearly in a monocular (one-eyed) manner, rather than in the binocular (two-eyed) way. This suppression is known as amblyopia ex-anopsia, and it can become so marked that the suppressed eye may become completely blind. It also appropriately is known as "lazy eye." Sometimes this may be corrected by covering the better eye with a patch, so that the child is forced to use his lazy eye. (*See* AMBLYOPIA.)

Congenital cross-eyes are usually the result of an inherited abnormality of the muscles which move the eyeball (extraocular muscles). Childbirth injuries to the brain sometimes may also be a cause. Other eye problems, such as farsightedness or nearsightedness, which also may exist at the time of birth, complicate correction of cross-eyes.

Blows to the eye, other injuries, or disease such as diphtheria or meningitis, also may cause cross-eyes, temporarily or permanently. Brain damage, such as cerebral hemorrhage (stroke), may also result in cross-eyes. In addition, almost any disease which causes extreme weakening can be accompanied by cross-eyes, simply because the muscles of the eye—much like other muscles of the body—are quite easily fatigued.

The chances of complete recovery from strabismus due to injury or disease are usually quite good. Normal use of the eyes may return with correction of the systemic disease or repair of the damaged eye tissue. But if the cross-eye condition is present at birth, or if the cross-eyes develop later but as the result of a defect present at birth, then the condition will rarely clear up by itself. The earlier treatment is begun, the better the chances for success. In addition to the use of patches to prevent lazy eye, other treatments may be used, usually in combination. Eyeglasses aid by bending the incoming light rays so that the images of the two eyes converge (come together) for proper focus.

Surgical operations for correction of strabismus should be done while the child is quite young. After he has passed the age of six or seven, the defect usually becomes permanent. Operations for strabismus in older children or adults are usually performed in order to obtain a cosmetic improvement. In other words, the operation may not aid the person's sight, but will give the eyes a better appearance. This is important, for cross-eyed children are often misunderstood or even teased cruelly by classmates. Like cross-eyed adults, they may suffer sufficient embarrassment to cause emotional illness.

Another method of treatment is to use orthoptic exercises. These are eye exercises specifically used to correct strabismus by retraining the eye muscles so that fusion (coordination of the images seen by the two eyes) may be obtained. The exercises are performed under the guidance of trained medical personnel called orthoptists. Orthoptics is quite scientific and must be care-

fully supervised to be successful. Parents who develop amateur exercises for their cross-eyed child may simply be indulging in useless activity while the child gradually loses his eyesight.

Not all persons with strabismus are aided by orthoptics. The exercises may be of value only if combined with an eye operation, corrective glasses, or both. The exercises usually re-educate the brain to compensate for defects in eye muscles, rather than training the muscles themselves. Once fusion is obtained, it can last a lifetime with reasonable care.

In addition to exercises, the eye may sometimes be treated by pleoptics. This consists of using flashes of light to train the eye to use certain of its areas for vision.

Early screening for detection of amblyopia ex anopsia offers a child the chance to have normal vision in the future. "Lazy eye" tests should be given between the ages of three and a half and five.

Paddock Crescent Newspapers

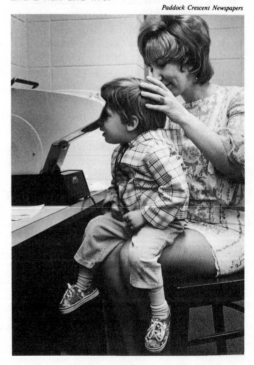

WARNINGS OF STRABISMUS. Parents should remember that the signs of strabismus may not always be noticed by casual observation of the child's eyes. This is especially true in "mild" cases where the eye is not very far away from its normal position—yet enough to give a double image.

Watch also for these things: the child rubbing his eyes often; closing or covering one eye; excessive blinking, frowning, or unexplained stumbling; irritability when reading; tilting or bending the head when looking at an object. If they do not indicate cross-eyes, these symptoms very likely will reveal other eye problems.

Unusual difficulty or reluctance to participate in games with other children could be a sign of visual defects. Obviously, however, this also could relate to other unnoticed physical or emotional problems.

Report such questionable activities to your family doctor or pediatrician unless you have good evidence that it really is strabismus. In this case have your child's eyes checked promptly by an ophthalmologist (eye specialist). Even if your child seems to have normal sight, it is wise to give him a general checkup by an eye doctor once each year. Unnoticed strabismus and other eye disorders can be dangerous and should be detected and treated as early as possible for the greatest success. (*See also* EYE; EYE CARE; EYEGLASSES; EYESIGHT.)

Croup. When babies or children have a severe sudden attack of laryngitis with harsh coughing and choking at night, the problem is popularly known as croup.

The larynx is the voice box. In babies and children it is particularly small and easily becomes irritated and inflamed, even when no infection is present. The tissues and parts adjoining the larynx also tend to enlarge from retention of fluid in the tissue itself. These swollen tissues tend to close off the breathing passage, making the child choke and cough. (*See* CHOKING; COUGHING; LARYNX.)

At night, during sleep, this condition is particularly aggravated by nose and throat secretions which run down the throat and collect in the swollen larynx. The irritation apparently causes spasms (sudden muscular contractions) of the throat which result in repeated coughs with a metallic, crowing, or barking noise. There also is a harsh, vibrating sound when the child inhales. This probably is made by the air bubbling past the swollen tissues and phlegm in the larynx.

Breathing usually is difficult or labored. At times this can amount almost to suffocation, which is very frightening to the baby or child as well as to the parents. It is more likely to occur if an obstruction, such as a bit of foreign matter or a lump of phlegm, gets stuck between the swollen parts of the throat. The breathing can become slowly more difficult, with gradual increase of swelling and accumulations, or it can change suddenly and become alarmingly worse. The child becomes pale, restless, anxious, contracts his rib cage, and is eventually exhausted. This can sometimes result in suffocation and collapse of the child unless emergency steps are taken. Doctors in rare cases have to perform a tracheostomy, surgically opening a hole directly through the wall of the throat into the windpipe below the larynx, in order to admit tubes to restore breathing and to drain or pump away the accumulated fluids. In most cases, however, this is not necessary.

The coughing, throat irritation, and increasing breathing difficulty can be aided by several simple home measures. Any child who is coughing or having difficulty breathing should inhale steam. Have a vaporizer operating next to him at night—before croup starts or the problem becomes serious. In severe cases put up a sheet as a tent over the bed to direct the vaporizer fumes toward him all night. You also can have a child sit in a closed bathroom while you steam it up heavily by running hot water in the tub or shower.

A good preventive is to maintain humidity in the house as a whole throughout the winter, preferably with a humidifier large enough to supply the entire house. Some authorities recommend as high as 50 percent relative humidity for good living and working conditions. (*See* HUMIDITY.)

Croup patients also should be given emetics to induce vomiting of phlegm and other accumulations which are difficult to digest. Doctors may use ipecac syrup in small amounts every ten or fifteen minutes until vomiting starts.

Hot wet packs over the throat also may help ease the discomfort. You can use a washcloth wrung out of water just hot enough that it won't burn or hurt. But keep rewarming it. (Electric heating pads should be avoided for small children and babies.)

Occasionally, when necessary, physicians may prescribe a mild sedative, such as phenobarbital, in small amounts to help relieve muscular spasms and tension. Sometimes antibiotics or sulfa drugs may be used.

Laryngitis and croup also can be caused or prolonged by emotional reactions, even in a baby. The throat becomes tense or irritated as the result of excess pressure, exasperation, or upset at home or school. (*See* CHILD BEHAVIOR.) A mother's tension also is easily transmitted to her child, who feels it when she handles and cares for him.

Crying. The characteristic vocal expression of emotion, accompanied by tears, is commonly referred to as crying. It is usually a perfectly normal response to grief or to happiness. Certain abnormal emotional disorders also may precipitate crying.

The newborn infant's cry serves to inflate his lungs, clear the secretions from his throat, and clean his eyes after his trip through the birth canal. The newborn cries on and off for no apparent reason, although hunger and pain always seem to stimulate crying. The more individual care an infant receives, the less he will cry. Excessive and prolonged crying is an indication for a careful physical examination to rule out an organic disease.

Adults suffering from depression or other emotional disorders may cry easily or often.

Tear production usually accompanies crying. Tears are manufactured by the lacrimal glands contained in the upper outer portion of each eye. These glands are supplied by nerve fibers from the autonomic nervous system. (*See* NERVOUS SYSTEM.) Secretion of tears can be initiated by emotional stimuli and by activation of special nerve receptors in the eyelids. Therefore, irritating substances (onions, strong chemicals) can also induce lacrimation.

Tears as normal body secretions have several important functions. They (1) lubricate the eyelid so that it can glide easily over the eye, (2) provide an ideal surface for the cornea (outer layer) of the eye so that it can accept light rays, and (3) wash away harmful chemicals and bacteria. Tears contain a special enzyme called lysozyme, which is capable of killing bacteria.

Cryotherapy. The use of *extremely* cold temperatures to treat various diseases is called cryotherapy. Liquid nitrogen is used to cool a needle or probe to about $-200°$ C. This probe is then applied to various body lesions to either heal or eradicate them. Severe nosebleed (epistaxis) is often treated in this manner. (*See* NOSEBLEED.) The wen or sebaceous cyst resulting from a clogged sebaceous gland can sometimes be eliminated with cryotherapy. (*See* SEBACEOUS GLANDS.)

A very important use for cryotherapy has been developed recently in the field of eye surgery. The retina of the eye can become separated from the surrounding structures and cause blindness (a retinal detachment). By using the extremely cold needle in a surgical procedure (cryosurgery), the retina can be held down to the surrounding sclera.

(*See* EYE.) The probe is touched to the edge of the retina and to the sclera, resulting in a small scar. This scar tissue holds the retina in place.

Another recent application of cryosurgery is in the field of cancer surgery. Here the cold probe is applied to the cancerous lesion, resulting in the destruction of the lesion. This procedure has not been in use long enough for proper evaluation, but it may prove useful in the treatment of certain easily accessible tumors and some benign tumors. (*See* CANCER.)

Cryptomenorrhea.   If a woman has an obstruction of the lower genital canal which blocks the flow of menstrual blood, she is said to have cryptomenorrhea. (*See* MENSTRUAL FAILURE.) The tissues in the area sometimes become distended as the blood backs up. A physician can usually correct this condition by creating an opening and allowing the blood to drain. Most commonly the condition is caused by an imperforate hymen.

Cryptorchism.   Failure of the testes to descend from the abdomen to the scrotum during fetal development is termed cryptorchidism, or cryptorchism. (*See* UNDESCENDED TESTICLES.)

Curettage.   The process of scraping out the lining of the uterus is known as curettage. This procedure is done using a curet, a curved instrument with a sharp or serrated edge. Samples of the scrapings are sent to a laboratory to be studied for clues to uterine conditions. (*See* D & C.)

Curvature of the Spine.   The normal spine is not straight but has a characteristic front-to-back curvature. The shape of this curve varies with a person's age and development. At birth, the curve is shaped like the letter "C," with the open side toward the front and the rounded side toward the

back. As the infant learns to hold his head up, sit alone, and stand erect, this C curve becomes modified. The final shape of the spine is that of two letters "S" stacked on top of each other. In the cervical (neck) area, the curve is open toward the back; in the thoracic (chest) area, it is open toward the front; in the lumbar (low back) area, it again opens toward the back; and finally in the pelvic (hip) area it opens toward the front.

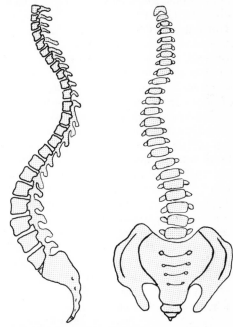

Abnormal curvature of the spine, with a hollowing of a portion of the back, is called lordosis, as shown in the side view at left. A curve to the side (*right*) is called scoliosis.

This normal curvature can be made abnormal in two ways: it can be exaggerated or reduced. An exaggeration of the thoracic curve results in kyphosis, or "hunchback." An exaggeration of the normal lumbar curve is lordosis or "swayback." A reduced curve is usually seen in the lumbar area, and is called "flatback."

There is no normal side-to-side curve of

the spine. If one does occur, this is called scoliosis. Scoliosis can theoretically occur anywhere in the spine, but is usually found in the thoracic and lumbar areas.

Curvatures of the spine are divided into two major groups: functional and structural. A functional curve can be corrected by a change in the body's position. A structural curve is present no matter what position the body is in; it indicates permanent change in the shape of bones or in the length of muscles, tendons, and ligaments. (*See* KYPHOSIS; LORDOSIS; POSTURE; SCOLIOSIS; SPINE.)

Cushing's Disease and Syndrome.
Excessive production of glucocorticoids by the adrenal cortex is called *Cushing's syndrome*. Mose cases are due to an increase in the number of cells in the adrenal cortex, with or without the formation of a tumor there. The term *Cushing's disease* is applied to the same disease complex, associated with a benign tumor of the pituitary gland.

The increased secretion of hydrocarbons and other glucocorticoids produces changes in the distribution of body fat, which decreases around the patient's abdomen and increases in his face and neck ("bull neck"). There is a large and continuous loss of protein from the body, manifested by skin changes and weakened bones (osteoporosis). Blood glucose (sugar) is increased and there may be glucose in the urine (diabetes) in spite of increased insulin secretion.

The face is florid and the thinned abdominal skin has long streaks. In women, there is a loss of menses and libido, possibly frank masculinization. Mild retention of sodium and loss of potassium may occur— but much less severe than if there were an excessive aldosterone secretion. (*See* ALDOSTERONE.)

Diagnosis is made on the basis of puffiness of the skin, masculinizing effects, increased blood pressure, higher than normal glucose levels in the blood, and high amounts of excreted steroids in the urine. Cushing's disease is treated by partial removal of the cortex portion of the adrenal glands, leaving enough tissue to maintain adequate functioning.

Cutaneous.
The scientific name for the skin is cutis; cutaneous means of, or pertaining to, skin. For example, cutaneous surface refers to the surface of the skin. (*See* SKIN.)

Cuts.
Gashes in the skin made by a sharp-edged object such as a knife or broken glass are known as cuts. All cuts, even very small ones, must be carefully treated to avoid infection. They should be thoroughly cleansed with soap and water, then covered with an adhesive bandage or sterile gauze. (*See* FIRST AID.)

If a cut bleeds profusely, as it often does when blood vessels have been severed, pressure must be applied to control the flow of blood. Strong antiseptics should be avoided, but diluted tincture of iodine, metaphen, and other mild antiseptics can be applied to destroy surface bacteria. If the wound is deep or dirty, the victim should consult a doctor or be taken to the nearest hospital. If it is a deep cut, the doctor must frequently determine whether or not a tendon has been severed, as tendon repairs must be made as soon as possible after the accident.

Cuts that do not penetrate into underlying fat may be dressed with an antibiotic ointment. If the wound reaches the fat, it usually requires suturing, or sewing together, to help the healing process and avoid unsightly scars. An injection of tetanus antitoxin may be administered as a preventive against lockjaw (tetanus). (*See* TETANUS.)

Cyanide.
Any salt of hydrocyanic acid is called a cyanide, the most common being potassium cyanide. A small amount of potassium cyanide, taken by mouth, can produce death in minutes. When a strong

acid is added to a potassium cyanide solution, it forms hydrocyanic acid, the vapors of which are highly poisonous, with an odor of bitter almonds.

Cyanides are poisonous because they stop the oxidative processes in the body cells. The only effective treatment of an otherwise lethal dose is an intravenous injection of sodium nitrate solution. A patient who has taken a less than lethal dose can recover without permanent complications if his recovery is aided by artificial respiration. (*See* POISONING.)

Cyanosis.   Blueness of the skin is called cyanosis. It indicates that the protein hemoglobin of the blood is not carrying its normal quantity of oxygen. When the oxygen concentration in hemoglobin is within normal limits, the blood appears red, but when it is low, the hemoglobin turns purple.

Low oxygen in the blood is a significant sign of a problem of blood circulation or of the lungs. Nearly every major heart or pulmonary disease can result in cyanosis, so the cause of the blueness should be promptly sought. It may occur, for example, in pneumonia, asthma, lung collapse (atelectasis), some poisonings, congenital heart defects, bronchitis, tuberculosis, suffocation, and tetany. Frequently only a physician can pinpoint the cause. Some mild cyanosis, such as on exposure to the cold, represents no major emergency, but does show that there is a slowing of the circulation in the blood capillaries.

Cyanosis will vary depending on a number of factors: the degree of the oxygen deficiency, the rate of blood circulation, the color of the skin to begin with, and the thickness of the skin. Thus you may not notice cyanosis readily in a deeply tanned person unless you look at his lips or fingernails, where the skin is thin.

Infants born with cyanosis are commonly called "blue babies." They may be suffering from a congenital heart defect, from hyaline membrane disease with atelec-

tasis, or from problems that bring about suffocation (asphyxia). (*See* HYALINE MEMBRANE DISEASE.)

Cystic Fibrosis.   Children inherit cystic fibrosis from both parents who carry a defect in their genes as a recessive characteristic. (*See* GENETICS.) The disease is a disorder of the mucous, salivary, and sweat glands. Normal mucous secretions flow easily, but in cystic fibrosis they are thick and sticky and block lung passages and ducts in the pancreas. The problem also is known as C/F, for short, as well as "pancreatic cystic fibrosis," or fibrocystic disease.

Cystic fibrosis makes its presence known as early as the first few weeks after birth or much later, even after many years. Usually the lungs are involved first. The thick mucus collects and plugs air passages, and interferes with mechanisms designed to clear out dust and bacteria. Complications may appear rapidly or slowly. Bronchial tubes (air passages of the lungs) are obstructed, and alveoli (tiny air sacs of the lungs) trap air, as in emphysema. (*See* EMPHYSEMA; LUNGS.) Staphylococcus and other bacterial infections find the impaired lungs fertile places for development, and complicate the disease. Portions of the lung may collapse. Without therapy to loosen the mucus and help the patient cough it up, permanent damage may be done to the lungs.

The blocking of ducts in the pancreas results in insufficient flow of the enzymes necessary for proper digestion. One result is that food passes through the system without being properly broken down; a common symptom is bulky feces with a fatty content and a foul odor. The child often is hungry and eats more than a normal individual, yet cannot get enough nourishment. He may fail to gain weight or to grow as he should.

Some patients with cystic fibrosis also have dysfunctions of the liver, outward protrusion of the rectum (prolapse), hard masses of fecal material in the intestines, and abdominal pains due to the digestive disorders.

One child in ten or twenty with pancreatic cystic fibrosis is born with thick black material (meconium ileus) in the small intestine. The resulting blockage can be fatal unless rapidly corrected by surgery. (*See* MECONIUM ILEUS.)

There is excessive salt loss through perspiration in cystic fibrosis patients, particularly when the child has a fever or the weather is hot. The salt must be replaced in the system, or abdominal and circulatory problems may cause collapse and even death. Determining the amount of salt in a person's sweat is one of the best diagnostic tests for cystic fibrosis.

The child with pulmonary (lung) cystic fibrosis will tend to cough. He may also have noises in his chest (rales), and develop a barrellike chest or "pigeon breast" (the breastbone projects forward as on a bird). Lack of sufficient oxygen uptake by the blood due to the malfunction of lungs may cause cyanosis (bluish skin color) and other more far-reaching complications of circulation and the heart.

Some children with cystic fibrosis tend to have nasal polyps and sinusitis. (*See* POLYPS; SINUS.) These symptoms may alert the physician to investigate whether the child has cystic fibrosis. Lung problems are determined by X ray.

There is no cure yet for cystic fibrosis. Early recognition and treatment of the problem is important, however, as measures can be taken to arrest the progress and complications of the disease. Techniques for spraying medication to loosen the mucus and aid its expulsion are effective. Tents over the bed, which maintain a misty atmosphere, help free the lungs of the mucus, as do home humidifiers and breathing exercises. Physical activity is better than confinement to bed for most patients, as activity helps loosen mucus. Placing children in a proper reclining position and manipulating the body with the hands is used by physical therapists to aid mucus removal. Antibiotics are used to fight infection.

With newer methods of treatment, cystic fibrosis no longer is the dread disease it was years ago. Some patients who have been treated are now living normal adult lives. Numerous treatment centers have been established as the result of efforts of the National Cystic Fibrosis Research Foundation of New York City.

About four thousand new cases a year are reported in the United States. In addition it has been estimated that from 2 to 5 percent of the population may be carriers of the defective genes that produce cystic fibrosis in offspring. These persons are not ill with the disease themselves, but may pass it on to their children.

Cystitis. Any condition which causes inflammation (swelling) of the bladder, with or without infection, is known as cystitis. This term thus covers an extremely wide range of bladder problems, either acute (sudden and severe) or chronic (recurrent and long-term).

Cystitis usually is secondary to infection elsewhere in the urinary tract, such as in the kidneys, prostate gland, or urethra. (*See* URINARY TRACT PROBLEMS.) Inflammation of the bladder can also result from injuries to the organ, such as by blows to the outside of the lower abdominal region, and by foreign objects (rare) or calculi inside the bladder itself. A form termed "honeymoon cystitis" also is found among some women a few days after sexual intercourse. (*See* BLADDER.) Bladder inflammation and infection are very common among children and infants. However, they usually are brought to the doctor's attention in relation to bedwetting and breakdown of toilet training. (*See* BEDWETTING.)

In most adults and children the bladder is so elastic that it is not injured by distension (overfilling). But in extreme cases small blood vessels may be injured in the bladder walls. Cracks may appear in the mucous membrane lining of the organ. There may be edema (watery swelling of the tissues) which spreads over the bladder interior. These conditions make it easier for infection to set in.

Prevention is highly recommended—particularly for patients subject to infection or inflammation of the genito-urinary system. In hospital care, catheterization is used as a preventive as well as a cure. A simple preventive measure patients can use is to empty the bladder as soon as possible whenever they feel the impulse to urinate. Retention of urine in the bladder also retains bacteria and gives them a better chance to gain an infective hold before they can be expelled with the urine.

For additional information about the causes, symptoms, and treatment of cystitis, see the separate article on URINARY TRACT PROBLEMS.

Cystocele.   When the bladder protrudes into the vagina through a hernia, it is called cystocele. For further information on the causes and treatment, see VAGINAL HERNIAS.

Cystoscope.   The instrument doctors use to examine the urinary tract is called a cystoscope. Direct visual examination of the urinary tract with a cystoscope is termed cystoscopy. (*See* URINARY SYSTEM; URINARY TRACT PROBLEMS.)

Cysts.   A saclike formation is called a cyst. Some cysts are normal openings in the body. Unless you are in the medical profession, however, you are unlikely to hear the term unless it refers to an abnormal small sac which is filled with fluid or a semifluid. This article will describe only this type.

Cysts may appear in many parts of the body, but more often are found on the skin or the mucous membranes, the skinlike lining of body passages. Frequently they crop

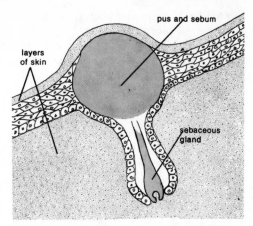

Infections of the sebaceous glands often appear as lumps on the skin. These are cysts which may contain a mixture of sebum, cell debris, and pus, and may grow to the size of a grape or even larger. In the drawing above, a cyst has closed off the pores of the skin and obstructed flow from the sebaceous gland.

up, for reasons not often known, in the passages of female organs, such as the ovaries. Some of these cysts are related to fluid increase by the corpus luteum after ovulation (release of an egg) or during early stages of pregnancy.

Most cysts of the body disappear spontaneously (without treatment). Others are burned off with heat, electricity, or chemicals in a process called cautery. (*See* CAUTERY.) Cutting surgery may remove others. Some disappear after treatment of an underlying disease.

A pilonidal cyst is one containing hair that is found near the excretory outlet, the anus. (*See* PILONIDAL CYST.) Cysts of the sebaceous glands are common. (*See* SEBACEOUS GLANDS.) Esophageal cysts may be troublesome because they interfere with breathing and swallowing processes. They also secrete an acid material which may provoke ulcers in the esophagus or intestinal tract. (*See* ESOPHAGUS.) Other cysts are identified by adjectives signifying their location or type, such as: mucous cyst, filled with mucus; cutaneous or dermoid cyst, located in the skin; and necrotic cyst, containing dead (necrotic) tissue.

A tumor is something like a cyst, but differs in that it is composed of solid tissue rather than a fluidlike substance. (*See* TUMORS.)

Cytology. The study of cells from the body is a branch of biology known as cytology. Its name originates from the Greek words "kytos" (cell) and "logos" (knowledge or science).

The example of cytology best known to the public is the Pap smear test, which is used to detect abnormal or cancerous cells of the female sexual organs. (*See* PAP SMEAR TEST.) Cytologic smears from other parts of the body also are used for cancer detection. These smears are studied under a microscope, sometimes stained with dyes that are absorbed only by the type of cells

the technicians wish to identify. Blood tests and biopsies (small slices of tissue surgically removed from the suspected organ or tissue area) also are studied for the cells they contain.

Cytotechnology. The specialty within medical technology that deals with the science of cytology—the study of cells, their origin, structure, and functions—is known as cytotechnology. Cytotechnologists, those who work in this specific laboratory field, are trained to recognize minute abnormalities in color, size, and shape of the cell substances that signal the presence of disease. Often, while the team in surgery waits, technicians prepare tiny sections of the patient's body tissue for microscopic examination to help determine a diagnosis on which surgeons and other physicians can act.